Endoc
M

System requirement:

- **Windows XP or above**
- **Power DVD player (Software)**
- **Windows media player 10.0 version or above (Software)**

Accompanying Photo CD ROM is playable only in Computer and not in DVD player.

Kindly wait for few seconds for Photo CD to autorun. If it does not autorun then please do the following:

- Click on my computer
- Click the **DVD drive labelled JAYPEE** and after opening the drive, kindly double click the file **Jaypee**

Endocrine Surgery Made Easy®

Amit Agarwal
Additional Professor
Department of Endocrine Surgery
Sanjay Gandhi Postgraduate Institute of Medical Sciences
Raibareli Road, Lucknow, India

Anshan
Tunbridge Wells
UK

JAYPEE BROTHERS
MEDICAL PUBLISHERS (P) LTD.
New Delhi

First published in the UK by

Anshan Ltd
in 2009
6 Newlands Road
Tunbridge Wells
Kent TN4 9AT, UK

Tel: +44 (0)1892 557767
Fax: +44 (0)1892 530358
E-mail: info@anshan.co.uk
www.anshan.co.uk

ISBN 13 978-1-848290-36-5

British Library Cataloguing in Publication Data
A catalogue record for this book is available from the British Library

Printed in India by Ajanta Offset & Packagings Ltd., New Delhi

To

my father ***Sri JK Agarwal***
whose far-sighted vision inspired us to set high goals
and
my mother ***Mrs Suman Agarwal***
who selflessly and tirelessly supports our every venture

Foreword

Evolution of the surgery of endocrine organs is a fascinating journey extending over hundreds of years.

The first credible description of goiter surgery was provided in 1170 by Roger Frugardi of Salerno. Pierre-Joseph Desault of Paris described a successful thyroidectomy in 1791 at the time of the French Revolution. The adrenal glands were first depicted by Bartholomaeus Eustachius in 1552. These events and many others too numerous to list were all long before the recognition and acceptance of the concept of 'internal secretion' into the circulation by the ductless glands.

Evidence for the importance of internal secretion came from many sources not the least being the clinical observations by Thomas Addison in 1855 of the consequences of adrenal gland destruction and those of Theodor Kocher describing 'cachexia strumiprivi' after total thyroidectomy. The significant revolution in physiological thinking and knowledge came with Bayliss and Starling's remarkable discovery of 'secretin' in 1902. Starling proposed the name 'hormone' for this chemical messenger although the term 'endocrine' had been proposed earlier by Édouard Laguesse of Lille.

Initially, endocrines diseases were recognized because of deficiency of hormone but soon syndromes due to hormone excess were reported. Surgery was now developing not only for tumors and hyperplastic organ enlargement but also for diseases caused by excessive hormone secretion.

Theodor Kocher of Berne operated on thousands of goiter cases and achieved remarkable success in reducing thyroidectomy mortality from approximately 40% to ultimately 0.2%.

For this and other major contributions to surgery, pathology and physiology, he was awarded the Nobel Prize in 1909. Other pioneers in the endocrine field were similarly recognized and recipients of this award included Frederick Banting, Edward Kendall and Charles Huggins.

General anesthesia, antisepsis and hemostasis, the latter resulting primarily from surgical instrument development, permitted the treatment of more complex and dangerous endocrine disorders such as pheochromocytoma (Cesar Roux, 1926) and insulinoma (William Mayo, 1927).

The discovery and synthesis of thyroxine and cortisol made hormone replacement a reality and paved the way for safe thyroid, adrenal and pituitary surgery.

Antithyroid drugs facilitated safe preoperative preparation of the toxic patient and radioactive iodine provided an alternative definitive treatment to surgery.

It was becoming clear that surgery of the endocrine organs required not only excellent surgical technique but also a firm scientific foundation.

Hormone assays and later radioimmunoassay, invented by Yalow and Berson, initiated an era of precise evaluation of hormonal abnormality. Advances in radiological techniques, especially cross-sectional imaging with CT and MRI, and the use of radioisotopes were pivotal to the accurate localisation of endocrine tumours.

Biochemical and histopathological discoveries such as Pearce's APUD concept all underlined the scientific basis of the speciality. Today molecular biology and genetics also play a crucial role.

Further impetus has been recently derived from the remarkable explosion of endoscopic and minimally invasive surgical techniques.

There is no doubt that in spite of a somewhat protracted and tortuous development, endocrine surgery has now come of age with its recognition and acceptance as a true surgical speciality in its own right.

It is difficult to determine at which point exactly this event occurred but it is probably between the 60's and 70's when surgeons began to regard the endocrine system as a whole, appreciated the need to work closely with other disciplines (endocrinologists, biochemists, radiologists, pathologists, nuclear medicine specialists, basic scientists, etc.) and also began to publish books and journals devoted to the subject. Postgraduate courses in endocrine surgery started to appear and very soon National and International Associations were born.

It is against this background that the present textbook *Endocrine Surgery Made Easy* has been written. Although there are many textbooks of endocrine surgery available, this present book is no ordinary text. It has been written by a single, highly experienced endocrine surgeon working in a sophisticated Indian Endocrine Institution of International renown.

The book which is superbly illustrated has the somewhat unusual format of 'questions and answers' with an enormous number of illustrative clinical cases all personally managed by the author. The endocrine topics covered are extensive, comprehensive and detailed forming an excellent basis for the instruction of general surgeons with an interest in endocrine surgery and also for the more specialised endocrine surgeon.

The format of the text is certainly in keeping with the educational axiom 'assessment drives learning'.

Endocrine Surgery Made Easy is an outstanding text and promises to be a most valuable contribution to the speciality and will undoubtedly benefit patient care. I commend it enthusiastically to all endocrine surgeons.

Malcolm H Wheeler MD, FRCS
Formerly Professor of Surgery
University Hospital of Wales, Heath Park
Cardiff, Wales, UK

PREFACE

The inspiration of this book came from the queries that I received from general surgeons and my trainees in practice whenever they were called upon to manage an endocrine case. This book is thus meant to help the undergraduates (who always want to know that extra bit beyond their textbooks), the postgraduates (who want help with the endocrine cases for examination purposes), the general surgeon (who needs a simplified diagnostic and management protocol for the occasional endocrine case that he comes across), for the Mch endocrine trainee (who needs to have an overview for the final examination) and for the specialist endocrine surgeon (who may need to refresh his knowledge). However, looking up a textbook of Endocrine Surgery, of which many good ones are available, could be a daunting task. Thus, this handbook was envisaged for a quick reference and I hope the readers would find it useful.

Amit Agarwal
amitsgpgi@rediffmail.com

ACKNOWLEDGEMENTS

I am indebted to the Director, SGPGIMS and I feel privileged to be a part of a premier institute like SGPGIMS, a center of excellence which provides world class training and a disciplined approach which made this work possible. I would like to acknowledge with thanks the contribution of Dr Sushil Gupta, Additional Professor in the Department of Endocrinology for his prompt and ever-ready support in managing most of these cases and for his valuable input. I would like to thank Prof PK Singh, Head of the Department of Anesthesia and his colleagues for their important and indispensable role in managing these complex cases. I am greately indebted to my faculty colleagues Prof Rakesh Kapoor, Dr SK Agarwal, Dr Ashok Kumar and Prof Shaleen Kumar for their valuable advice from time to time. I am also thankful to Dr S Gambhir and Dr PK Pradhan from the Department of Nuclear Medicine for thier help with the nuclear scans and Dr Manoj Jain for the Department of Pathology for his help with the microphotographs. I am also thankful to members of the Indian Association of Endocrine Surgeons as well as International Association of Endocrine Surgeons for their encouragement. I am thankful to my teacher Prof SK Mishra for his constant critique and to all my residents including Dr Anand Kumar Mishra, Dr Nikhil SIngh and Dr Ranjith Sukumar, to name few, for their contribution in managing cases and their constant questioning. I am also thankful to my family—my father-in-law Mr Hari Mohan and mother-in-law Mrs Sudha Mohan for their inspiration, my brother Alok Agarwal for his support, my wife Dr Vijaya Mohan for being a pillar of strength and my children Arpit and Vedant who tolerated my long absences from home.

I would especially like to thank Prof MH Wheeler for sparing his valuable time to write the foreword for my book. A special word of thanks for my publishers M/s Jaypee Brothers for their excellent formatting and printing of the book and in suggesting an appropriate title for my work. Last but not the least I must thank all my patients for putting faith in me and for trusting me with their lives.

Contents

Section 1—Thyroid Disorders

Benign Thyroid Disorders

1. Solitary Thyroid Nodule 3
2. Euthyroid Multinodular Goiter 9
3. Toxic Multinodular Goiter 17
4. Toxic Adenoma 23
5. Thyroid Cyst 29
6. Graves' Disease 33
7. Graves' Ophthalmopathy 45
8. Juvenile Graves' Disease 53
9. Graves' with Periodic Paralysis 57
10. Hyperthyroidism in elderly with Heart Disease 61
11. Amyloid Goiter 65
12. Thyroglossal Cyst 71
13. Painful/Nodular Hashimoto's Thyroiditis 79
14. Subacute Thyroiditis or De Quervain's Thyroiditis 85
15. Large Goiter 93
16. Marine–Lenhart Syndrome 99
17. Linguarl Thyroid 103
18. Dyshormonogenetic Goiter 107
19. Retrosternal Goiter 113
20. Post-thyroidectomy Stridor 127

Malignant Thyroid Disorders

21. Papillary Carcinoma 133
22. Papillary Microcarcinoma 145
23. Occult Papillary Carcinoma Presenting as Cervical Lymph Node Enlargement 151
24. Locally Invasive Papillary Carcinoma 157
25. Differentiated Thyroid Carcinoma with Lung Metastases 165
26. Tall Cell Variant of Papillary Carcinoma (TCV) 171
27. Follicular Variant of Papillary Carcinoma 177
28. Completion Thyroidectomy 183
29. Thyroid Cancer in Children 191
30. Follicular Neoplasm 197
31. Hurthle Cell Neoplasm / Carcinoma 201
32. Follicular Carcinoma Presenting with Bone Metastases 207
33. Sporadic MTC 217
34. Multiple Endocrine Neoplasia Type 2A (MEN 2A) 233
35. Persistent Hypercalcitoninemia 243
36. Anaplastic Carcinoma: Diagnostic and Therapeutic Challenge 249
37. Thyroid Lymphoma 257

Section 2—Parathyroid Disorders

38. Primary Hyperparathyroidism 265
39. Primary Hyperparathyroidism with Pancreatitis 281
40. Familial Isolated Hyperparathyroidism (FIHPT) 287
41. Parathyroid Crisis 295
42. Persistent Hungry Bone Syndrome Following Parathyroidectomy 301

Section 3—Adrenal Disorders

43. Conn's Syndrome 309
44. Occult Ectopic ACTH Syndrome 323
45. Overt Ectopic ACTH Syndrome 333
46. Benign, Functioning Adrenal Adenoma 343
47. Adrenocortical Carcinoma Presenting as Adrenal Incidentaloma 349
48. Metastatic Adrenocortical Carcinoma 359
49. Functioning Adrenocortical Carcinoma in Children 365
50. Adrenocortical Carcinoma Presenting as Cushing's Syndrome in Adults 373
51. Sporadic Pheochromocytoma 379
52. Hereditary Pheochromocytoma: Von Hippel Lindau (VHL) Disease 403
53. Unusual Presentation of Pheochromocytoma: Patient Presenting with Hemiparesis 415
54. Unusual Presentation of Pheochromocytoma: Fainting during Micturition 423
55. Pheochromocytoma Presenting with Glycosuria 431
56. Pheochromocytoma Presenting as Orthostatic Hypotension 435
57. Pheochromocytoma Presenting as Unexplained Shock 441
58. Extra-adrenal Pheochromocytoma 445
59. Paraganglioma 451
60. Normotensive Pheochromocytoma 457
61. Adrenal Incidentaloma 461
62. Bilateral Adrenal Masses 471
63. Cushing's Syndrome due to Bilateral Adrenal Lesions 477

64. Adrenal Cyst 485
65. Adrenal Myelolipoma 489

Section 4—Endocrine Pancreas Disorders

66. Organic Hypoglycemia: Insulinoma 495
67. Inculinoma and Hyperparathyroidism as Part of MEN-1 515

Section 5—Other Endocrine Disorders

68. Gonadal Dysgenesis 523
69. Klinefelter Syndrome with Gynecomastia 527
Index *533*

Section 1

THYROID DISORDERS

BENIGN THYROID DISORDERS
MALIGNANT THYROID DISORDERS

Chapter 1

Solitary Thyroid Nodule

CASE STUDY

A 40-year-old male presented to us with progressively increasing swelling for last 2 years. He had no compressive symptoms. On examination he has found to be having a large left sided thyroid nodule which was moving on deglutination. It was firm in consistency and its lower border was palpable. There was no deep cervical lymphadenopathy. The right lobe of thyroid was just palpable and was normal in consistency. He was evaluated by serum TSH, FNAC and Ultrasonography. Based on clinical examination and the three investigations, a diagnosis of benign, euthyroid solitary thyroid nodule was made. In view of large size of the nodule he was advised to undergo surgery. An uneventful hemithyroidectomy was performed and the histopathology confirmed a colloid nodule.

QUESTIONS

What points should be sought in clinical evaluation of solitary thyroid nodule (STN)?

Assessment of risk of malignancy is one of the main aims of the clinical evaluation. However, clinical evaluation is imperfect in predicting thyroid malignancy in a given case of solitary thyroid nodule but can provide some clue:

- Slow growing nodule with history of recent increase in size suggests malignancy.
- Recent development of pressure symptoms like difficulty in swallowing, development of hoarseness, and breathlessness suggests malignancy.
- Sudden onset of neck pain suggests a benign process and is due to hemorrhage in a benign cyst.

- Enlargement during pregnancy.
- History of childhood radiation increases the risk of malignancy (PTC).
- Thyroid nodule in a child is more likely to be malignant as compared to an adult.
- Family history of benign goiter suggests a benign nodule in an index case.
- Family history with reference to familial MTC + familial PTC has to be sought.
- Symptom of hyperthyroidism (suggests AFTN) or hypothyroidism (suggests Hashimoto's thyroiditis)

How will you evaluate solitary thyroid nodule?

A patient with STN requires three investigations as part of initial work-up.

i. ***Serum TSH:*** This should be the initial laboratory investigation as TSH assays are very sensitive in detecting thyroid dysfunction. Only those patients with low TSH require further evaluation by free T4, T3 and radio-iodine scanning.

ii. ***FNAC:*** It is a simple and safe procedure with very high diagnostic sensitivity.

iii. ***Ultrasonography:*** It should be used routinely in the initial evaluation of a patient with solitary thyroid nodule. Besides general advantages, the specific utility of USG in thyroid assessment is:
   - It reliably distinguishes solid from cystic lesions.
   - It detects five times as many nodules as thyroid palpation.
   - It can also measure the thyroid volume.
   - It has high morphologic resolution and can reliably suggest malignancy.

How will you interpret the cytology report?

All solitary or dominant thyroid nodules that are palpable and/or suspicious on USG should be subjected to FNAC. Cytology by FNAC is a simple, safe procedure that is performed on OPD basis without local anesthesia. Adequate biopsy can be obtained in 90-95% cases (less in cases of cystic nodules) while sensitivity in experienced hands is > 95%. FNAC results can be categorized as:

i. ***Benign:*** Seen in 80% cases.
ii. ***Malignant:*** Seen in 5% cases.
iii. ***Suspicious/indeterminate:*** Most commonly given for follicular neoplasm.
iv. ***Inadequate/non-diagnostic smears:*** 5-10% such cases should be reaspiration (preferably under US guidance) and would result in confirmed diagnosis in > 50% cases.

How will you manage a patient of solitary thyroid nodule?

The various modalities available are:

i. Surgery
ii. Levothyroxine suppressive therapy
iii. Other treatments

Surgery

The indications are:

- Malignancy
- Suspicious/indeterminate cytology
- Pressure symptoms
- Cosmesis

Except for malignancy, almost all benign solitary thyroid nodules are treated by hemithyroidectomy. Postoperative thyroid replacement is given if the serum TSH (measured at 6 week and at 3 months) rises; routine postoperative TSH suppression to avoid recurrence in the contralateral lobe is of doubtful value.

Levothyroxine suppressive therapy

Though it is still a routine practice to advise thyroxine suppresive therapy, its benefit is questionable. Less than 20% patients will have a decrease in nodule volume by more than 50%. Also, the degree of TSH suppression that is required to produce reduction in size puts the patient on increased risk of complications. Further, cessation of therapy would result in regrowth of nodule.

Other treatments

Percutaneous injection of ethanol, thermal ablation and cryoablation have been tried but they have doubtful value and are not universally acceptable.

Chapter 2

Euthyroid Multinodular Goiter

CASE STUDY

A 55-year-old man presented with history of goiter for last 5 years and difficulty in breathing for last 6 months. There was no history of sudden increase in size. He was a resident of endemic goiter area. He did not have any difficulty in swallowing. On examination he was found to be having grade 2 goiter, which was firm and nodular. There were no hard areas and no deep cervical lymphadenopathy. USG revelaed multiple hypoechoic areas in both lobes and his thyroid function tests were within normal limits. FNAC was suggestive of colloid goiter. Plain X-ray neck revealed retrotracheal extension which was confirmed on CT scan. He was advised to undergo surgery and an uneventful total thyroidectomy was performed. Intraoperative findings revealed enlarged thyroid gland weighing 350 gm with grade 3 tubercle of Zuckerkandl and cut section showed multiple nodules.

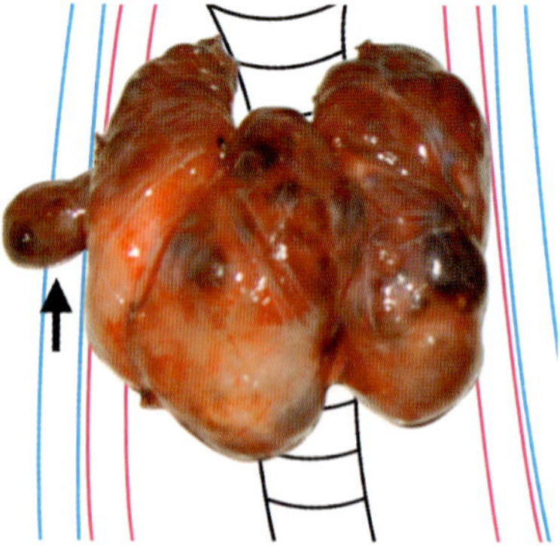

Fig. 2.1: Gross specimen showing multiple nodules along with tubercle of Zuckerkandl (arrow)

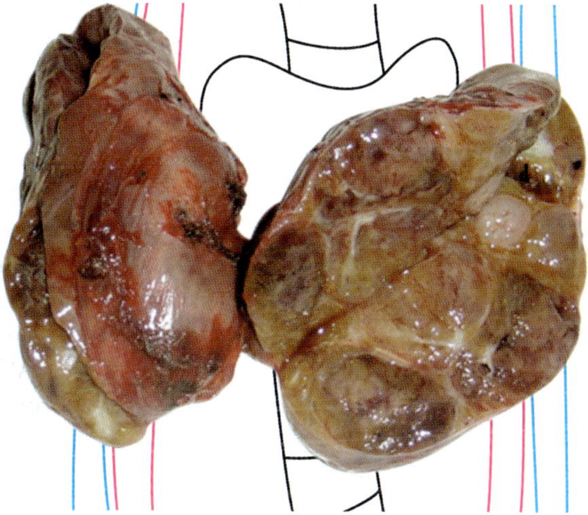

Fig. 2.2: Cut section of thyroid lobe showing multiple nodules

QUESTIONS

How do you define multinodular goiter?

A multinodular goiter is defined as thyroid enlargement with follicles that are morphologically and functionally altered.

What is the etiopathogenesis of MNG?

The etiopathogenesis is multifactorial. The underlying mechanism is discordant growth of heterogeneous cell cohorts. The various factors are:

i. Iodine deficiency
ii. Naturally occurring goitrogens
iii. Genetic factors

iv. Dyshormonogenesis
v. Circulating growth factors like TSH, EGF, IGF

What is the role of iodine deficiency?

In presence of iodine deficiency the body compensates by:

i. Decreased urinary iodine excretion
ii. Decreased hormone production
iii. Enhanced peripheral conversion of T4 to T3
iv. Preferential production of T3
v. Gradual increase in iodine clearance by thyroid cells

What clinical features one should look for?

i. History of compressive features like dysphagia, dyspnea
ii. *History of change in voice:* though uncommon it may occur due to pressure effect of large nodules or sudden hemorrhage
iii. *Pain or sudden increase in size of goiter:* due to hemorrhage or may signify malignant change within the goiter
iv. Features of hyper- or hypothyroidism
v. *Family history of goiter:* dyshormonogenesis
vi. On examination one should look for the grade of goiter, variegated consistency, position of trachea, any retrosternal extension, any lymphadenopathy and general features of hyper- or hypothyroidism

How will you evaluate a case of MNG?

i. *Thyroid function Tests:* to identify subclinical or overt thyrotoxicosis. Subclinical thyrotoxicosis is defined as suppressed TSH in presence of normal free T4 and T3.

ii. *FNAC:* especially of dominant nodule or those with a different consistency from other nodules
iii. USG
iv. ***Plain films of the neck and chest:*** to look for tracheal position, retrotracheal extension, incipient compression, calcification and retrosternal extension
v. *CT/MRI:* better delineation of goiter, airway and vessels
vi. ***RAI scan:*** role has now diminished. Useful only for toxic patients with a dominant nodule
vii. PFT with flow-volume loop studies to pick up cases with incipient obstruction of upper airway

Why should MNG be treated at all?

i. Goiter may give rise to local discomfort
ii. Large goiters may cause mechanical obstruction of the upper airway
iii. Goiters have an annual growth potential of 20% which can complicate any treatment
iv. Patient may develop subclinical toxicity with its potential for osteoporosis and atrial fibrillation, particularly in the elderly
v. Overt thyrotoxicosis can occur in 5-10% within a 5-year period
vi. Thyroid cancer may be present in MNG in 5-10% cases
vii. MNG may have a retrosternal component with its potential for complications
viii. Patient's concern with respect to cosmesis

What is the role of thyroxine suppressive therapy?

There is lack of evidence from prospective clinical trials demonstrating the value of thyroxine in MNG. In a recent trial, thyroxine produced goiter reduction in only 1% of cases. Furthermore, thyroxine therapy in doses sufficient to suppress TSH may have adverse side effects – significant bone mineral loss and development of toxicity with its increased risk of atrial fibrillation.

What is the role of radio-iodine therapy?

RAI therapy can cause goiter reduction by 40-60% within two years including decrease in compressive symptoms. However, it does have its share of complications – hypothyroidism in 20-45% within the first year; rare cases of radiation thyroiditis and development of autoimmune hyperthyroidism (Graves' disease) which is the most important complication occurring several months after therapy in 5% of cases. It has been estimated that the lifetime risk of radiation induced carcinoma in extrathyroidal tissue in people 65 years of age or older who are treated with high doses of RAI is similar to the mortality rate associated with bilateral subtotal thyroidectomy (BST).

What should be the choice of surgical procedure for MNG?

Surgical options for MNG include–bilateral subtotal thyroidectomy (BST), Dunhill procedure (total lobectomy on one side and subtotal lobectomy on the other), and total thyroidectomy.

There is considerable debate about the ideal surgical procedure. The overall consensus is that the incidence of complication rates following thyroid surgery by experienced surgeons is low. Although the incidence of transient hypoparathyroidism increases with the extent of the resection, permanent complication rates are similar for all three procedures. Further, there is a risk of recurrence with BST, both in the short as well as long term, and therefore, total thyroidectomy may be the operation of choice for euthyroid MNG.

Can you decrease goiter recurrence rates after STT?

Several large, though uncontrolled, studies have yielded no convincing evidence that thyroxine therapy after STT is effective. Therefore, routine thyroxine therapy after surgery for MNG cannot be advised.

Chapter 3

Toxic Multinodular Goiter

CASE HISTORY

A 30-year-old female presented with history of goiter for last 7 years along with prominence of eyes. She had been diagnosed as a case of hyperthyroidism and was put on anti thyroid medication for last 7 years. She also had hoarseness of voice for last 3 years. On examination she was found to be having grade 2 multinodular goiter along with bilateral exophthalmos and lid lag. She had all signs of toxicity which was confirmed on subsequent investigations. Her anti-thyroid medications were increased and once the thyroid function tests became normal she was put on collosal iodine for 14 days and then taken up for total thyroidectomy. Her postoperative period was uneventful. Histopathology

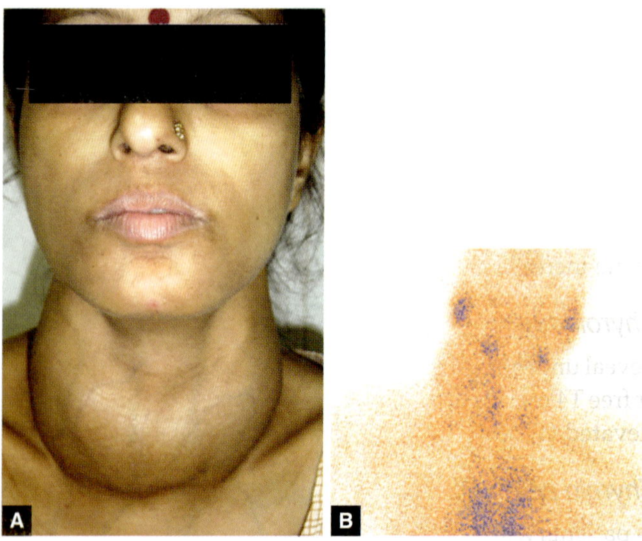

Figs 3.1A and B: (A) Patient with large toxic goiter (B) Nuclear scan showing both hot and cold areas in toxic MNG

revealed multiple nodules in both lobes and isthmus along with areas of cystic degeneration.

QUESTIONS

What is the pathogenesis of toxic MNG?

It is more common in iodine deficient regions.There are more than one autonomous thyroid nodules with extranodular tissue suppression. There is diffuse hyperplasia of thyroid follicular cells functioning independently of TSH regulation.

How do you make a diagnosis of toxic MNG and differentiate from Graves' disease?

Usually seen in elderly with apathetic hyperthyroidism. It usually arises in patients with multinodular goiters of long duration. It can present either as subclinical thyrotoxicosis or as overt thyrotoxicosis. Thyrotoxicosis may develop quite suddenly after exposure to iodine-containing contrast or excess dietary iodine. Cardio-vascular manifestations like tachycardia, congestive heart failure and atrial fibrillation are more common as compared to Graves' disease because of the increased age of the patients of toxic MNG.

Thyroid function tests

Reveal undetectable or suppressed TSH. Some times the total or free T4 may be normal but total or free T3 is almost always elevated (T3 thyrotoxicosis).

Thyroid scan

In patients with toxic MNG , there is a heterogenous pattern with some focal areas of enhanced uptake and areas of decreased uptake. Technetium pertechnetate is preferred over radio-iodine scanning. The 24-hour RAIU studies are no longer performed but if done are normal or slightly elevated.

Ultrasound

Reveals nodules in both lobes with cystic degeneration

FNAC

The role is limited because the cytology of active nodules is difficult to interpret as they may simulate papillary carcinoma. However, a rapidly enlarging nodule may be aspirated.

Imaging

A CT scan may be required to assess retrosternal or retrotracheal compression which is commonly seen in large toxic MNG.

Can toxic MNG be associated with Graves' disease?

Toxicity in patients with multinodular goiter may also be the result of Graves' disease, which can develop within a multinodular goiter or be the primary cause of nodule formation. In such a situation the technetium scan would reveal that the internodular tissue is not suppressed. Such toxic mutlinodular goiter patients may also have the eye signs associated with Graves' disease.

What are the management options?

Anti-thyroid medications

Antithyroid medications are required life long because unlike the usual spontaneous remission in Graves' disease, the hyperthyroidism in Toxic MNG is indefinite. They are also used in preparing patients for surgery or in patients undergoing radioiodine therapy to control symptoms.

RAI

Although it is the preferred treatment in many centers due to its ease of administration and being free of any serious complications, there are several disadvantages. Several doses may be required. Uptake is often relatively low, requiring almost twice the dose needed in Graves' disease. Also, the volume reduction is only 40-45% and large goiters would persist even if the patient has become euthyroid. In contrast to surgery, only 50% become euthyroid within 3 months of radioiodine therapy. Side effects are being increasingly recognised like Graves' disease (4%), hypothyroidism (14% within 5 years) and the theoretical risk of radiation-induced malignancy and ophthalmopathy.

Surgery

It is the treatment of choice in toxic MNG particularly if goiter is large, patients have obstructive symptoms, if there is concern of carcinoma or if there is substernal extension. Surgery results in immediate euthyroidism and the patient is freed from the large goiter volume and its associated cardiac manifestations. Unlike Graves' disease, Lugols' or Collosal iodine should be avoided in the preparation for surgery, as this may significantly worsen thyrotoxicosis. The preferred operation is either a total thyroidectomy or a bilateral procedure like lobectomy on one side and subtotal lobectomy on other side.

Chapter 4

Toxic Adenoma

CASE STUDY

A 34-year-old female patient presented with swelling on the right side of neck for last 6 months along with history of oligomenohrrea, palpitation, increased sweating and intolerance to heat. On examination she was found to be having a pulse rate of 120/min with moist palms and fine tremors in hand. Local examination revealed 6 × 5 cm neck swelling which was moving with deglutination and arising from left lobe of thyroid. Right lobe of thyroid was not palpable and there were no enlarged deep cervical lymph nodes. Her thyroid function tests revealed suppressed TSH and elevated T4 and T3. Nuclear scan showed diffuse increased uptake in left lobe with absent right lobe. She underwent left hemithyroidectomy and her post-operative

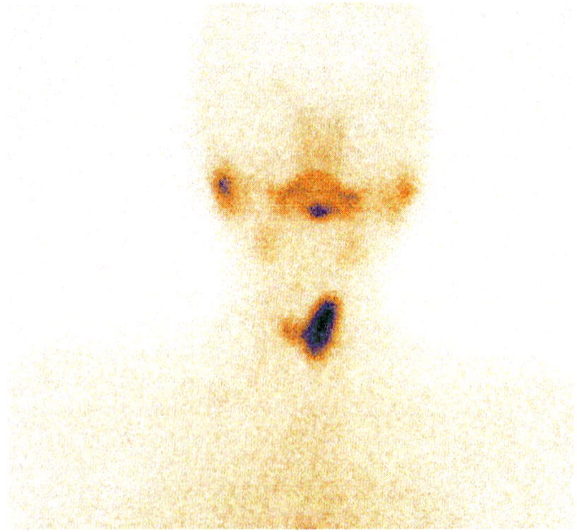

Fig. 4.1: Nuclear scan showing increased uptake in left lobe with no uptake on right side: suggestive of toxic adenoma

period was uneventful. A repeat scan done 6 months later showed almost complete recovery of the opposite lobe of thyroid.

QUESTIONS

How do you diagnose toxic adenoma (AFTN)?

Clinical features

The patient may not have the clinical signs or symptoms of thyrotoxicosis, if he is having subclinical or mild hyperthyroidism. The patient may give history of a long-standing thyroid nodule and that only recently he or she may have developed symptoms of hyperthyroidism. On physical examination there is a solitary nodule usually more than 3 cm. The contralateral thyroid lobe may not be palpable because of TSH suppression.

Laboratory diagnosis

Thyroid function tests reveal suppressed TSH and elevated T4. It is important to determine T3 also, because in some cases in which the nodule is secreting primarily T3, the levels of T4 would be normal (T3 toxicosis). Conventionally the next step in the algorithm of work-up of a thyroid nodule is a fine needle aspiration cytology but finding of a suppressed TSH should alter this algorithm and the next step instead should be a nuclear scan. On a nuclear scan, a toxic adenoma will appear anywhere in the spectrum from warm to hot depending upon the degree of suppression in the surrounding thyroid tissue. The presence of a thyroid carcinoma in an AFTN is rare.

Ultrasound

Ultrasound does not add any more useful information to the diagnosis of toxic thyroid nodule.

Differential diagnosis

This includes relapse of hyperthyroid Graves' disease in remnant thyroid tissue after thyroid surgery or toxicity in thyroid dysgenesis.

What are the management options?

Treatment with antithyroid drug is in of no use because after discontinuation of medication, relapse invariably occurs. The three modalities of treatment include:

Surgical management

Because of the variable results with radioiodine therapy-either recurrent thyrotoxicosis or hypothyroidism, many clinicians choose surgery as the treatment of choice for toxic adenoma, especially in young patients and those with larger (> 3 cm) nodule or nodules with areas of necrosis and hemorrhage. The minimum and adequate operation is hemithyroidectomy and not nodulectomy. Patients are made euthyroid before surgery through the use of antithyroid drugs and beta-blockers. However, because of the autonomy of the toxic nodule, cold iodine should not be used to prepare the patients for surgery as is done in Graves' disease. The advantages of surgery include—low rates of recurrent hyperthyroidism (although autonomy may remain), low rates of complications in skilled hands and rapid return to euthyroidism. Surprisingly, permanent hypothyroidism may occur in 5% patients because of co-existent thyroid disease.

Radio-iodine therapy

It is cheap, safe and effective. As the size of nodule increases, the amount of I^{131} needed to deliver 30,000 rads increases. However, persistence or recurrence of hyperthyroidism may occur in 10.2% (range, 0% to 41.4%) and hypothyroidism may occur in 11.7% (range, 0% to 58.3%). In many patients who are clinically euthyroid after radioiodine therapy, autonomy may still be present as shown by the persistence of hot nodule in post therapy scans. Radioiodine is absolutely contraindicated in pregnancy and lactating mothers. It is generally recommended that pregnancy be discouraged for 4-6 months after therapy and until normal thyroid functions are resumed.

Percutaneous ethanol injection

This treatment modality is rather recent and involves intranodular injection of ethanol with ultrasound guidance. Euthyroidism is achieved in 65 to 85% of patients by 12 months after treatment. Injections are repeated 2 to 12 times at weekly intervals. When compared to radioiodine therapy the cure rates are similar, however, the rates of hypothyroidism and recurrence are lower, and the nodules shrink to a greater degree. The main adverse effects could be dysphonia (thought to be caused by pressure or chemical damage to the RLN from ethanol leaking form the thyroid), significant local pain, fever, hematoma, and transient and sometimes extreme worsening of the thyrotoxicosis.

Chapter 5

Thyroid Cyst

CASE STUDY

A 27-year-old male patient presented with history of gradually increasing swelling in front of neck for last 4 years. On examination it was found to be a cystic swelling arising from the left lobe of thyroid with gross deviation of trachea to the right side. He also gave history of prior aspiration from the swelling 3 months back following which the swelling considerably decreased in size but did not disappear completely. Infact it again increased in size to the present dimensions. USG revealed a large cystic lesion of the thyroid and diagnostic US-guided FNAC was suggestive of benign cystic lesion of thyroid. He was taken up for surgery and, a well encapsulated 12 × 10 × 9 cm cyst arising from the left lobe of thyroid was found. Left hemithyroidectomy was

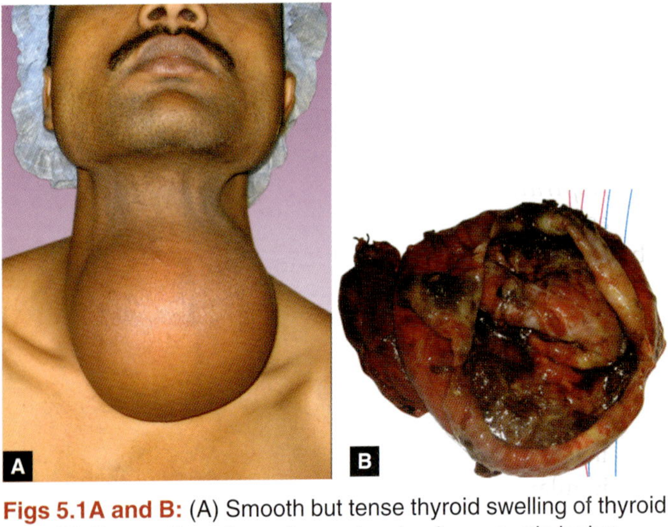

Figs 5.1A and B: (A) Smooth but tense thyroid swelling of thyroid cyst (B) Cut-section of specimen showing large cystic lesion

performed and cut section revelaed a large cyst with almost 500 ml dirty brown fluid and weighing 588 grams. The postoperative period was uneventful and the histopathology was that of a benign thyroid cyst.

QUESTIONS

What are thyroid cysts?

This category of thyroid lesions includes both pure thyroid cysts as well as solitary thyroid nodules which are predominantly cystic or nodules which have undergone degenerative changes. Even though the incidence of malignancy in cysts is slightly lower than solid lesions, nonetheless all thyroid cysts should undergo diagnostic aspiration by FNAC. In cases of complex cysts, ultrasound-guided aspiration should be done from the solid part of the cyst or from the wall of the cyst.

How would you manage a thyroid cyst?

The various options of management are:

a. ***Aspiration:*** Thyroid cysts are easily managed by aspiration but recurrence is very common
b. ***Levothyroxine suppression:*** May delay the recurrence especially when cyst is aspirated after few weeks of levothyroxine therapy; nonetheless the risk of relapse is significant
c. ***Ethanol sclerotherapy:*** This is an emerging option but the safety and efficacy is doubtful and complications include seepage resulting in RLN injury and internal jugular vein thrombosis

d. *Surgery:* Is indicated when the cyst recurs after these modalites. Also indicated as first line therapy in large cysts (> 4 cm) as the risk of relapse is high in these lesions.

How would you differentiate between thyroid and parathyroid cyst?

Parathyroid cysts are often mistaken for more common lesion such as thyroid cyst because there are no clinical and radiological differentiating features between the two. Parathyroid cyst can only be suspected when clear colorless fluid is aspirated from the cyst because the aspirate from thyroid cyst is usually cloudy, gelatinous or bloody. The diagnosis can be confirmed by an elevated PTH (carboxy-terminal or midmolecular PTH assays) in the aspirate which is always higher than the serum PTH. A minimum of 1 ml of aspirate is needed for the assays and should be sent without adding saline.

What is the management of parathyroid cyst?

Since most parathyroid cysts are nonfunctional and are almost never malignant, aspiration may be therapeutic as well. However, they may recur and may require multiple aspirations. If repeated aspiration is unsuccessful, if a functional cyst is present or when the cyst is large, surgical excision is the treatment of choice.

A parathyroid cyst is usually smooth, and has a shiny, semitransparent thin wall. It is loosely attached to the thyroid gland and can be dissected off the thyroid easily.

Chapter 6

Graves' Disease

CASE STUDY

A 28-year-old woman presented with complaints of palpitations, weight loss, increased sweating and heat intolerance for last 4 months. On examination she was found to be having a pulse rate of 100/min., moist hands, fine tremors in hands, brisk reflexes and a staring look with lid lag and a diffuse, smooth grade 2 goiter. A clinical impression of Graves' disease was made. Her thyroid hormonal profile confirmed the findings of hyperthyroidism; USG thyroid revealed enlarged thyroid gland without any nodules and eye examination confirmed proptosis. She was started on methimazole in doses of 30 mg/day and continued on this medication for 12 months. On achieving euthyroidism her medications were stopped

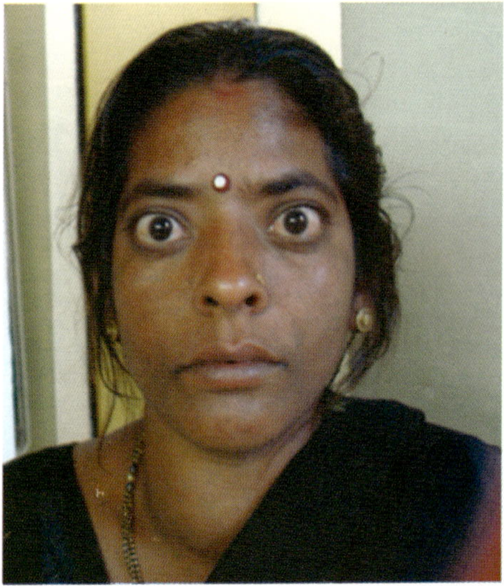

Fig. 6.1: Goiter with ophthalmopathy

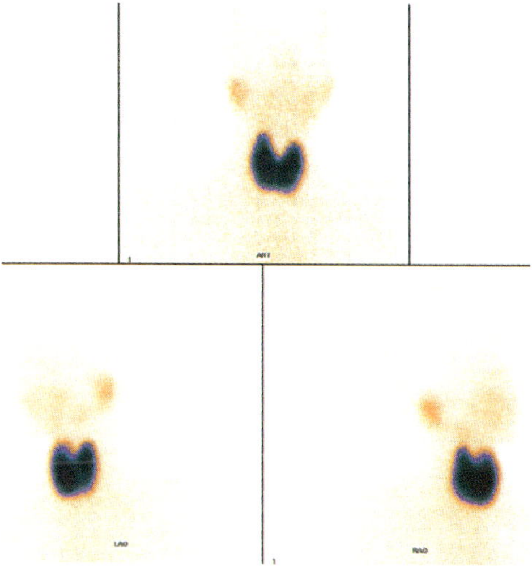

Fig. 6.2: Nuclear scan showing increased uptake as suggested by convex borders of thyroid lobe and suppressed salivary tissue uptake

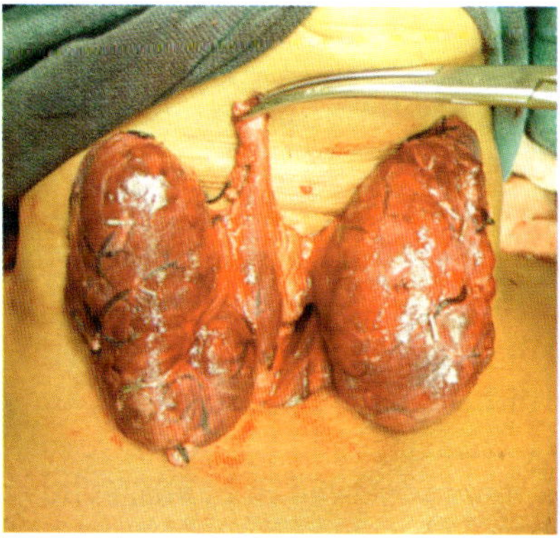

Fig. 6.3: Specimen of total thyroidectomy showing a prominent pyramidal lobe

but she relapsed within 1 month. Following this, she was again put on anti-thyroid medication and was advised definitive treatment in the form of surgery in view of her eye disease which had been progressing despite her medical treatment. After achieving euthyroidism and after keeping her on collosal iodine for 12 days she underwent an uneventful total thyroidectomy.

QUESTIONS

What is Graves' disease?

It is an autoimmune disorder characterized by excessive production of thyroid hormones (hyperthyroidism), diffuse enlargement of thyroid (goiter) and quite often associated with eye involvement (Graves' ophthalmopathy). It results from interaction of thyroid stimulating antibodies (TsAb) with thyroid stimulating hormone receptor (TSHR).

What are the clinical features of Graves' disease (GD)?

Graves' disease is five times more commonly seen in women of reproductive age group. The most common clinical features are a triad of palpitation, heat intolerance and weight loss along with a diffuse goiter. Other symptoms could be nervousness, increased sweating, tachycardia, dyspnea and diarrhea. Prominent signs are presence of skin changes (warm, thin and moist skin with palmar erythema), nail changes (soft, friable nails with onycholysis), tremors (fine distal tremors observed in hands, eylids and tongue), ophthlamopathy, atrial fibrillation and brisk tendon reflexes.

Pretibial myxoedema

This refers to the diffuse thickening of the pretibial skin usually seen in Graves' disease patients who have eye disease also. Edema is due to the deposition of hyaluronic acid.

Thyroid acropachy

It is a harmless manifestation seen in patients with severe and long standing GD particularly those having eye disease as well. It refers to the clubbing and/or soft tissue swelling of the distal part of the digits.

How do you make a diagnosis of GD?

Hormonal assay

An elevated total T4 and/or total T3 along with suppressed TSH is sufficient to make a diagnosis of GD. Measurement of Free T3 and Free T4 is optional.

Antibody measurement

Thyroid peroxidase antibody (TPOAb) is detectable in > 90% of GD patients but it does not have a diagnostic utility. However, measurement of TRAb could be useful in patients with eye disease without biochemical hyperthyroidism.

Thyroid scan

Previously RAI uptake studies were done but are now no longer required to make a diagnosis of GD. It may be useful in a situation where one needs to differentiate GD from thyrotoxic phase of subacute thyroiditis. Thyroid scan can be done to complement the diagnosis of GD and may also show up cold areas in patients with GD with co-existing nodules.

What are the management options?

The three approaches for the management of GD are:

a. Medical management
b. Surgical management
c. RAI therapy

Medical management

Antithyroid drugs are usually the first line therapy.

- ***Drugs:*** Commonly used drugs are the thionamides (carbimazole and methimazole) and Propyl Thiouracil (PTU).
- ***Mode of action:*** The antithyroid action of methimazole (MMI) is by inhibition of iodine organification as well as coupling of iodotyrosines. In addition, they have also a immunomodulatory effect of uncertain clinical utility. PTU also acts by inhibiting iodine organification but has an additional action of inhibiting peripheral conversion of T4 to T3. Methimazole is 10 times more potent than PTU.
- ***Starting dose:*** The starting dose is usually 20-30mg/day of MMI and 200-300 mg/day of PTU. The advantage of giving MMI is that it can be given as a single daily dose, thus improving compliance whereas PTU has to be given in three divided doses. Usually it takes 4-6 weeks to have some effect, hence the thyroid function tests are repeated after 6 weeks of starting and thereafter every 6 weeks till the patient achieves euthyroidism. Once euthyroidism is achieved, it is maintained with minimum effective dose by titration according to thyroid function tests done at 3-6 months interval. The antithyroid medications are continued for 12-18 months. During this period 40-60% patients

would go into remission and would not require any further medication. However, in another 40-60% patient, relapse would occur following cessation of antithyroid medication after achieving euthyroidism. Relapases are more common in younger patients, those with large goiter, smokers and those with high pretreatment T3 levels. The side effects of antithyroid drugs could be minor like fever, rash urticaria and arthralgia but do not require discontinuation of treatment (though preparation could be changed). Major side effect is the development of agranulocytosis which is seen in 0.5% and is dose related for MMI but not for PTU.The risk is higher in those receiving > 40 mg/day of MMI. Once agranulocytosis develops, the antithyroid medication has to be stopped immediately. This side effect is more common in elderly patients and develops within 3-4 months of starting treatment. It may develop suddenly, the first sign being URI with fever. Hence, the patients are instructed to get the blood counts before starting treatment and to repeat if they develop fever/URI. Both MMI and PTU are hepatotoxic as well and both cross placenta and may cause fetal hypothyroidism. The latter can be avoided by giving reduced doses of antithyroid drugs to a patient of GD who becomes pregnant. MMI may cause congenital anomalies hence PTU is preferable for a pregnant patient. However, breastfeeding is not contraindicated during antithyroid treatment.

- ***Other drugs:*** Beta blockers are the other group of drugs that are commonly used in the management of GD. They are useful in ameliorating manifestations of hyperthyroidism that result from excessive sympathetic activity such as tachycardia, palpitation, tremors and anxiety. They act faster than thionamides in providing symptomatic relief and also can be used for rapid preparation of patients for surgery.

RAI therapy

Provides definitive management of GD as 80-90% patients become euthyroid after RAI therapy, although it may take 6-8 weeks to achieve this. Usually euthyroidism is achieved by single dose, but 25% patients may require a second dose and 5% may require even a 3rd dose. The most common regimen that is followed is the standard fixed dose regime and most patients require 2-3 mCi of I^{131} (1 mCi delivers 70-90 rad). The biggest drawback of RAI therapy is that it causes permanent hypothyroidism in majority of patients. It is wise to give a short course of antithyroid medication prior to giving RAI therapy so as to prevent worsening of thyrotoxicosis that may occur due to leakage of the thyroid hormone from the destructive process caused by RAI therapy. RAI is absolutely contraindicated in pregnancy and lactation and is relatively contraindicated in children and adolescents. Potential long-term risks of development of malignancy have not been found to be substantiated in adults unlike children and adolescents. Though still controversial, RAI therapy may worsen eye disease particularly in smokers and those who have infiltrative eye disease.

Surgical management

The advantages of surgical management are:
- It results in immediate euthyroidism
- Early or immediate pregnancy can be planned following surgical treatment unlike RAI therapy

- It results in predictable hypothyroidism after total thyroidectomy
- It can be performed with minimum morbidity and virtually no mortality by experienced surgeons
- There is no risk of worsening of eye disease; infact surgery may result in regression of eye disease in substantial proportion of patients. Also avoids the use of steroids in treating eye disease
- Surgery provides adequate management of co-existing malignancy
- Also provides tissue for histology
- It is the only effective therapy in specific situations like retrosternal goiter, large goiters and those with uncontrolled hyperthyroidism
- It is the safest option for pregnant patients requiring management of GD
- Avoids possible long-term risks of RAI particularly in children and adolescents.

However, disadvantages of surgery include complications like RLN injury, hypoparathyroidism (their incidence is low in experienced hands), need for general anesthesia with inherent risks, neck scar (can be avoided by endoscopic thyroidectomy), recurrent hyperthyroidism (can be avoided by total thyroidectomy).

Surgical procedure: A variety of surgical procedures can be performed with their own advantages and disadvantages:

- *Sub-total thyroidectomy:* Involves bilateral procedure with an attempt to leave minimal tissue (usually 3-4 gm on either side). The advantage is that it may avoid potential complication like RLN injury or hypoparathyroidism. However, most studies have now shown that the incidence of these complications is not higher if a total thyroidectomy is performed. The disadvantage of STT is that it results in late and unpredictable hypothyroidism, the incidence being 40-60% at 1 year and 80% at 10 years. The incidence of recurrent hyperthyroidism is also substantial.

- *Dunhill procedure:* This is a bilateral procedure in which hemithyroidectomy is performed on one side with subtotal lobectomy on the other side in an attempt to minimize the complications
- *Total thyroidectomy:* This is the preferred surgical procedure even for a benign disease like GD as it can be performed safely by experienced surgeons. The incidence of recurrent hyperthyroidism is virtually nil and it results in resolution of eye disease in substantial number of patients.

Pre-operative preparation:

- All patients should be euthyroid before surgery (hormonal estimation in patients may show a suppressed TSH with normal T3 and T4. Such paients should be considered euthyroid as TSH takes 2-3 months to normalize)
- Patients should be put on inorganic iodine for 10-14 days prior to surgery to reduce the vascularity and make the gland firmer so that it is easier to handle during surgery. The commonly available iodine is collosal iodine which is a supersaturated solution of potassium iodide and is given in doses of 2-5 drops three times a day with water or fruit juice (it contains 48 μg iodide/drop).

Rapid preparation for surgery: There are certain situations where hyperthyroidism is not being controlled and the patient may need to be subjected to immediate/early surgery for achieving euthyroidism. In such situations, rapid preparation in 4-5 days can be done by:

- high doses of beta blockers with or without glucocorticoids
- oral ipanoic acid (500 mg twice daily).

Chapter 7

Graves' Ophthalmopathy

CASE STUDY

A 24-year-old female presented with relapse of symptoms of hyperthyroidism following cessation of anti-thyroid medication. She was apparently asymptomatic 5 years back when she developed a stairing look of her eyes and tremors of hands along with significant loss of weight. She was diagnosed as a case of hyperthyroidism and was put on anti-thyroid medication (methimazole, 30 mg/day). The treatment was then stopped after continuing for 3 years following which she developed relapse of her previous symptoms. Her presenting complaints included gritting sensation in her eyes, inability to close her eyes during sleep, tremors, nervousness and increased sweating. On examination she was found to be having bilateral exophthalmos with lid lag and convergence weakness. Ophthalmometry revealed proptosis—22 mm on both sides and her clinical activity score was 8 while her NO SPECS class was 4. She had grade 2 diffuse firm goiter. CT scan of the orbit confirmed bilateral proptosis and thickening of medial and

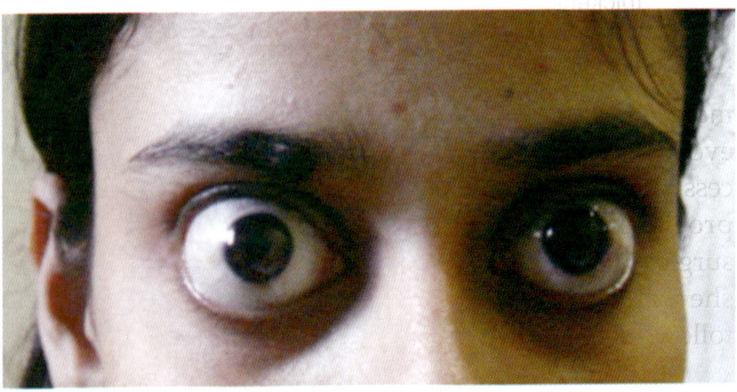

Fig. 7.1: Bilateral exophthalmos

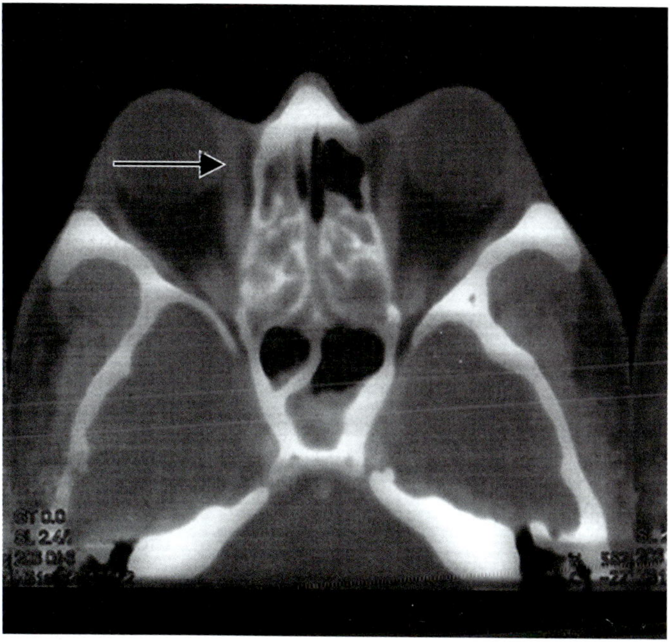

Fig. 7.2: CT of orbit showing bilateral proptosis and thickening of medial rectus in mid portion (arrow)

inferior rectus muscles. She was restarted on antithyroid medication and was advised local measures for relief of her eye symptoms. Since she had multiple relapses following cessation of anti thyroid medication and her eye disease was progressively increasing, she was advised to undergo surgical ablation of thyroid. After achieving euthyroidism, she underwent an uneventful total thyroidectomy and follow-up visits revealed that her eye disease had stabilized.

QUESTIONS

What is the incidence of Graves' eye disease and how would you confirm the presence of eye disease?

Over 20-25% of individuals with GD have clinical involvement of the eyes known as thyroid-associated ophthalmopathy (TAO) or Graves' ophthalmopathy (GO). In 10% of patients with GO, hyperthyroidism develops later.

Symptoms described by patients with GO include a gritty sensation in the eyes, sensitivity to light, increased tearing, double vision, blurring of vision, and feeling of pressure sensation behind the eyes.

Physical examination may reveal:

a. extraocular muscle dysfunction
b. proptosis (forward protrusion of eyes)
c. periorbital and eyelid edema
d. conjunctival chemosis (swelling) and injection (redness)
e. lid lag and lid retraction (stare)
f. exposure keratitis (corneal injury due to dryness)

How do you classify the severity of eye disease?

The intensity of eye inflammation is measured by using the Clinical Activity Score (CAS) while the severity of eye changes can be classified by using the NO SPECS system

*Clinical activity score (CAS)**

A score of 1 is given for each feature present.

Pain

- Painful, oppressive feeling on or behind the globe during last 4 weeks

- Pain on attempted up, side or down gaze during last 4 weeks

Redness

- Redness of the eyelid (s)
- Diffuse redness of the conjunctiva, covering at least one quadrant

Swelling

- swellling of the eyelid (s)
- chemosis
- swollen caruncle
- increase by 2 mm or more in proptosis during a period of 1-3 months

Impaired function

- Decrease in eye movements in any direction of 5 degrees or more during a period of 1-3 months
- Decrease in visual acuity (1 or more lines on Snellen chart, using a pinhole) during a period of 1-3 months

**Mouris MPet al. Clin Endocrinol (Oxf)1997;47(1):9-14.*

*"NO SPECS" Classification**

Class 0: no symptoms or signs
Class 1: Only signs (limited to upper lid retraction and stare, with or without lid lag)
Class 2: Soft tissue involvement (edema of conjunctivae and lids, conjunctival injection, etc.)
Class 3: Proptosis
Class 4: Extraocular muscle involvement (usually with diplopia)

Class 5: Corneal involvement (primarily due to lagophthalmos)

Class 6: Sight loss (due to optic nerve involvement)

* *Werner SC. J Clin Endocrinol Metab 1977;44:203-4.*

What are the management options?

Antithyroid drugs are usually the first-line therapy in patients with GO. However, relapses of thyrotoxicosis after discontinuation of treatment with antithyroid medications are frequent and may result in exacerbation of the orbital inflammation. In such cases rapid ablative or definitive therapy is usually advisable followed by the appropriate supportive/local treatment of GO.

Definitive therapy can be achieved either by RAI or Surgery. However, there is evidence, albeit weak, that GO can possibly worsen with RAI treatment. The eye disease improves in 75% of patients treated with surgery, in 60% treated with medically, and in only 25% of patients treated with RAI.

Surgery also avoids the potential toxicities of corticosteroids.

What are the local measures for symptomatic relief?

a. Frequent instillation of methylcellulose-containing eye drops to prvent drying
b. Taping the eyelids shut at night to prevent nocturnal corneal drying
c. Elevation of the head during night to prevent dependent edema
d. Use of tinted lenses or sunglasses with side cover may assist in decreasing photophobia

e. Cessation of smoking
f. Topical use of guanethidine eye drops to correct lid retraction has variable effectiveness

What are local management options ?

Immuno-modulatory therapy

a. Corticosteroids have both anti-inflammatory and immunomodulatory effects and may inhibit the synthesis and release of glycosaminoglycan by fibroblasts. They provide rapid relief from the pain, injection and conjunctival edema. However, regression in proptosis and ophthlamoplegia occurs to a lesser extent and these may exacerbate after drug withdrawl.
b. Cyclosporin
c. Somatostatin analogue therapy
d. Plasmapheresis
e. Orbital radiotherapy

Surgical treatment of Graves' ophthalmopathy

Only a small proportion of patients with GD would require operative intervention. The three most common procedures are:

- Orbital decompression to relieve optic neuropathy or proptosis
- Extraocular muscle surgery to reduce diplopia
- Eyelid procedures to treat retraction and cosmetic disfigurement.

Chapter 8

Juvenile Graves' Disease

CASE STUDY

A 15-year-old girl presented with history of goiter for last 2 years, prominence of eyes and significant weight loss. She was diagnosed to be a case of Graves' disease and put on antithyroid medication. However, she continued to be toxic and did not go into remission. She was then taken up for surgery after preparation with collosal iodine. She underwent total thyroidectomy and her postoperative period was uneventful. She developed biochemical hypocalcemia which was treated with oral calcium and vitamin D which were tapered off in next 4 months. She has subsequently gained weight and her school performance has improved.

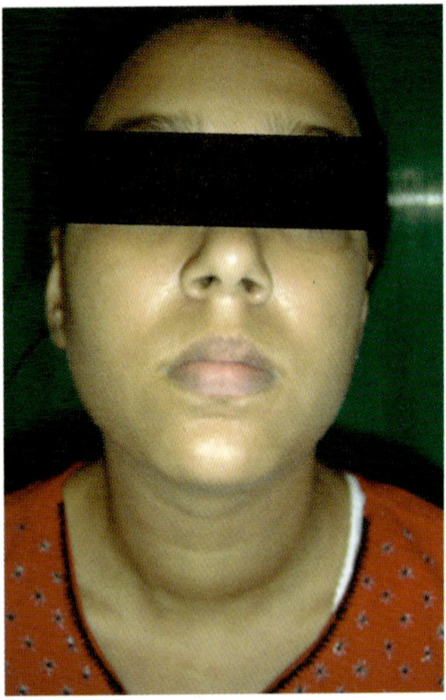

Fig. 8.1: 15-year-old girl with goiter

QUESTIONS

What is the incidence of Juvenile Graves' disease and what is the clinical presentation?

Graves' disease (GD) is a rare disease in childhood and adolescence, though it is the commonest cause of hyperthyroidism in this age group. The incidence of juvenile GD is 3 in 100000. Most children with GD have a family history of some type of autoimmune thyroid disease and it is more common in children with Down's syndrome than in normal children.

The clinical features of thyrotoxicosis are similar to those in adults: commonest features being goiter, tachycardia, nervousness and exophthalmos. The manifestations of Graves' eye disease are more common but less severe and are also likely to respond to treatment. Most children would have exophthalmos, wide palpebral fissures and a staring look. The eye disease in adolescents is not immunologically mediated but is a direct result of thyrotoxicosis and hence remits when the thyrotoxicosis is treated.

What is the initial management of this disease ?

The ideal treatment of GD in adolescents remains controversial. Most European Investigators favor antithyroid drug treatment as the initial treatment of choice. The recommended initial dose of MMI is 0.5 to 1.0 mg/kg daily given once or twice daily while the dose of PTU is 5-10 mg/kg given in three divided doses. Compliance is better with MMI as compared to PTU as fewer tablets per day are needed with MMI. Higher doses should be avoided because the frequency of side effects is dose dependent. Hepatic toxicity is a rare but potentially lethal complication of mainly PTU therapy. After 4-6 weeks when clinical and biochemical improvement occurs, either the dose should be tapered or thyroxine can be added (block and replace regime) to avoid the development of hypothyroidism.

However, medical therapy has a high failure rate in children and adolescents with remission rates of 34-36%. A high risk for recurrence of GD in the first year after cessation of treatment and after previous relapses has been recognized. Possible indicators of failure or recurrence include younger age, those with large goiters, high level of TSH receptor antibodies and those with a high T3 to T4 ratio.

Do adolescents require definitive therapy—RAI or Surgery ?

RAI has proved to be effective in children with hyperthyroidism, but its long-term safety with respect to radiation oncogenesis and gonadal damage has not been conclusively established. Most people would prefer to treat these children with antithyroid drugs for 3-4 years until the age of 18-20 when radioiodine treatment or surgery is more suitable. However, in experienced centers surgical results are very good and hence surgery can be offered as the definitive therapy for these adolescents particularly those with large goiters and poor compliance.

Chapter 9

Graves' with Periodic Paralysis

CASE STUDY

A 34-year-old man, resident of Nepal and teacher by profession presented with history of episodic generalized weakness. None of these episodes were accompanied by respiratory or bulbar involvement and there was no history of sensory involvement or residual weakness after the attacks. There was no history of diuretic intake. On detailed history taking, he was asymptomatic 10 years back when he noticed weakness of both lower limbs at night which resolved in the morning and on consultations with a local doctor he improved symptomatically. Two years later he again developed weakness. When examined by a doctor he was found to be having signs and symptoms of hyperthyroidism with a goiter and was put on antithyroid medication. Four years later on discontinuation of

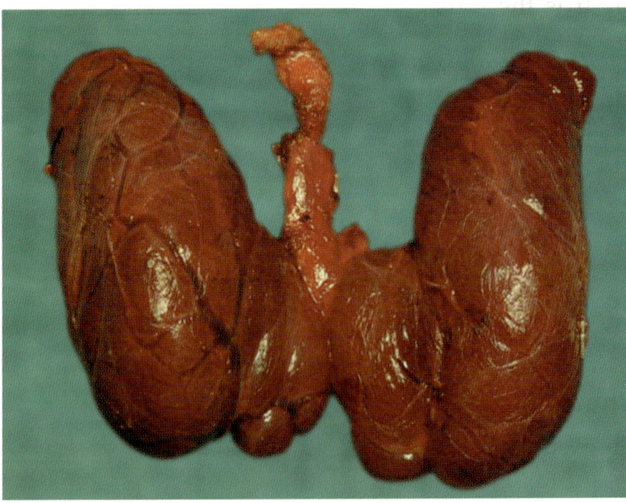

Fig. 9.1: Total thyroidectomy specimen in a patient with periodic paralysis

antithyroid medication he again developed generalized weakness and on admission to a hospital was found to be hypokalemic and was put on oral potassium supplements. He was subsequently referred to us when the diagnosis of Thyrotoxic periodic paralysis due to uncontrolled Graves' disease was made. After achieving euthyroidism he was referred for definitive therapy in the form of surgery. He underwent total thyroidectomy. At last follow-up of 2 years he is doing well and did not experience any further attack of periodic paralysis.

QUESTIONS

What are the clinical features of thyrotoxic periodic paralysis (TPP)?

i. It is the most common acquired cause of periodic paralysis
ii. It typically affects the Orientals
iii. It is predominantly a disease of males unlike thyrotoxicosis which is seen more commonly in females
iv. Usual age of onset is second to fourth decade
v. Family history is rare
vi. Graves' disease is the most common cause of hyperthyroidism in affected patients
vii. However, findings of a hyperthyroid state may be very subtle.

What is the management of TPP?

i. Acute attacks may respond to oral or intravenous potassium; however, recurrent attacks are not prevented by prophylactic potassium administration

ii. Treatment of underlying thyrotoxicosis abolishes attacks
iii. Non-specific beta blockers may reduce the frequency and severity of attacks
iv. Avoid precipitating factors like extreme exertion, alcohol, and heavy carbohydrate ingestion
v. Unlike familial periodic paralysis, acetazolamide is not helpful in preventing attacks and may infact precipitate an attack of paralysis in TPP
vi. Correction of the hyperthyroid state is the most definitive treatment of TPP. This can be achieved either by RAI therapy or Thyroidectomy. Surgical management in the form of total thyroidectomy ensures freedom from further attacks and may be preferred over RAI therapy for this subset of thyrotoxicosis.

Chapter 10

Hyperthyroidism in Elderly with Heart Disease

CASE STUDY

A 58-year-old lady presented with history of goiter for last 10 years and recent onset of palpitation, sweating, nervousness and diarrhea. She had also suffered from right hemiparesis form which she had almost fully recovered. On examination, she was found to be having grade II goiter. She was also noted to be having atrial fibrillation with a pulse rate of 165/min. On enquiry it was revealed that she had been on anti-thyroid medication but has been taking it irregularly. The thyroid function test report that she was carrying revealed hyperthyroidism. The patient was admitted and immediately put on beta-blockers along with methimazole and collosal iodine in doses of 5 ml three times a day. She reverted back to sinus rhytm after 4 days of intensive treatment. She was also put on anticoagulant therapy. Once her condition stabilized, she was discharged on antithyroid medication with advice to undergo definitive management of thyrotoxicosis either by radio-iodine therapy or surgery. The patient opted for thyroidectomy which was performed uneventfully.

QUESTIONS

What are the cardiovascular disorders that can result from Thyrotoxicosis?

The various cardiovascular disorders associated with thyrotoxicosis are:

- sinus tachycardia
- systolic hypertension
- ventricular systolic and diastolic dysfunction
- dysarhythmias.

What is the commonest cardiovascular disorder associated with thyrotoxicosis?

The commonest disorder is Atrial Fibrillation (AF) and the frequency of AF in hyperthyroid patients ranges from 10-15%.

What is the emergency management of AF associated with thyrotoxicosis?

The commonest drug that is used to control AF is beta blocker like propanolol or a short acting agent like esmolol. Other drugs that can be used are calcium channel blockers or digoxin (especially in patients with concomitant heart failure). If these drugs fail to control AF, then amiodrone can be used but only in conjunction with antithyroid drugs.

What is the risk of thromboembolism in AF associated with Thyrotoxicosis?

The frequency of thromboembolism in thyrotoxic AF is greater as compared to that in non-thyrotoxic AF not associated with rheumatic fever. The risk is especially greater in elderly persons and those with history of hypertension and diabetes. However, the decision to start anti-coagulant therapy should be based on presence of validated stroke risk factors only.

What is the definitive management of such a patient?

After control of AF with beta blockers or other drugs, patients should be put on antithyroid medications till euthyroidism is achieved. Sometimes rapid control of hyperthyroid state is required such as in patients with heart failure or unstable angina. This can be achieved with inorganic iodine followed by definitive therapy such as RAI or surgery.

Chapter 11

Amyloid Goiter

CASE STUDY

A 63-year-old female who was a known case of end stage renal disease and hypertension was referred from Nephrology for complaint of progressively increasing goiter for last 2 years. On examination there were no features of hyper or hypo-thyroidism and she had a grade 2 goiter which was nodular and firm without any lymphadenopathy and moving with deglutition. Thyroid function tests were suggestive of euthyroid goiter. FNAC was suggestive of hyperplastic nodule/follicular neoplasm. Ultrasound revealed multiple hypoechoic areas. She underwent total thyroidectomy and a 230 gm multinodular goiter was removed. The cut section revealed fatty infiltration with calcific and fibrotic areas with multiple nodules. Microscopy revealed an encapsulated tumor (follicular adenoma) along with extensive deposition of acellular, eosinophilic and congophilic material admixed with mature adipose tissue. A histopathological diagnosis of amyloid goiter was made.

QUESTIONS

What is Amyloid Goiter (AG)?

Amyloid goiter is defined as a symptomatic mass or clinically detectable thyroid enlargement because of amyloid deposition. It occurs in association with both primary and secondary amyloidosis. The predisposing disorders associated with secondary amyloidosis include chronic inflammatory diseases (like rheumatoid arthritis, familial Mediterranean fever, giant lymph node hyperplasia and Muckle-Wells syndrome), neoplasms, and hereditary disorders.

How can you make a preoperative diagnosis of AG?

The preoperative diagnosis of amyloid goiter should be suspected in a patient with known systemic amyloidosis or with a long-standing predisposing disease who presents with a rapidly growing diffuse goiter associated with euthyroid state. Hypothyroidism is rarely seen in amyloid goiter. Since AG may cause localized pressure symptoms like dyspnea or hoarseness, it is important to exclude anaplastic carcinoma or lymphoma both of which are associated with a rapidly enlarging thyroid with local pressure symptoms.

Thyroid function tests

The majority of patients with AG are euthyroid despite the extensive involvement of the thyroid gland.

CT scan

When diffuse decreased density of the enlarged thyroid is recognized on CT, amyloid goiter should enter into differential diagnosis. The diffuse decreased density on CT is thought to represent large amount of adipose tissue often found in amyloid goiter.

FNAC

FNAC is of limited value and may sometimes be misleading

In the absence of secondary amyloidosis, multiple myeloma and plasmacytoma should be considered and bone marrow aspiration biopsy and laboratory studies should help in making a correct diagnosis.

How do you classify AG?

Amyloidosis is classified on the basis of biochemical nature of amyloid protein deposits. In primary amyloidosis, with or without multiple myeloma, the major fibrillar protein is amyloid L (AL) based on the light chain components of immunoglobulins. In secondary amyloidosis, the fibril subunit is amyloid A (AA). Immunohistochemical staining for AA is more sensitive and specific than AL. Amyloid L comprises the light chain fragment of Ig demonstrating positive staining with either kappa-or lambda-light chain antibodies. Secondary amyloidosis accounts for majority of cases (50-80%) of AG.

Can you differentiate between primary and secondary amyloidosis and why this is important?

Potassium permanganate treatment of Congo-red stained sections may be helpful in differentiating amyloid A from other type of amyloid AL. Confirmation of the specific type of amyloid is valuable in assessing the overall prognosis because patients with secondary amyloidosis have better overall survival than patients with primary amyloidosis.

What are histological features of AG and what is the role of immunohistochemistry?

On light microscopy, amyloid deposition appears as a extracellular amorphous and eosinophilic material spread in a diffuse pattern throughout the gland and distorting the follicular architecture. Presence of mature adipose tissue is an important finding. Further confirmation of amyloid material is done by Congo red and crystal violet stains. Congo red imparts a unique apple green bifringence when sections are polarized under light microscopy. With crystal violet staining metachromasia is seen. Negative calcitonin immunoreactivity in AG would help to distinguish from Medullary thyroid carcinoma

What are various fat containing lesions of the thyroid?

Thyroid lesions containing adipose tissue are unusual. These include: adenomas, amyloid goiter, nodular hyperplasia, Graves' disease and sometimes in normal thyroid.

Chapter 12

Thyroglossal Cyst

CASE STUDY

A 40-year-old lady presented with complaint of painless swelling in front of neck for past 2 months only and which had been progressively increasing. There was no history of compressive symptoms or those suggestive of hyperthyroidism or hypothyroidism. On examination, the swelling was found to be subhyoid in location, firm and moving well on deglutination. Thyroid was normally palpable. The swelling also moved upwards on protrusion of tongue. A clinical diagnosis of thyroglossal cyst was made. Ultrasound revealed normal thyroid in the normal position and a rounded hypoechoic swelling in the subhyoid location. Aspiration revealed mucoid fluid showing fair number of inflammatory cells predominantly polymorphs admixed with macrophages on proteinaceous background with no atypical cells, consistent with thyroglossal cyst. She was taken up for Sistrunk's operation, and a 4 × 3 cm cyst was excised along with the tract and the central portion of hyoid bone. On cut-section, the cyst was found to be filled with thick turbid fluid. The postoperative period was uneventful and the sections from the cyst wall showed fibrocollagenous tissue lined partly by stratified squamous epithelium and partly by flattened epithelium. The fibrocollagenous tissue showed infiltration by mild chronic inflammatory cells and thyroid follicle was seen, consistent with a benign thyroglossal cyst.

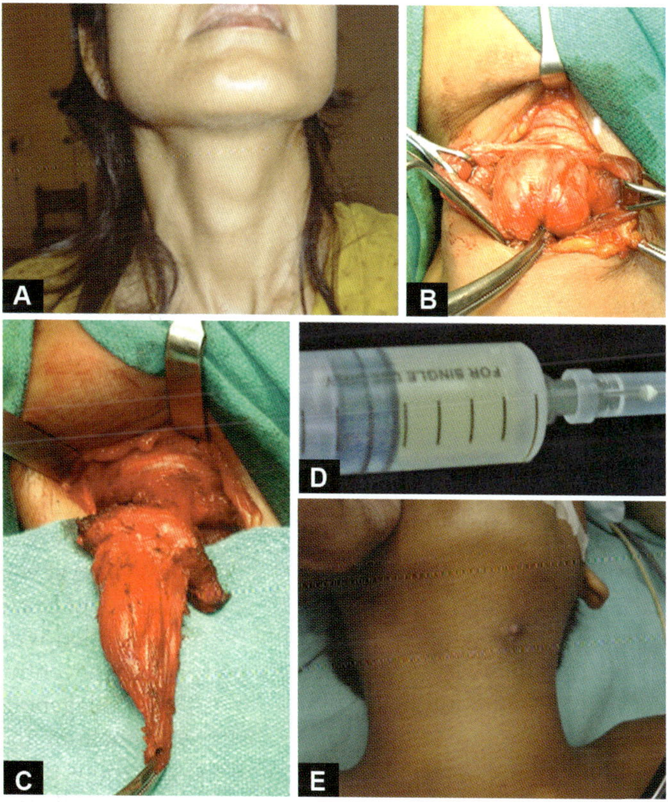

Figs 12.1A to E: (A) Anterior neck swelling in an infrahyoid location (arrow) (B) Intra-operative picture of Thyroglossal cyst (C) Central portion of hyoid bone excised (D) Mucoid aspirate from the cyst (E) Thyroglossal fistula in another patient

QUESTIONS

What is a thyroglossal duct cyst (TDC), and what is its embryological basis ?

TDC is a collection of fluid in the distal most portion of a persistent thyroglossal duct. Thyroglossal duct in turn is the persistent tract that forms as the thyroid gland descends from the foramen caecum down to the lower neck during the development phase. Normally the duct disappears before birth. The thyroglossal duct has a S-shaped configuration: initially it lies in an anterior plane, then passes through the hyoid bone and then in its distal course lies on a posterior plane in relation to hyoid bone. The tract also tends to arborize, particularly in its proximal portion.

What are clinical features of TDC?

i. It is the most common cause of midline mass in the cervical region
ii. Usually comes to clinical attention in children or young adults but sometimes can be seen in adults also
iii. Most commonly presents as an asymptomatic soft, cystic midline swelling. Most commonly it is situated in an infrahyoid location in between the hyoid and thyroid gland. Rarely in 10-20% it is in a suprahyoid position or eccentrically located, more commonly to the left of midline
iv. It moves with deglutination or on thrusting the tongue forward
v. Sometimes pressure upon the swelling can result in bitter taste (dysgeusia) due to release of discharge through the communication with the foramen caecum.

vi. Due to previous inadequate surgery, either as a result of misdiagnosis or due to incomplete surgery, patients may present with a thyroglossal fistula or sinus
vii. Patients may also present with an infected thyroglossal cyst

How will you evaluate such a case?

The clinical diagnosis of TDC can be complemented by a USG of the neck which would reveal a cystic space occupying lesion (SOL) in an infrahyoid location along with an intact thyroid in the normal location. In the past RAI scans were done to identify ectopic thyroid tissue in the cyst and to prevent removal of the only existing thyroid tissue. Sometimes aspiration can be done which would confirm the presence of cloudy and mucoid fluid which does not contain thyroid follicular cells. CT and MRI may give additional information only when carcinoma associated with the cyst is suspected. Fistulogram can be ordered in cases of thyroglossal fistula/sinus which would help to delineate the branches of the thyroglossal duct.

What is the differential diagnosis of TDC?

i. ***Midline epidermoid cyst:*** There would be no history of previous repeated infections
ii. ***Lymph node enlargement:*** Lymph node does not move on protrusion of tongue
iii. ***Branchial cyst:*** It is situated more laterally. Also the sinus tract of branchial cyst extends upwards towards tonsillar fossa.

Why should TDC be operated?

i. The cyst has a tendency to become infected due to lymphoid tissue in its lining and repeated infections makes surgery difficult and predisposes to inadequate surgery and recurrences
ii. For cosmetic reasons
iii. In case of recurrent infections
iv. Rarely papillary thyroid carcinoma can develop
v. In cases of thyroglossal fistula or sinus

What is the histological picture of TDC?

The TDC is usually lined with epithelial cells with thyroid follicles in the cyst wall along with lymphoid infiltrate.

What is the operative management and how can you prevent/reduce recurrences?

Even today, the gold standard is the classical SISTRUNK operation. The key points are:

i. Resection of the central portion of hyoid bone
ii. To remove a cuff of tissue, usually 1-1.5 cm in between the foramen caecum and hyoid bone, in an attempt to incorporate numerous small branches of the thyroglossal duct which are common in the suprahyoid region.
iii. Specimen should include a small cuff of tongue muscles (geniohyoid and genioglossus)
iv. Avoid rupture of the cyst as this would make dissection difficult

Operative Procedure

A horizontal incision is given across the cyst, platysma is incised in the line of incision and flaps are raised. Strap muscles are retracted and the cyst is dissected all around; care is taken so as not to transect the duct superior to the cyst. The duct is followed upto the hyoid bone. The central portion of the hyoid bone is separated by cutting on either side by a bone cutter. In the suprahyoid portion of dissection, no attempt is made to visualize the thyroglossal duct but instead a cuff of tissue, around 1-1.5 cm is excised upto the foramen caecum incorporating a portion of tongue muscles. The last part of dissection is facilitated by putting index finger of left hand in the mouth of the patient and pushing the tongue down.

In cases of thyroglossal fistula or sinus, an elliptical incision is given all around the opening. Dissection can be facilitated by injecting a small amount of methylene blue to delineate the aroborization of the thyroglossal duct.

Chapter 13

Painful/Nodular Hashimoto's Thyroiditis

CASE STUDY

A 45-year-old female patient presented with complaints of swelling in anterior neck noted only 4 months back and since then progressively increasing in size, more so in last one month. She also complained of fever on and off with chills and rigor for last 3 months and dysphagia, dry cough and pain in the swelling for last one month only. No history of heat tolerance, loose stools, tremors, pedal edema, diplopia, change in voice or dyspnea was noted. Her menstrual history was normal. On examination, she was pale with no cyanosis, icterus or clubbing, no tremors and a regular pulse rate. Thyroid was enlarged 2.5 times, multinodular and hard in consistency with tenderness but there was no deep cervical lymphadenopathy and lower border was palpable. Respriatory, cardiovascular, GIT systems were normal. Sensory and motor examination was normal. In view of short history of rapid enlargement of thyroid, presence of dysphagia, hard multinodular goiter a strong suspicion of malignancy (lymphoma, SCC, Anaplastic, Reidel's thyroiditis) was kept and she was evaluated as follows:

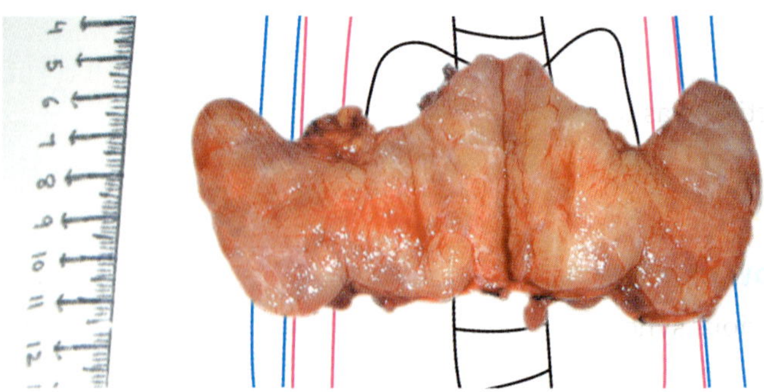

Fig. 13.1: Total thyroidectomy specimen showing fibrotic thyroid in the case of Hashimotos' disease

FNAC:	Lymphocytic thyroiditis
TFT:	Euthyroid
TMA:	Positive
USG thyroid:	Multinodular goiter, hypoechoic to hyperechoic space-occupying lesions with increased internal vascularity on Doppler.
USG abdomen:	Mild hepatomegaly but no enlarged para-aortic nodes or splenomegaly
CXR:	Normal
Barium swallow:	Normal

A diagnosis of painful Hashimoto's thyroiditis was made and the patient was started on Prednisolone in doses of 10 mg thrice a day for 2 weeks and then tapered to 20 mg and subsequently 10mg once a day. However, after initial relief in pain, she again started having severe pain when the steroids were tapered and hence thyroxine suppressive therapy was started but there was no relief in pain. Steroid were re-started in doses of 10 mg once a day and continued for one month and then tapered gradually. But again she started having severe pain because of which the dose of steroids was again increased. In view of multiple relapses on tapering doses of steroids, the patient was taken up for total thyroidectomy; the specimen weighed 80 gm and cut section was homogeneous but with a fibrotic texture.

QUESTIONS

How can you classify Hashimoto's disease?

Various synonyms have been used for Hashimoto's disease (HD) such as chronic thyroiditis, chronic autoimmune thyroiditis, chronic lymphocytic thyroiditis. There are 4 subtypes of HD depending on the stage:

i. *Subclinical:* In the early stage the patients are euthyroid and either do not have a goiter or may have a small goiter
ii. *Chronic:* Thyroid function tests are variable; goiter becomes firm and larger
iii. *Chronic Hashimoto's thyroiditis:* This is the classical Hashimoto's disease with a large firm goiter and transient hypothyroidism
iv. *Atrophic thyroiditis:* Thyroid atrophies due to destructive thyroiditis and fibrosis and permanent hypothyroidism results.

In addition there is a variant of HD known as painful HD. The reason for thyroid tenderness in patients with HT remains unexplained. One of the contributory factors could be thyroid capsule distention resulting from rapid thyroid growth.

How do you establish the diagnosis of HD?

i. *Clinical observation:* Diffuse goiter, often lobulated (hence confused with multinodular goiter), soft to firm in consistency, usually non-tender but rarely overtly painful and tender. Presence of pain suggests either a painful variant of HD or development of lymphoma
ii. *Thyroid function tests:* Variable depending upon the stage of disease
iii. *Serology:* Positive thyroid antibodies- anti Tg antibody and anti TPO antibody
iv. *FNAC:* Required when goiter is rapidly increasing in size or goiter is very hard or when suspicion of development of B-cell lymphoma is suspected.

What is the differential diagnosis of HD?

The two differential diagnosis are:

Graves' disease

Duration of symptoms is usually more than 3 months. 30% will have eye signs; T3/T4 ratio is >20; anti TSH-R antibody is positive; TSH-binding immunoglobulin is positive and RAIU is high.

Subacute thyroiditis (SAT)

It is important to differentiate HT from SAT, the latter being the commonest cause of painful thyroiditis, because the clinical course and treatment options and response are different. Patients with HT may run a long, variable course and they are likely to have multiple relapses whenever an attempt is made to withdraw steroids. On the other hand, patients with SAT respond dramatically to steroids and pain and swelling resolves within 72 hours with a sustained remission on stopping steroids after a week. On histology, patients of HT do not show giant cells and granulomas which are characteristic of SAT.

Features	HT	SAT
Prior goiter	Usual	Rare
Prior AITD	Usual	No history
Pain/tenderness	Infrequent	Frequent and extreme
Goiter	Present	Present
Thyrotoxicosis	Variable	Yes
RAIU	Variable	Very low
MCAB	Strongly positive	Negative or weak
Pathology	Fibrosis, lymphocytes	Giant cells, polymorphs, granulomas
Steroid response	Partial and transient	Dramatic and sustained
Risk of long-term hypothyroidism	Yes	Rare
Treatment	Thyroxine, NSAIDs, steroids, rarely thyroidectomy	NSAIDs, steroids, rarely thyroidectomy

What is the treatment of HT?

The usual treatment of HT is thyroxine replacement and NSAIDs. However, patients of painful variant of HT may not respond significantly to NSAIDs while response to steroids may be partial and temporary and whenever the steroids are stopped, patients are likely to experience relapses. Thyroidectomy in such a situation offers the greatest likelihood of sustained and complete pain relief. Because of this reason total thyroidectomy is advocated. As the thyroid gland is likely to be small and fibrosed, the risk of surgery is increased and hence thyroidectomy by an experienced thyroid surgeon is advocated.

What is the histopathological picture of HD?

Section from thyroid show thyroid follicles of variable sizes arranged in lobules separated by thick fibrovascular septa. The follicles are lined by cuboidal to flattened epithelial cells having uniform round normochromic nuclei and moderate to abundant amount of eosinophilic cytoplasm. Variable amount of colloid is present in the follicles. Plenty of lymphoid follicles, few with germinal centers are interspersed in between the follicles. There is destruction of thyroid follicles also due to lymphoid infiltrate. Few multinucleated giant cells may also be seen.

Chapter 14

Subacute Thyroiditis or De Quervain's Thyroiditis

CASE STUDY

A 40-year-old male presented with severe pain in front of the neck for 15 days along with difficulty in swallowing. He also gave history of excessive sweating and tremulous-ness. He also had difficulty in climbing stairs and had fever with chills and rigor. On examination he looked ill, anxious and uncomfortable. He had tachycardia with PR of 124/min, but was normotensive. His hands were hot and moist with fine tremors. Local examination revealed a mild thyromegaly which was exquisitely tender and firm to hard in consistency.

A clinical impression of thyroiditis was made and based on the following investigations a diagnosis of subacute thyroiditis was made.

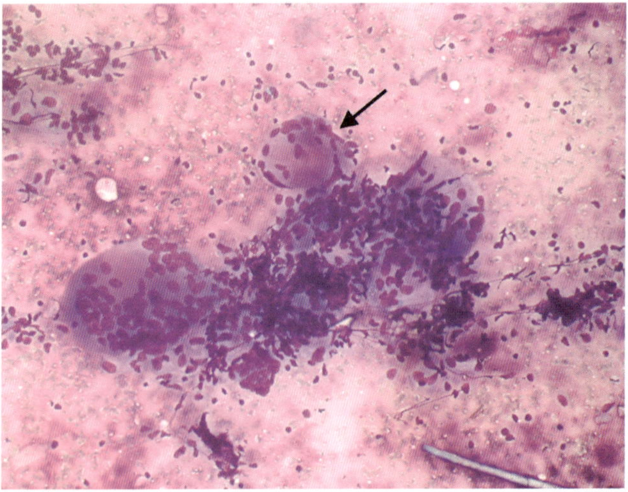

Fig. 14.1: FNA from a case of subacute thyroiditis showing histiocytic giant cells (arrow) and dirty background (MGG stain)

Thyroid Function Tests

Proportionately elevated T4 and T3 and suppressed TSH
- *T4:* 225 ng/ml
- *T3:* 5.12 ng/ml
- *TSH:* undetectable

Thyroid Scan

Whole of the gland showed very poor radiotracer concentration. Background and salivary activity was normal. Suggestive of thyroiditis

TPO Antibodies

Very low titeres were present. Patient was put on beta blockers and non-steroidal anti-inflammatory drugs to which he responded.

QUESTIONS

How do you describe this clinical entity?

It is well-defined clinical entity characterized by spontaneous, self-limiting, usually painful inflammatory lesion of the thyroid gland. It is the most common cause of painful thyroid. This disorder has several synonyms, some reflecting misconceptions: pseudo-granulomatous thyroiditis, subacute granulomatous thyroiditis, giant cell thyroiditis, subacute painful thyroiditis.

What is the etiopathogenesis?

It is not an autoimmune disease.
- A viral etiology has often been implicated.

- This condition is often preceded by a prodromal phase characterized by skeletal aches and pains, malaise, fatigue or frank URTI
- Its highest seasonal occurrence concides with peaks of summer enterovirus infections.

How do you make a clinical diagnosis?

The characteristic feature of SAT is pain- in the region of thyroid, sometimes radiating to the angle of jaw, or to the ear on affected side or the anterior chest. Swallowing, moving the head or coughing may aggravate the pain.

Rarely, SAT may have a dramatic presentation with marked fever, severe thyrotoxicosis and obstructive symptoms caused by severe thyroid inflammation and edema

Most also complain of malaise (which can be sometimes extreme), mayalgia, fatigue and feverishness).

In acute or early phase, symptoms of hyperthyroidism may be seen in the form of tremulousness, weight loss, heat intolerance or rapid heartbeat.

Atypical presentation

Rarely SAT may present as a painless solitary thyroid nodule and may be misdiagnosed as papillary cancer.

On examination

Most patients appear flushed and uncomfortable on examination. The thyroid gland may be only slightly to moderately enlarged but is usually tender, sometimes exquisitely so, and firm to hard in consistency.

Physical signs of hyperthyroidism are often demonstrable.

What is the differential diagnosis?

Causes of painful thyroid

- Subacute thyroiditis
- Subacute granulomatous thyroiditis
- Acute suppurative thyroiditis
- Acute hemorrhage into a cyst
- Acute hemorrhage into a benign or malignant nodule
- Painful Hashimoto's thyroiditis
- Radiation thyroiditis
- Rapidly growing anaplastic carcinoma
- Thyroid lymphoma

What is the course of the disease?

The duration for which this self-limiting disease may last, may vary from 2 to 5 months. Recurrences are very rare. In the initial acute or early phase, there is pain and thyrotoxicosis caused by follicular destruction and leakage of preformed hormone from the gland. This phase usually lasts for 3-6 weeks.

This is followed by a phase of transient hypothyroidism in patients whom the SAT has persisted over the interval because the stored follicular colloid is depleted and the thyroid cells are virtually incapable of producing new hormone. Transient hypothyroidism may persist for months. Transient hypothyroidism may be subclinical or overt.

This is eventually followed by recovery or euthyroidism as the thyroid is repleted with colloid and thyroid function is restored though a variable amount of interstitial fibrosis may persist.

What are the diagnostic investigations you would order to establish the diagnosis of SAT?

ESR

During acute phase ESR is usually quite high and infact a normal ESR virtually rules out a diagnosis of SAT

Hematology

Leukocytosis, normochromic, normocytic anemia.

Thyroid function tests

Elevated T4 and T3; however, T3 is only proportionately elevated unlike GD where T3 is disproportionately elevated when compared to T4.

Serum Tg

Elevated: Infact, serum Tg remains elevated long after all other evidence of inflammatory process has subsided.

Thyroid autoantibodies

Absent or low titer

RAI uptake studies

Very low, 0-1%: SAT is one of the hyperthyroid conditions associated with high levels of circulating thyroid hormones but a very low RAI uptake.

RAI scan

Patchy or irregular distribution or no uptake (In Hashimoto's thyroiditis, uptake is more than SAT).

FNAC

Features of SAT include: epithelioid granulomas, multinucleate giant cells, follicular cells with intravacuolar granules and acute or chronic inflammatory changes. FNAC often shows large number of histiocytes which can be misinterpreted or can be misleading.

What are the microscopic changes?

The histopathological changes are distinct from Hashimoto's thyroiditis. The lesions are patchy in distribution. The follicles appear much larger with disruption of epithelial lining. Histiocytes congregate around masses of colloid producing giant cells but are infact pseudo-giant cells.

How would you manage such a case?

- *In mild to moderate cases:* Salicylates and NSAIDs.
- *In severe cases:* Prednisolone is the drug of choice in doses of 10 mg QID. Relief of symptoms occurs within 24 hours. Even then, full doses are continued for a week followed by tapering of the dose over 4-6 weeks and then discontinued altogether. In 20% patients, however, as tapering is done, recurrence of manifestations may occur thereby necessating a more gradual tapering of dosage. Before discontinuing steroids, RAIU studies should be done if the uptake is still low, inflammatory process is continuing, hence, steroids should not be discontinued.
- Ipanoic acid (Telepaque) may also be employed and is quite useful in achieving rapid control of severe thyrotoxicosis.
- Beta blockers are useful in controlling manifestations of thyrotoxicosis.
- Anti-thyroid drugs have no role in management of SAT.
- Thyroidectomy is required in an unusual situation of a very prolonged or protracted course with malaise and severe local pain continuing almost indefinitely.

Chapter 15

Large Goiter

CASE STUDY

A 44-year-old male presented with history of goiter for almost 30 years which has been progressively increasing for last 2 years but he did not have any compressive features. On examination he was found to be having a large diffuse goiter which was soft to firm in consistency. FNAC revealed a benign colloid goiter and CT scan did not reveal any significant compression in the neck and there were no deep cervical lymphadenopathy; however, there was significant retrotracheal extension which was also evident on the plain X-ray of the neck. He was taken up for surgery and total thyroidectomy was performed. Operative findings included a very short middle thyroid vein and large superior pedicle vessels. The trachea was found to be floppy and hence a prophylactic tracheostomy was done which was removed on the 6th postoperative day. The weight of the resected specimen was 2.5 kg and the histopathology was suggestive of follicular carcinoma with poorly differentiated areas.

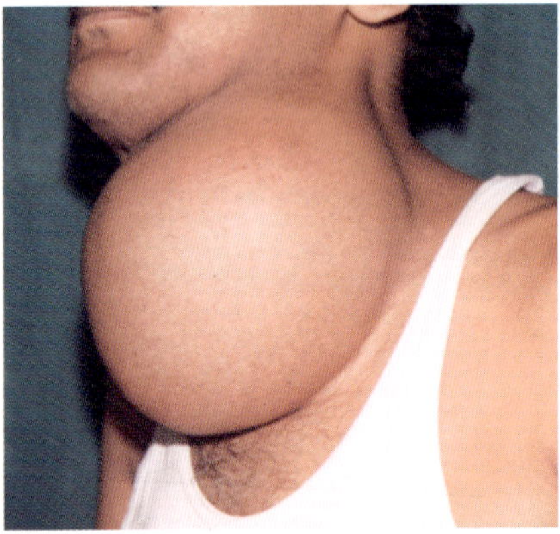

Fig. 15.1: Clinical photograph showing large goiter

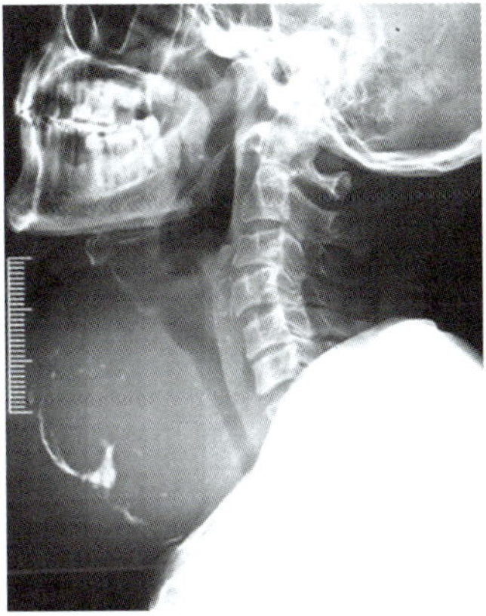

Fig. 15.2: Plain X-ray showing calcification in goiter and anteroposterior compression of trachea

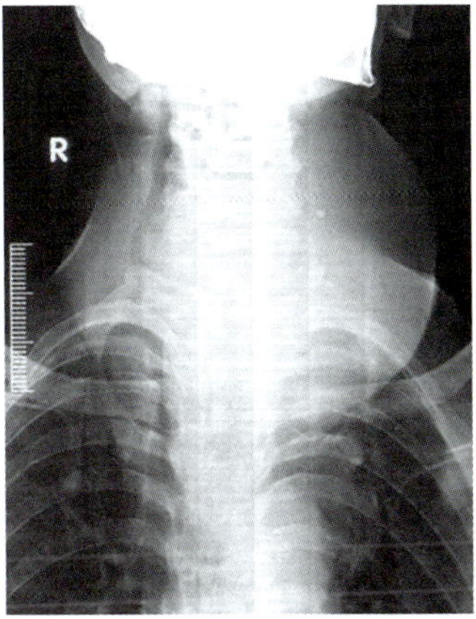

Fig. 15.3: Side-to-side compression and deviation of trachea

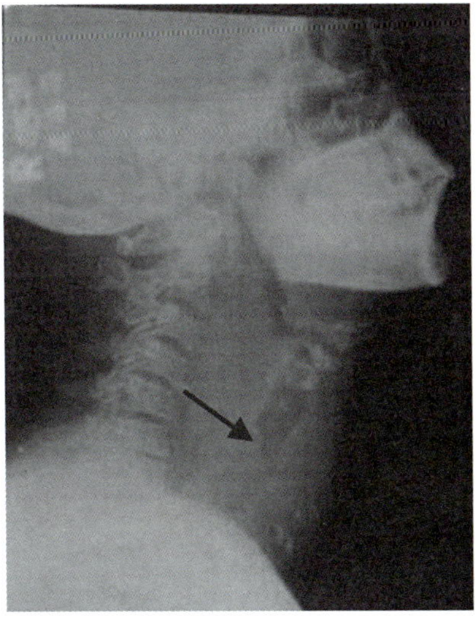

Fig. 15.4: Plain X-ray neck showing retrotracheal widening (↔)

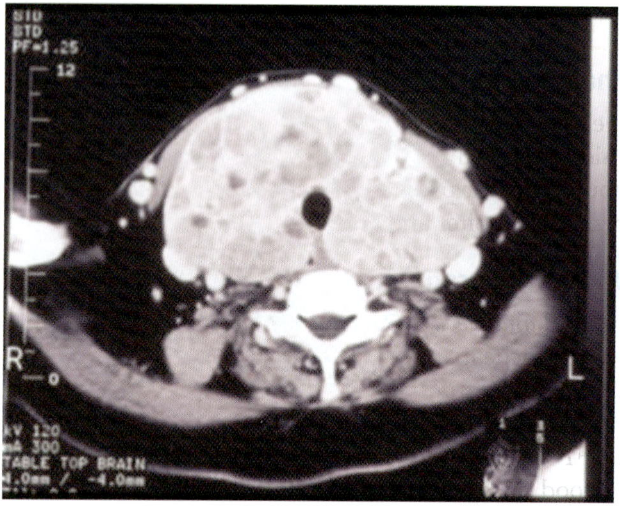

Fig. 15.5: CT neck showing retrotracheal extension

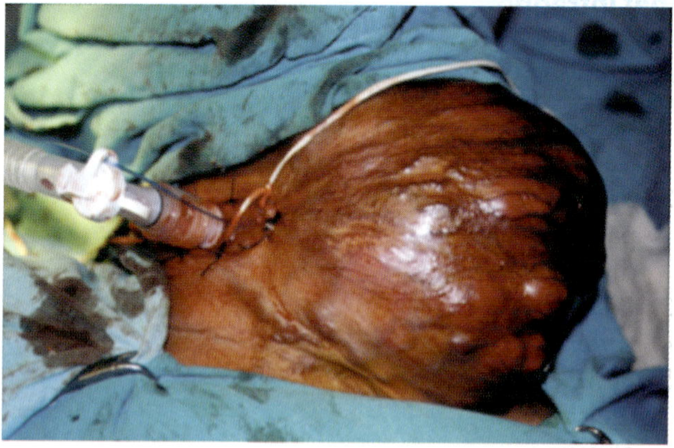

Fig. 15.6: Preoperative tracheostomy in a patient with large goiter

QUESTIONS

What is the clinical presentation of large goiters?

One should elicit history of rapid growth, duration of goiter which is usually several years and on examination one should look for presence of stridor/dyspnea, firm or hard areas in the goiter and any retrosternal extension.

What preoperative work-up is required?

1. *C-XR and Neck X-ray:* to look for tracheal compression, retrotracheal extension
2. *CT neck:* to study the relationship of goiter with internal jugular vein, strap muscles, carotid artery.
3. PFT
4. Blood donation
5. Pre-anesthetic check-up.

What intraoperative problems are to be anticipated while operating upon large goiters?

1. *Intubation:* In large goiters sometimes intubation may be difficult requiring fiberoptic support or if it fails tracheostomy may need to be done.
2. *Ryle's tube:* Always ensure that RT is put before the patient is draped as intraoperatively the esophagus is difficult to delineate
3. *Incision:* Should be liberal
4. *Anterior jugular veins:* Should be ligated in continuity
5. *SCM:* Always mobilize the flaps in the corner and also the sternomastoid muscle until the IJV is clearly seen; always cut the strap muscles routinely
6. *Middle thyroid vein:* Is short and broad; one may need to apply vascular clamp over the middle thyroid vein (MTV) before it is cut.

7. ***Superior pedicle:*** contains large vessels and has to be dealt carefully.
8. ***Tubercle of Zuckerkandl:*** Large goiters tend to have significant size tubercle of Zuckerkandl which may be going behind the trachea and should be carefully mobilized.
9. ***Parathyroids:*** Usually the inferior glands become devascularized when the thyroid gland is mobilized out of the gutter and should be dissected out for autotransplantation later, early in the course of dissection before they become ischemic.
10. ***RLN:*** In large goiters the RLN may be closely adhrerent to the thyroid lobe and infact be pulled up with the lobe.
11. ***Look for tracheomalacia:*** In large and long-standing goiters the incidence of tracheomalacia is very high and hence one should keep a high degree of suspicion. Always palpate the trachea and then ask the anesthetist to withdraw the endotracheal tube and look for collapse of a segment of trachea.

What precautions are to be taken in postoperative care?

After surgery for large goiters, one can give 200 mg of hydrocortisone to take care of laryngeal edema which can develop due to extensive dissection. Also one should be beware of tracheomalacia which should be suspected if the patient appears to be hypoxic, clinically (presence of stridor or if the patient is very irritable) or on ABG.

Chapter 16

Marine-Lenhart Syndrome

CASE STUDY

A 44-year-old male presented with history of thyromegaly for past 20 years, more or less static in size with no compressive features. He had symptoms of thyrotoxicosis and on examination was found to be having a soft thyromegaly with a discrete nodule of 5 × 5 cm in the lower pole of left lobe. There were no eye signs. Thyroid function tests revealed an elevated T4(275.1), elevated T3 (4.63) and a suppressed TSH (<0.15). Technetium scan revealed a hyperfunctioning thyroid nodule corresponding to the palpable nodule with reduced background and salivary activity and reduced uptake in the rest of the gland. FNAC from the nodule was suggestive of colloid nodule. An impression of Marine-Lenhart syndrome was made and the patient underwent total thyroidectomy. The histopathology revealed a follicular adenoma.

QUESTIONS

What are the different situations in which Graves' disease can be associated with nodule formation?

There are four situations in which GD can be associated with nodule formation:

i. ***GD with solitary nodule:*** Nodule is palpable on clinical examination and is usually cold on isotope scan. The concern in such a case is associated malignancy as the risk of malignancy in such a case is approximately 23% which is greater than the rate seen in general population. FNAC in such a nodule with a background of hyperplastic tissue in GD is usually a follicular lesion; hence even with a benign cytology the presence of carcinoma cannot be entirely ruled out. In such a situation, perhaps surgical management is more suited than RAI.

ii. ***GD with autonomous functioning nodule (Marine-Lenhart syndrome).***

iii. ***GD with multiple thyroid nodules:*** nodules are clinically palpable and confirmed on ultrasonography and isotope scan. In such a situation the technetium scan would reveal that the internodular tissue is not suppressed. Such Toxic multinodular goiter patients may also have the eye signs associated with Graves' disease.

iv. ***Patchy GD:*** Nodules are not clinically palpable nor identifiable on ultrasonography but on isotope scan there is mottled uptake. It is due to nodular autoimmune thyroid disease and are usually associated with Hashimoto's disease (Hashitoxicosis).

What is Marine-Lenhart syndrome?

GD with autonomously functioning nodule is known as Marine-Lenhart syndrome. The syndrome was initially described in 1911 by Marine and Lenhart and is now considered a distinct subentity of GD. Its occurrence is rare. A technetium scan may show increased homogenous uptake throughout the gland with an area of intense focal uptake in the right lobe corresponding to the palpable nodule. However, sometimes the scan picture may be of diffuse uptake typical of GD but with less activity in the nodule which becomes intense after ablation of the tissue with RAI. Patients with this syndrome generally are radio-resistant and require a higher dose of radioactive iodine (usually 25 mCi) for ablation compared to patients with GD without functioning adenomas. For this reason surgical management is a valid option.

Chapter 17

Lingual Thyroid

CASE STUDY

A 28-year-old lady presented with an enlarging mass at the back of the tongue. She was otherwise asymptomatic with no history of dysphagia, dyspnea, dysphonia, or bleeding from the mass. On examination she was found to be signs of hypothyroidism along with a friable globular swelling at the foramen caecum. Subsequent investigations were as follows:

- ***TSH:*** 12.5.
- ***Thyroid scan:*** Hot spot in the oral cavity with no functioning thyroid tissue in the neck.
- ***Ultrasound:*** absence of thyroid in the normal anatomical location in the neck
- She was subsequently put on thyroid hormone suppression. Three months later the mass reduced in size and her TSH normalized.

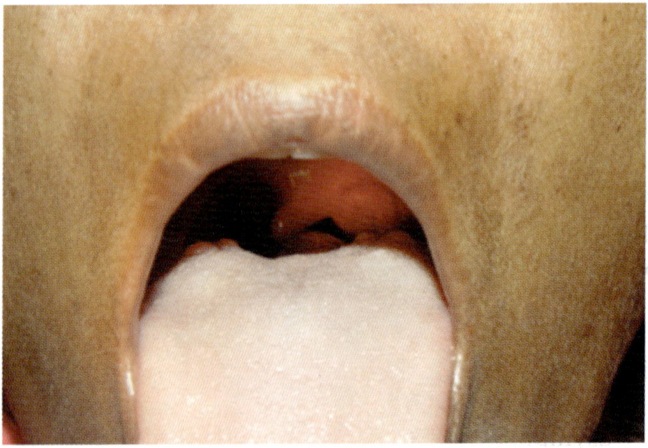

Fig. 17.1: Lingual thyroid at the base of tongue

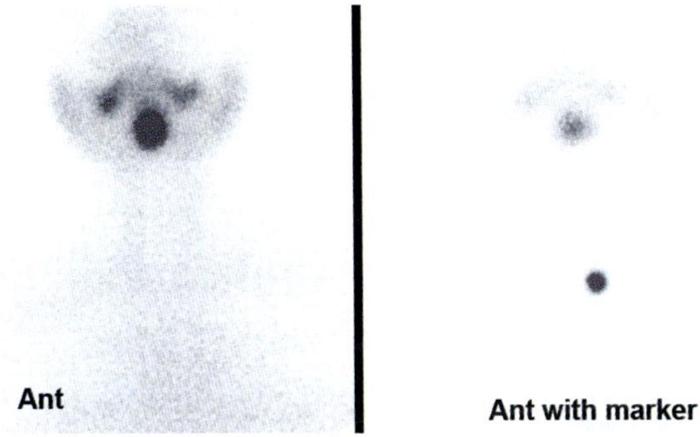

Fig. 17.2: Nuclear scan showing absence of normal cervical thyroid but uptake seen in oral cavity

QUESTIONS

What is the embryological basis of lingual thyroid?

The thyroid originates from the foramen caecum at the base of the tongue. The thyroid anlage descends as the thyroglossal duct, in the midline of the neck, reaching its normal position anterior to the trachea and larynx. Lingual thyroid occurs when there is no descent of the thyroid.

What is the clinical presentation?

Though lingual thyroid is rare, it is the most common location for functioning ectopic thyroid tissue.

i. Majority of cases occur in young women of age group 18-40 years.
ii. Commonest presentation is as discovery of an incidental mass on the back of tongue in an asymptomatic patient.
iii. However, patients can also present with dysphagia dyspnea, dysphonia or as bleeding from the mass.

iv. Symptoms may precipitate with hormonal fluctuations, e.g. during menstrual cycle or pregnancy.
v. Patients are frequently hypothyroid; hypothyroidism may cause the lingual thyroid to enlarge and become symptomatic.

How will you evaluate such a case?

Lingual thyroid tissue is associated with an absence of the normal cervical thyroid in almost 75% of cases, hence an ultrasound of the neck and radio-isotope scanning is essential to establish that the lingual thyroid is the only functioning thyroid tissue in the patient. Thyroid function tests are done to establish the presence of hypothyroidism.

What are the management options?

The usual management of such a condition is thyroid hormone suppression to reduce the size of the lingual thyroid and also to correct the hypothyroidism. Surgical excision is rarely required- in cases of failure of suppressive therapy to reduce the size, ulceration, hemorrhage or suspicion of malignancy. During surgery the thyroid tissue may be auto-transplanted as the incidence of malignancy is very low.

Chapter 18

Dyshormonogenetic Goiter

CASE STUDY

Parents of a 9-year-old girl complained of growth failure and developmental delay since infancy. She was born to G8, partially supervised, with no antenatal or prenatal complications. It was a home delivery with no history of birth asphyxia. All developmental milestones were delayed with head holding at 10 months, sitting at 10 months and speech at 1.5 years. She did not attend school and she did not receive any other medications. There was no history of constipation. A mild neck swelling was noticed since birth which has since then progressively increased to grade 2 goiter. Family history of thyroid disorders in two other siblings was noted. In one sibling the speech was also delayed. On examination both siblings have grade 2 goiter which is soft, diffuse and without any nodules. Possibilities of thyroid hormone resistance, iodine deficiency goiter or dyshormonogenesis were kept. Both the siblings with goiter were evaluated as follows:

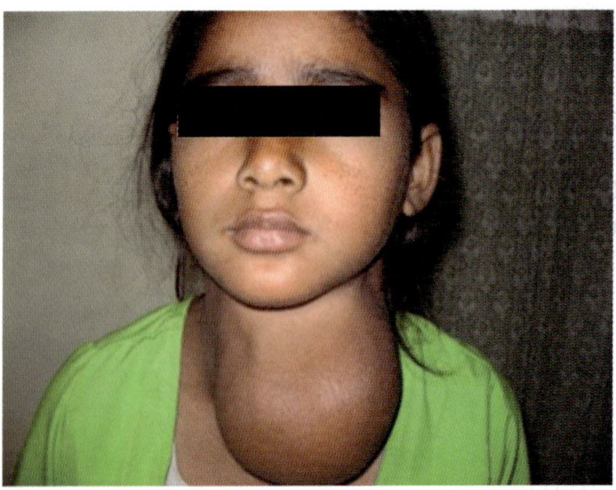

Fig. 18.1: Young girl with large goiter and signs of hypothyroidism

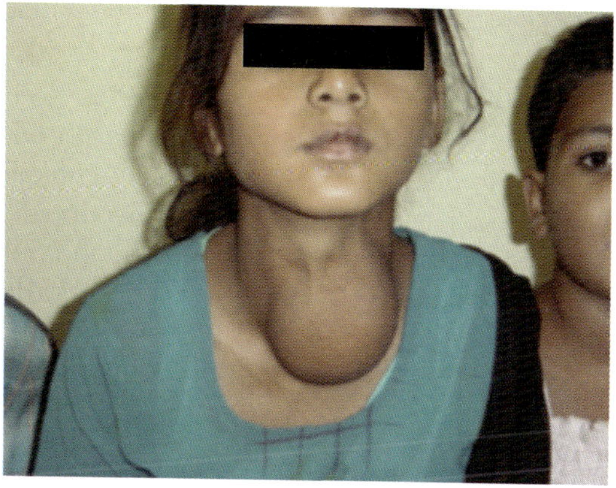

Fig. 18.2: Decrease in goiter size following thyroxine administration

Investigations	Sibling 1	Sibling 2
Free T4	8.5	9.14
T3	1.96	1.56
TSH	> 60	> 60
TPO	3.73	< 12
Perchlorate discharge test	Positive for organification defect of thyroid gland	Positive for organification defect of thyroid gland
Pure tone audiometry	B/L normal hearing	B/L normal hearing
Post thyroxine replacement TSH	1.10	5.76

Based on the above investigations, a diagnosis of Dyshormonogenetic goiter was made and both siblings were put on thyroxine replacement following which the TSH normalized and the goiter size decreased.

QUESTIONS

What is dyshormonogenetic goiter?

It is a rare, often familial condition and genetically inherited. It results from iodide organification defects, characterized by substantial release of iodide from the thyroid after administration of perchlorate. Unrecognised and untreated children develop hypothyroid goiter. It results from mutation in Promoter or structural TPO gene leading to partial or total inactivation.

Normal physiology

Iodide transported into the thyroid gland is oxidized by H_2O_2, catalyzed by NADPH oxidase, and bound to tyrosine residues in TG. Subsequently iodinated tyrosine residues couple to form iodothyronine residues, mainly T4. Both iodination and coupling are catalyzed extracellularly by TPO at the apical border of thyrocyte. Total inability to oxidize iodide can almost completely result from mutation in TPO.

What are the five genes involved in thyroid hormonogenesis?

These are:

i. Thyroid peroxidase (TPO)
ii. Sodium Iodide Symporter (NIS)
iii. Thyroid oxidase ($THOX_2$)
iv. Pendrin (PDS)
v. Thyroglobulin (TG)

What are clinical manifestations of dyshormonogenetic goiter?

Clinical manifestations depend upon the extent of defect (as shown by the percholarate discharge test). If the defect is severe or complete children present with hypothyroidism and goiter. The goiter is initially diffuse but may become nodular later. Children will be euthyroid when the defect is mild and compensated. The diagnosis of Dyshormono-genetic goiter should be suspected when the patient comes from a non-endemic area, the goiter is present since birth, and there is no maternal history of intake of goitrogenic substances during pregnancy.

How do you establish the diagnosis of dyshormonogenetic goiter?

The definitive diagnosis is established by the perchlorate discharge test. The physiologic basis of this test is as follows: The trapping of iodine within the thyroid gland is by an active transport mechanism mediated by NaI symporter (NIS). Iodine is then rapidly bound to thyroglobulin and retained inside the gland. Iodine that is not bound to Tg can be released from the gland by ions such as thiocynate or perchlorate (ClO_4).

Test

Radioiodine is administered and counts are obtained every 10 to 15 min. Two hours later, high dose of $KClO_4$ (1g) is administered orally and repeated counts are obtained for next two hours. In normal individuals, radioiodine accumulation in the thyroid gland ceases after administration of the iodide transporter inhibitor, and little or no loss of the accumulated thyroidal radioactivity occurs. An organification defect is indicated if a loss of 5% or more occurs. Thus, intrathyroidal radioiodine loss after the administration of an inhibitor of iodide trapping measures intrathyroidal iodide that is not protein bound and indicates the presence of an iodide-binding defect

What is the role of surgery in dyshormonogenetic goiter?

Surgery is indicated only for cosmesis, relief of compressive features or if malignancy is suspected. However, FNAC may give an erroneous diagnosis of malignancy of follicular neoplasm because of florid epithelial hyperplasia which may be seen as a result of continuous TSH stimulation.

Chapter 19

Retrosternal Goiter

CASE STUDY

A 65-year-old female patient presented with history of breathlessness and hoarseness of voice for last 10 days. She also had a neck swelling for last 20 years with no history of recent increase in size. On examination she was found to be having inspiratory stridor and a large multinodular goiter whose lower border was not palpable; there was no cervical lymphadenopathy. Suspicion of retrosternal goiter was confirmed by a positive Pemberton's sign and chest X-ray which revealed mediastinal widening. MRI of neck and thorax showed multinodular goiter with retrosternal extension of the left lobe only upto the arotic arch. The cytology was suggestive of colloid goiter. The patient was admitted and supportive care was given in the form of continuous humified oxygen, steroids under antibiotic cover and propped up position for relief of her inspiratory stridor. She was then taken up for surgery. At operation first the right lobe was mobilized after division of strap muscles of

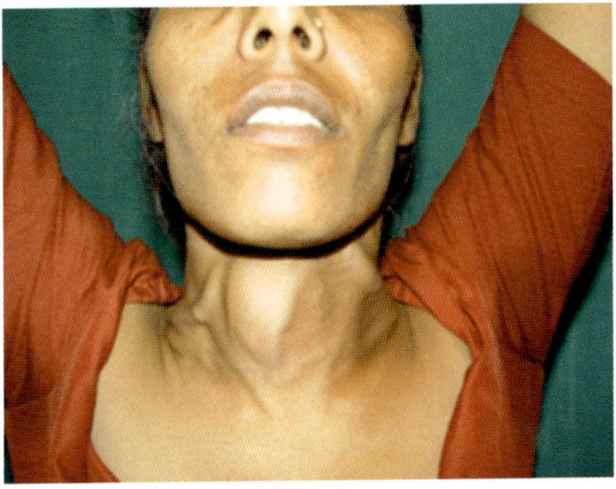

Fig. 19.1: Positive Pemberton's sign with engorged neck veins

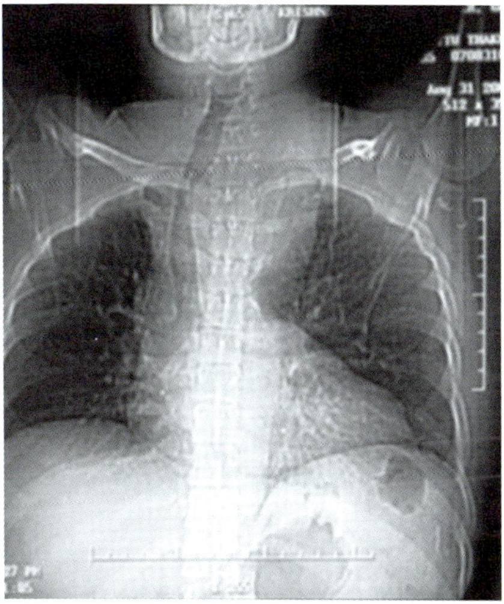

Fig. 19.2: Plain X-ray chest showing retrosternal extension with deviation of trachea

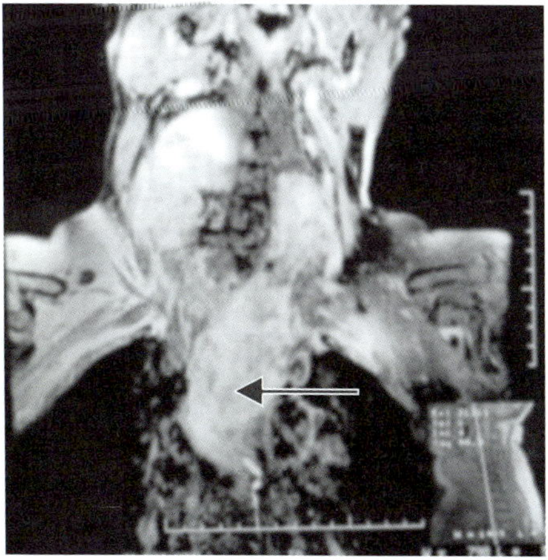

Fig. 19.3: MRI showing retrosternal extension upto aortic arch (arrow)

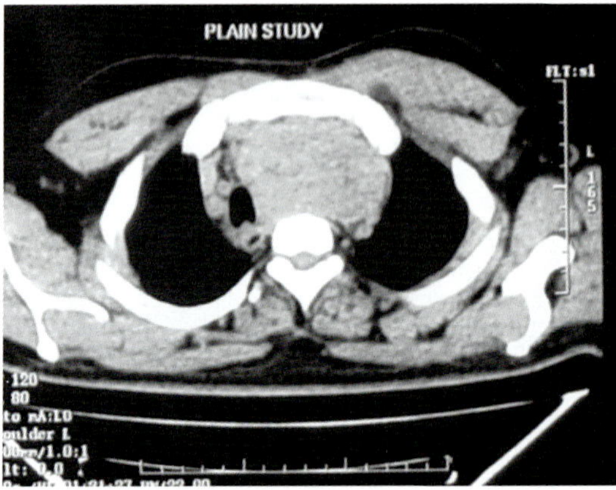

Fig. 19.4: CT of chest of another patient showing retrosternal extension just above the aortic arch

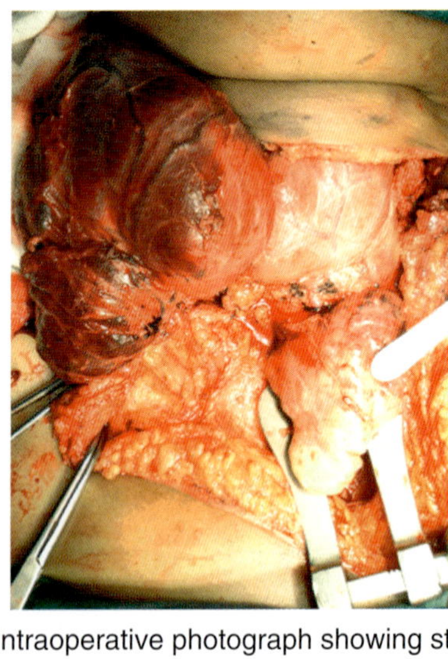

Fig. 19.5: Intraoperative photograph showing sternotomy to deliver the retrosternal portion of gland

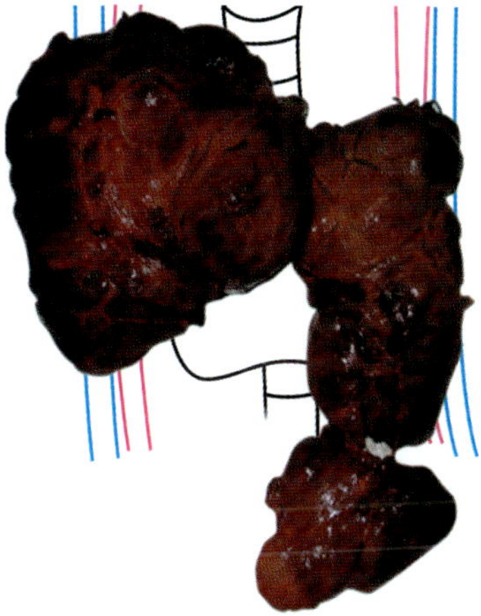

Fig. 19.6: Surgical specimen after sternotomy

both sides. The left lobe was then mobilized and superior pedicle was ligated. The left RLN was identified at its point of entry and further dissection was done anterior to the RLN keeping the nerve in view all the time. Since we were unable to reach below the left lobe, a decision of partial sternotomy was taken and the retrosternal portion of the thyroid was delivered. Since the tracheal was found to be floppy, tracheostomy was done. The specimen weighed 600 gm. The postoperative period was uneventful and the tracheostomy tube was removed on the 6th postoperative day. The histopathology was benign multinodular colloid goiter.

QUESTIONS

How does a patient of retrosternal goiter present?

i. *Asymptomatic:* 6-40% are asymptomatic and incidentally discovered on plain chest films. 20-30% have no palpable cervical goiter.

ii. *Respiratory symptoms:* Seen in 20-56%. It may range from mild to severe. Patient may have isolated dyspnea, dyspnea with cyanosis, suffocation, choking requiring immediate resuscitation. (In patients requiring intubation for acute airway compromise resulting from substernal goiter, surgery should be performed as soon as possible and the patient should not be weaned off from the ventilator before surgery, because this may be followed by acute asyphyxia). Patients may give a history that dyspnea or cough is worsened by lying flat or lying on one side. Sometimes the symptoms resulting from substernal goiters mimic those of bronchial asthma. Mechanism of airway obstruction: compression of trachea by a retrosternal goiter expanding between bony structures like spine, sternum and rib cage.

iii. *Symptoms of venous obstruction:* Seen in 10% cases. May result from partial or complete SVC obstruction, either due to pressure from a large benign retrosternal goiter or due to malignant infiltration by malignant goiter. Subclinical venous obstruction can be diagnosed by the Maranon's maneuver or Pemberton's sign – having the patient raise the arms above the head and observe facial plethora, distention of external jugular vein and superficial neck and upper chest veins. This sign is sometimes expanded to include some degree of respiratory discomfort also. SVC obstruction is an absolute indication for surgery and resolves completely after surgery.

iv. ***Hoarseness and RLN palsy:*** Resulting from stretching or entrapment of RLN. At times hoarseness may be present inspite of a functioning nerve, hence every attempt should be made to preserve the nerve.

v. ***Hyperthyroidism:*** More common in the elderly; cardiac effects like arrhythmias, congestive failure or ischemic heart disease carry a more serious implication.

vi. ***Dysphagia:*** May result from esophageal obstruction

vii. ***Rare symptoms:*** Hematemesis may result from downhill esophageal varices as a result of collateral circulation. Transient ischemic attacks can result from a " thyroid steal syndrome."

How do you classify the types of retrosternal goiter?

Various definitions and nomenclature such as intrathoracic goiter, substernal goiter, mediastinal goiter. Commonly accepted definitions are;

i. All goiters with a lower pole lying below the thoracic inlet.

ii. Those goiters in which at least 50% of the thyroid mass is below the thoracic inlet.

iii. Those goiters whose lower border radiographically reaches the transverse process of the fourth thoracic vertebrae.

iv. Those with a major intrathoracic component that required reaching into the mediastinum.

From a practical point of view I would like to classify retrosternal goiters as those whose lower pole lies below the thoracic inlet and they can be further classified on the approach used for delivery:

i. *Those that can be delivered from the neck:* Includes goiters whose lower pole extends into the anterior mediastinum below the thoracic inlet and up to the aortic arch on CT scan.
ii. *Those that require sternotomy (partial or full):* Includes goiters whose lower limit is below the aortic arch, goiters who are above the aortic arch but whose intrathoracic diameter is more than the thoracic inlet diameter and goiters with extension into posterior mediastinum.
iii. Isolated mediastinal goiter or completely intrathoracic goiter require thoracotomy or sternotomy.
iv. *Plain chest film:* Asymptomatic substernal goiters are picked up on routine AP or lateral films. Plain films provide an idea of the location of goiter in the mediastinum, degree of tracheal deviation, compression, or kinking as well as calcification in the goiter. It will also demonstrate macronodular lung secondaries. However, it should be kept in mind that airway compression is underestimated by as much as 40% on plain radiographs.
v. *CECT:* The extent and location of the substernal goiter is further defined on CT. It also documents the continuity or lack of it between cervical and substernal goiter. Airway compromise especially below the larynx is better correlated and demonstrated on CT. Similarly, the vascular supply of the mediastinal mass is better delineated on CT. The location in the mediastinum is exactly defined and helps the surgeon to be aware of the ventral RLN in cases of posterior mediastinal goiters. The inferior extent with relation to the aortic arch is defined and this helps to plan a sternotomy if required.

vii. *Flow volume loop studies:* Do not correlate very well with the degree of tracheal obstruction

viii. *Lung function studies:* These may help to document the functional impact of substernal goiters. The prcope-rative peak flow ratio (observed:predicted) is found to be significantly lower in patient with substernal goiters with a PPV of 90%. This reduced PEF usually improves after surgery. This test along with demonstration of failure of the peak air flow and forced expiratory volume to respond to bronchodilators, may be helpful in identifying those patients with respiratory disease and associated substernal goiters who are likely to benefit from surgery.

What are anesthesia considerations in surgery for substernal goiters?

Even though there may be extreme degree of tracheal deviation, intubation is rarely difficult. However, the surgeon and the anesthetist should be prepared for awake intubation if the intubation fails. All care should be taken that the intubation is successful in first attempt and is atraumatic to avoid any laryngeal edema which may prove fatal. A Ryle's tube should always be put.

What are the treatment options in retrosternal goiter?

i. *Suppressive therapy:* Is not effective and thus not recommended.

ii. *RAI therapy:* May cause exacerbation of compressive symptoms in a toxic substernal goiter, hence it is not recommended unless the patient is a poor operative risk.

iii. *Surgical therapy:* Retrosternal goiter should usually be removed if the patient is a good operative risk. Delay in surgical management may cause the goiter to increase in size leading to greater degree of compressive symptoms. The advantage of surgical therapy is that it resolves the compressive symptoms immediately; complication rates are low in experienced hands as > 90% of substernal goiters can be removed via the cervical route; a pathology report is available and any associated malignancy is adequately treated; underlying hyperthyroidism especially in elderly with risk of heart disease is effectively treated.

When is sternotomy required and what are its advantages?

Sternotomy, either partial or total split, is required only in 2-8% of cases. The indications are: when the diameter of the retrosternal portion of the goiter is more than the thoracic inlet or when the inferior limit of the retrosternal portion is beyond the aortic arch or in a case of isolated retrosternal goiter. The advantages over the lateral thoracotomy incision is that in sternotomy repositioning of the patient is not required; it provides excellent exposure for dissection under vision and the entire course of RLN can be demonstrated, preventing its injury.

What are the considerations in surgical delivery of retrosternal goiter from cervical route?

i. Generous skin incision
ii. Mobilization of SCM
iii. Division of strap muscles, at least on the side of the retrosternal component

iv. Sometimes performing surgery on the contralateral side first may allow increased mobility for delivery of the retrosternal portion
v. Control of middle thyroid vein
vi. Ligation of superior thyroid pedicle
vii. Identification of superior and if possible inferior parathyroid glands
viii. Attempt to identify the RLN before the delivery of the retrosternal portion. If the nerve is identified, one should stay anterior to the nerve always.
ix. Gentle pushing out (rather than pulling out) the retrosternal portion – this is done by gently breaking the loose adhesions surrounding the substernal portion of goiter with index finger in an incremental fashion keeping close to the thyroid all the time.
x. Toboggan technique (propagated by Charles Proye) This involves identification of the RLN at the point of entry into larynx and then sliding the hand down with palm up, to deliver the retrosternal portion, keeping anterior to the RLN all the time.
xi It is important to keep in mind that the RLN may be considerably displaced in retrosternal goiter.
   i. It may be intimately adherent to the posterior surface to the thyroid
   ii. It may be displaced medially
   iii. Or very rarely it may be ventral to the substernal portion of the goiter; this ventral RLN is prone to injury if not recognized well in time.

When do you require a postero-lateral thoracotomy?

Postero-lateral thoracotomy is required in cases of isolated posterior mediastinal goiter or crossed substernal goiter (usually on the right side). It is usually done in the 4th or 5th intercostal space. The lung is retracted and the goiter is identified, usually posterior to SVC and superior to azygos vein. The pleura over the goiter is incised and the goiter is gradually manipulated into the thoracic inlet for cervical delivery or is dissected out after ligating the thoracic supply of the mediastinal goiter.

Is the rate of complications more in surgery of retrosternal goiters?

The rate of complications may be slightly more as compared to surgery of cervical goiters. The following are the complications of surgery of retrosternal goiters:

i. ***RLN injury:*** May occur either because of inadvertent injury resulting from non-identification of the nerve or because of stretching during blunt dissection especially if the nerve is not identified before delivery of the retrosternal portion of the goiter.
ii. ***Parathyroid glands injury:*** Low threshold for autotransplantation is desirable especially for the inferior glands which are likely to become ischemic or may be removed with the specimen. Hence, it is very important that superior glands be carefully dissected and preserved *in situ.*
iii. ***Tracheomalacia:*** We have observed a higher rate of tracheomalacia in substernal goiters due to long standing compression. Best managed by intraoperative detection and a prophylactic tracheotomy
iv. ***Hematoma:*** Due to extensive dissection postthyroidectomy hematoma may result.

FACTS AND FIGURES

a. 30-40% are asymptomatic
b. In 20% patients there is no palpable mass
c. 90% of symptomatic patients have mainly respiratory symptoms like dyspnea, cough, hoarseness of voice
d. Obstruction of venous return occurs in only 10% of cases
e. Hperthyroidism can be seen in 35% of elderly patients with mediastinal goiter
f. Papillary carcinoma, either overt or incidental is seen in 3-15% of cases of retrosternal goiter
g. Majority of retrosternal goiters are benign multinodular goiters or follicular adenomas
h. Only 2-8% of retrosternal goiters require sternotomy
i. Only 7-10% are found to be bilateral
j. Only 7-10% are found in the posterior mediastinum
k. 8% of patients with retrosternal goiters may require emergent intubation.

Chapter 20

Post-thyroidectomy Stridor

CASE STUDY

A 32-year-old male patient presented with complaints of neck swelling for last 6 years. The swelling has been gradually increasing in size since then. There was no history of any change in voice, breathlessness or difficulty in swallowing. On examination he had a grade 2 goiter with a 15 × 15 cm globular, smooth swelling predominantly on the right side of neck. The trachea was grossly shifted to the left side. The lower border of swelling was palpable and there was no cervical lymphadenopathy. USG of the neck revealed a large cystic solitary thyroid nodule arising from lower pole of right lobe, 11.2 × 9.2 × 10.4 cm with approximate volume of 564 cc with few septations. There were multiple heterogenous nodules in the left lobe of thyroid, approximate 2 cm in diameter. Indirect laryngoscopy revealed gross shifting of glottis and vocal cords. The plain X-ray of neck showed gross deviation, compression and kinking of trachea.

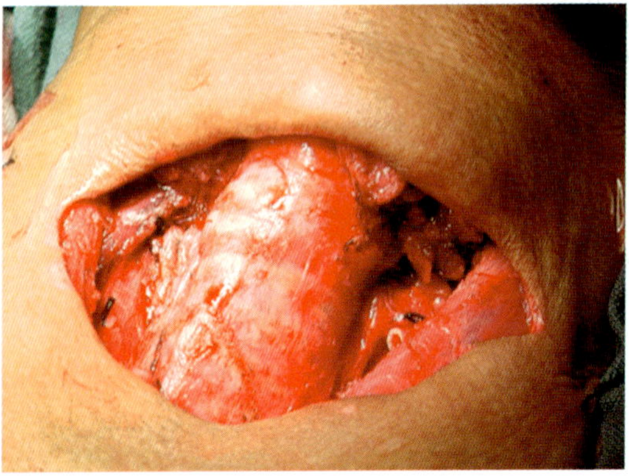

Fig. 20.1: Intraoperative photograph showing flattened trachea after partial withdrawal of endotracheal tube

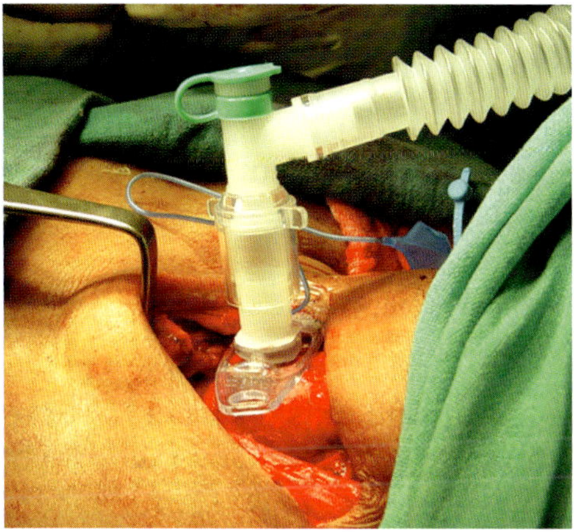

Fig. 20.2: Tracheostomy tube in place

FNAC of the thyroid was suggestive of thyroid cyst with colloid nodule. The patient was taken up for surgery and total thyroidectomy was performed after exposing and saving all the 4 parathyroids and RLN and external branch of superior laryngeal nerve. On palpation, the trachea was found to be very soft and floppy and obvious collapse of the anterior wall of tracheal wall could be seen after partial withdrawal of ETT; hence a prophylactic tracheotomy was done. The weight of the resected specimen was 1070 gram and the histopathology was benign multinodular goiter. The patient was decannulated on the 9th post-operative day.

QUESTIONS

How do you define tracheomalacia?

It is a condition where the diameter of trachea is reduced to less than half resulting in airway compression and stridor.

It usually results from loss of tracheal cartilage consequent to continuous and relentless compression by a long-standing goiter, particularly a large goiter.

What is the consequence of tracheomalacia?

A tracheomalacic trachea is prone to collapse following thyroidectomy and this results in acute airway obstruction in the immediate postoperative period and if not recognized well in time, can result in mortality.

What are the possible risk factors for development of tracheomalacia and can they be sought pre-operatively?

There are several clinical indicators which though not foolproof, should be sought preoperatively. These include- presence of stridor preoperatively, radiological evidence of tracheal compression, deviation, or kinking, long-standing goiter >10 years and large goiter or malignant infiltration of trachea, retrosternal goiter and difficulty in intubation.

How will you confirm a diagnosis of tracheomalacia following thyroidectomy before extubation?

Presence of one or more of the following criteria confirm the diagnosis of weakened tracheal rings and possible collapse.

i. Soft or floppy trachea on palpation— this should be done after partial withdrawal of ETT.
ii. Absence of peritubal leak on deflation of ETT cuff.
iii. Difficulty in negotiating the suction catheter after extubation.
iv. If the ETT is gradually withdrawn, one can actually see the collapse of trachea.

What are the causes of stridor following thyroidectomy

- Bilateral vocal cord palsy
- Glottic/subglottic edema
- Tracheomalacia

What are the various methods of management of tracheomalacia?

- Tracheotomy
- Prolonged nasal intubation
- Tracheopexy
- External fixation of tracheal cartilage—mesh, miniplate

In my hands the simplest and most effective method is prophylactic tracheotomy which promotes fibrosis in the next 5-6 days after which the patient can be decannulated.

What is the technique of tracheostomy?

The most floppy portion of trachea is chosen as the site of tracheotomy- it is usually at the junction of 2nd-3rd tracheal ring. AU shaped incision is made in the anterior wall of trachea with diathermy and size 6 or 7 tracheostomy tube is inserted and fixed. The anterior wall of the tracheal is then sutured to the lower thyroid flap which permits easy change of tracheostomy tube in the postoperative period. Regular tracheal toileting is done. It should be kept in mind that the tube gets blocked with secretions, hence it needs to be changed every alternate day. The tube is withdrawn for few minutes beginning on the 4th postoperative day and this interval is gradually increased till we are able to decannulate the patient usually on 7-8th postoperative day. In the long-term follow-up the incidence of tracheal stenosis consequent to tracheotomy is very rare.

Chapter 21

Papillary Carcinoma

CASE STUDY

A 19-year-old girl presented with complaint of gradually increasing swelling in front of her neck for last 9 months. She did not have any compressive features. On examination, she was found to be having a solitary thyroid nodule of the right lobe along with multiple, bilateral deep cervical lymphadenopathy. She was subsequently investigated as follows:

- USG: revealed multiple hypoechoic lesions in both lobes of thyroid along with microcalcifications. Multiple large lymph nodes were seen in either side of neck. Numerous tiny calcifications were also seen in lymph nodes.
- FNAC from the thyroid nodule as well as lymph nodes was suggestive of PTC.
- CT scan of the neck and mediastinum confirmed the findings of ultrasound. It did not reveal any infiltration of the jugular vessels nor did it reveal any superior mediastinal lymph nodes
- Thyroid function tests were within normal limits.

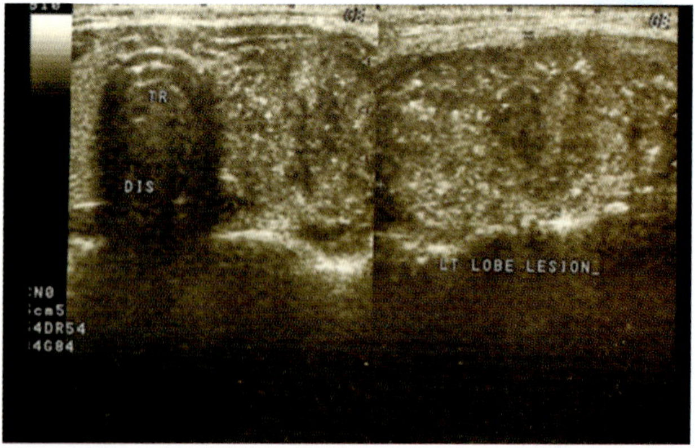

Fig. 21.1: Multiple punctate microcalcification in thyroid nodule

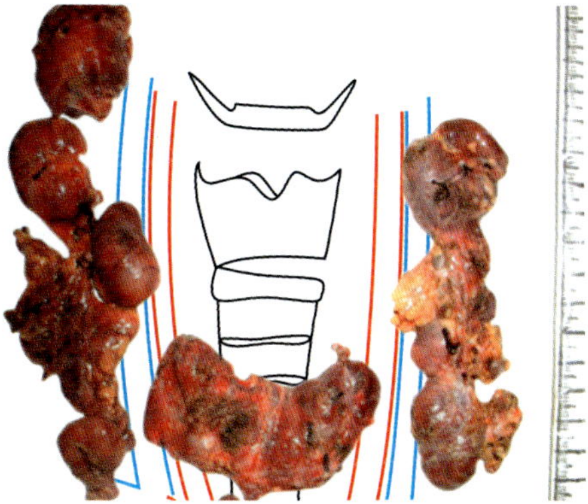

Fig. 21.2: Specimen of total thyroidectomy with bilateral modified neck dissection and central compartmental dissection

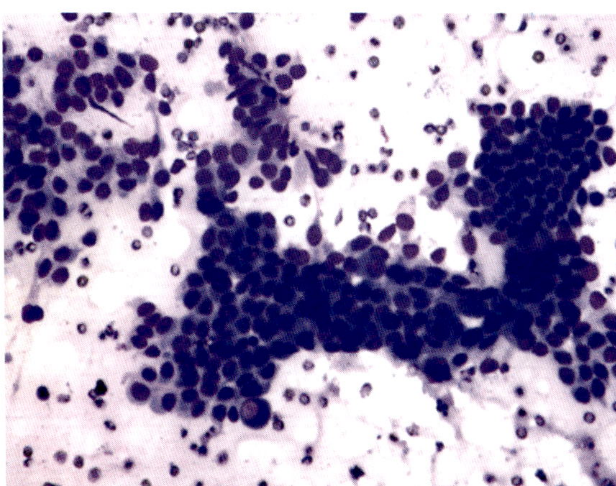

Fig. 21.3: Papillary carcinoma thyroid—characteristic nuclear features on FNAC smear (MGG stain)

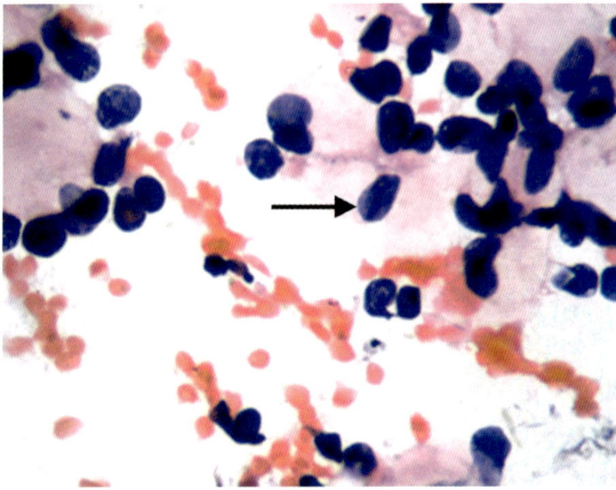

Fig. 21.4: Papillary carcinoma thyroid—nuclear grooving (arrow) on FNAC smear (PAP)

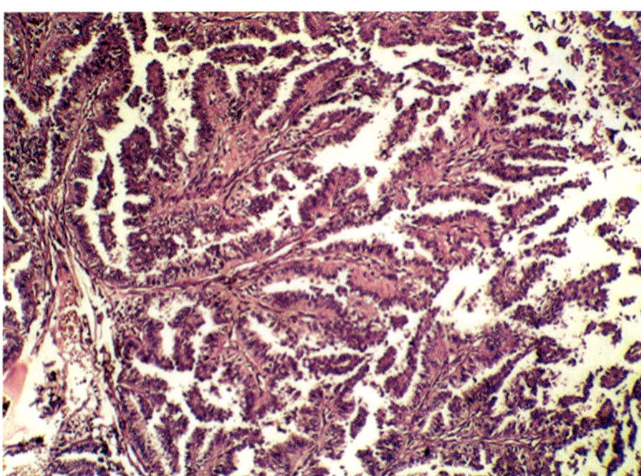

Fig. 21.5: Papillary carcinoma thyroid—arborizing papillae on histology (H and E stain)

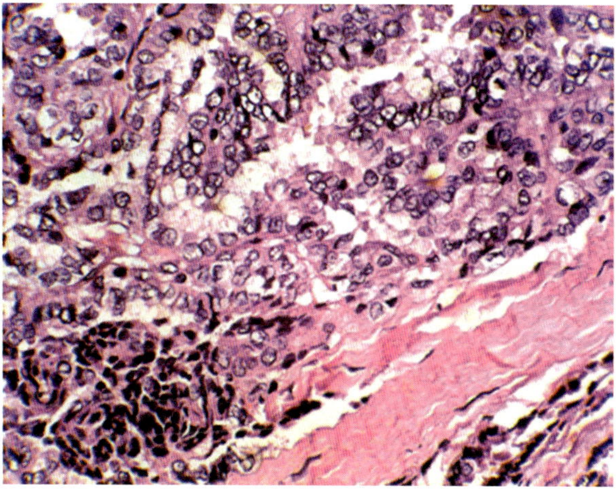

Fig. 21.6: Papillary carcinoma thyroid—distinct nuclear features (H and E stain)

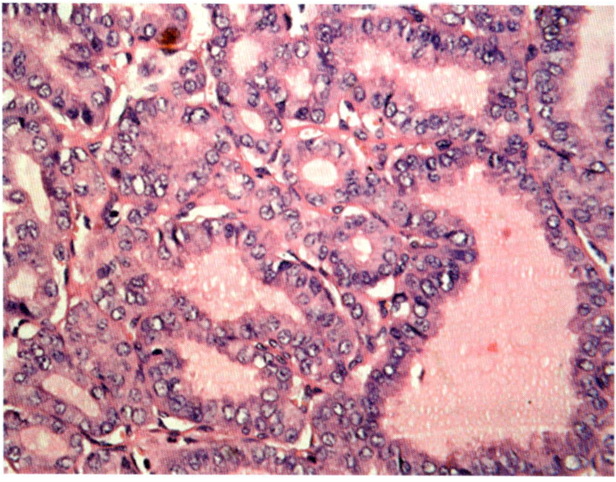

Fig. 21.7: Papillary carcinoma thyroid—ground glass nuclei (H and E stain)

She was taken up for surgery and total thyroidectomy along with full central compartmental dissection and bilateral modified neck dissection was performed. The postoperative period was uneventful and histopathology confirmed the diagnosis of papillary carcinoma; 7/7 lymph nodes of right neck, 8/9 of left neck and 3/6 of central compartment showed tumor deposits. She underwent whole body RAI scanning after 4 weeks of endogenous TSH stimulation which revealed increased uptake in the thyroid bed, superior mediastinum and bilateral lung fields. Thyroglobulin levels at this time were found to be elevated-460 ng/ml. She was treated with 125 mCi of RAI and is due for her next WBS in 6 months.

QUESTIONS

What is the distribution of different types of thyroid cancers?

The usual distribution of various types of thyroid cancers is as follows:

- Differentiated thyroid cancer (PTC and FTC): 94%
- Medullary thyroid cancer (MTC): 5%
- Anaplastic thyroid cancer (ATC): 1%

When should you suspect cancer in a patient presenting with solitary thyroid nodule?

- Commonest clinical presentation in a solitary thyroid nodule discovered by chance in an asymptomatic individual
- Can also present as a metastatic lymph node, particularly in children

- Rarely symptoms related to distant metastases to lung/ bone may be the presenting complaint
- Very rarely it presents with locally aggressive disease in the form of dyspnoea, dysphagia or hoarseness of voice.

How will you establish the diagnosis of PTC?

FNAC

The first and the most appropriate initial diagnostic procedure is FNAC. In experienced hands both false positive and false negative results are uncommon in PTC.

USG

Presence of microcalcification in thyroid is highly suggestive of papillary thyroid carcinoma

What is the etiopathogenesis of PTC?

The various predisposing factors are:

- Ionizing radiation: particularly to head and neck area and during childhood is a definte risk factor that predisposes to development of PTC (after the age of 15-20 years the risk is not significant)
- Nutritional iodine deficiency: not a well-studied risk factor but chronic stimulation by elevated TSH levels may predispose to thyroid hyperplasia and subsequent development of malignancy
- Genetic factors: familial PTC is reported in 5% of patients. Also, PTC is found to be present in several familial syndromes like Cowden's disease, Gardener's syndrome and familial adenomatous polyposis (FAP). In kindreds with FAP, the risk of development of PTC is >100 fold above general population.

What is the molecular biology of PTC?

In PTC, gene rearrangement of RET and TRK proto-oncogenes have been identified as causative events. RET rearrangement is seen in 50% PTC (however, it may also be identified in 50% of benign thyroid lesions as well). The novel rearrangement results in several chemeric oncogenes collective called as PTC. While RET/PTC 3 is the predominant rearrangement in radiation induced PTC (as seen in children affected by Chernobyl nuclear disaster), it is the RET/PTC1 which is the predominant rearrangement seen in typical PTC. More recently higher frequency of BRAF mutations have been detected in PTC as compared to other forms of thyroid cancer.

How would you prognosticate a case of PTC and what are the problems with these staging systems?

Several staging systems have been devised like AGES, AMES, MACIS, EORTC, TNM, etc. Most of these use age to separate low risk (mortality rate < 1%) from highrisk PTC (mortality rate > 40%).

Problems

- The problem with using age as risk stratification is that young patients have high rates of recurrence, therefore, cancer recurrence rate may be higher in low-risk patients as compared to high risk patients.
- On the other hand, TNM staging system gives undue importance to presence of lymph node metastases which does not affect the survival rates.
- Also, the usefulness of histological grade as a prognostic criteria is limited as most institutions do not report tumor grade in histology.

- The staging systems fail to accurately identify the small percentage of low-risk patients who may actually die of PTC.
- They are also imprecise in staging risk stratification prior to surgery.

What factors are associated with adverse prognosis in PTC?

Patient factors

- AGE > 45
- Male sex
- Family history of PTC

Tumor factors

- Large tumor size
- Extra-thyroidal extension
- Multicentricity
- Lymph node metastases
- High tumor grade
- Aggressive histological variants
- Distant metastases

Extent of surgery

- Limited surgery

What is the optimal management of PTC?

Management of PTC involves:

- Surgery, preferably total thyroidectomy
- Radio-iodine remnant ablation
- TSH suppression

What is the optimal extent of surgery for PTC?

- Total thyroidectomy is the preferred initial surgical procedure for most patients with PTC. Only in patients with a single focus of tumor which is <1.5 cm, hemithyroidectomy might be sufficient.
- Prophylactic hemi or full central compartmental lymph node dissection may be added for tumors >1.5 cm.
- Modified Neck Dissection is necessary for palpable lateral nodes. Even though microscopic metastatic disease in lateral nodes may be present in as many as 80% cases, there is no role of prophylactic lateral Neck Dissection. Similarly, berry-picking is an inadequate operation for palpable/positive lateral neck nodes while Radical Neck Dissection is seldom required in PTC.

What are the histological features of PTC?

- Predominance of papillary structures admixed with neoplastic follicles
- Papillae have a central fibrovascular core covered by a single layer of cells
- The characteristic nuclear changes include–nuclear grooving, pseudoinclusions, and typical pale optically clear nucleus with powdery chromatin. The nucleus of PTC has been named after the famous cartoon character as "orphan Annie eyes" because of eccentric empty looking nucleus
- 50% also show presence of psammoma bodies which are microscopic structures of concentric calcification

What is the role of radioiodine therapy?

The two objectives of RAI therapy are:

- Remnant ablation
- Therapy of distant metastases

Radioiodine remnant ablation (RRA)

This is defined as destruction of residual thyroid tissue following thyroidectomy. The aims/advantages of RRA are:

- Destroy any occult microscopic carcinoma within the remnant
- To allow detection and treatment of metastatic disease (In presence of thyroid remnant all the radioiodine would be taken up by the remnant and the metastatic disease even if present would not show up on RAI scanning).
- Facilitates the use of serum Tg as a tumor marker for recurrent or persistent disease.

Do all patients of DTC need RRA after thyroidectomy?

It has been convincingly shown that RAI therapy in high-risk PTC patients reduces both cancer recurrence and death. However, the benefit is not so clear in low-risk patients, e.g. young adult patients with small intrathyroidal tumor (< 1.5 cm).

What doses of RAI should be used for RRA?

- *For minimal uptake:* 29 mCi are used and this does not require hospitalization and isolation.
- *For significant uptake:* 50-100 mCi are required and for this patient has to be isolated for 2-3 days.

What are the side effects of RAI therapy?

Side effects of RAI therapy are dose-related:

- Radiation thyroiditis (most common)
- Sialoadenitis (dry mouth can be troublesome)
- Odynophagia

- Radiation cystitis
- Long-term carcinogenic risks like leukemia and development of other cancers have not been convincingly proven.

What should be the protocol for TSH suppression?

All patients require life long hormone replacement as well as TSH suppression, achieved by supra normal doses of thyroxine. However, the degree of TSH suppression is related to the risk category of the patient.

- For low-risk: TSH concentration is maintained between 0.1-0.5 mU/L.
- For high-risk: TSH concentration is kept below 0.01 mU/L.

This level of suppression is continued for first 5 years and thereafter the dose of thyroxine can be reduced to allow the TSH to rise to the next level so that for high-risk patients TSH is maintained between 0.1-0.5 mU/L.

How will you follow-up patients of PTC?

Postoperative surveillance should be tailored to the patients' level of risk. The investigations avilable for follow-up include—WBRAI scanning, serum thyroglobuluin, neck ultrasound, chest X-ray and above all clinical examination (to detect recurrences in thyroid bed and lateral neck nodes).

Chapter 22

Papillary Microcarcinoma

CASE STUDY

Scenario 1

Clinical presentation as solitary thyroid nodule < 1cm

A 28-year-old female patient presented with complaints of neck swelling since 6 months. There was no history of voice change. On examination she had a firm nodule in the isthmus measuring approx. 2 × 1 cm; the lobes of the thyroid were not palpable. There was no cervical lymph node enlargement. FNAC from thyroid nodule was positive for papillary carcinoma. USG neck revealed a hypoechoic ill-defined nodule (0.77 × 0.74 × 0.4cm). Her thyroid function tests were within normal limits. She was taken up for surgery and total thyroidectomy with central compartmental clearance was performed. The cut surface of isthmus showed a grayish white area measuring 0.8 × 0.5 cm. Rest of the

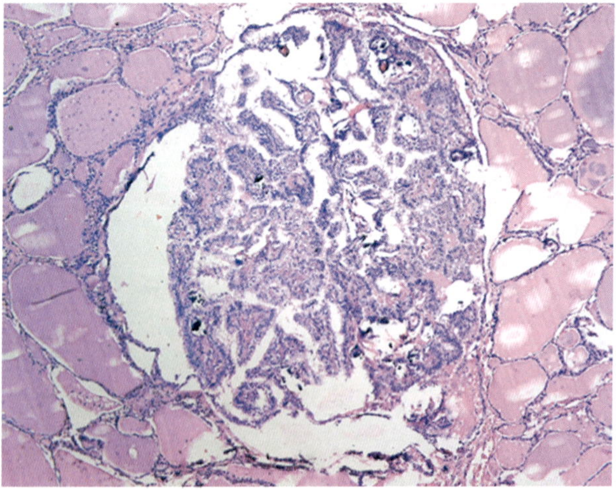

Fig. 22.1: Papillary microcarcinoma thyroid on histology (H and E)

thyroid was unremarkable. The lymph nodes of the central compartment were free of tumor. The final diagnosis was papillary microcarcinoma. The postope-rative period was uneventful and the patient was put on moderate TSH suppression. Serum Thyroglobulin estimation was done after 3 months and was found to be normal (< 4 mg/ml). Repeat stimulated Tg (patient was put off thyroxine for 3 weeks) was also found to be normal (< 4 ng/ml). She is on annual follow-up.

Scenario 2

Papillary microcarcinoma presenting as histological surprise

A 35-year-old female patient presented to the department of endocrinology with symptoms of hyperthyroidism that started 2 years back-palpitation, heat intolerance and tremors. She also complained of grittiness in both eyes along with increased lacrimation and peri-orbital puffiness. She never noticed any neck swelling. Her thyroid function tests done at that time were suggestive of hyperthyroidism and she was started on methimazole in doses of 20 mg per day. With treatment her symptoms improved but she took irregular treatment. She presented to our hospital because her eye symptoms worsened. On examination she was found to be having active eye disease-lid lag, positive Mobeius sign with periorbital edema and conjunctival injection. Her thyroid was 1.5 times enlarged, diffuse without thrill or bruit. She was also found to be having a thyroid nodule in lower pole of left lobe. A thyroid scan was asked for which revealed hyperfunctioning thyroid gland with hypofunctioning nodule in mid and lower part of left lobe. USG revealed complex cystic SOL with septae seen at lower pole of left lobe. Guided-FNAC was suggestive of colloid nodule. After achieving biochemical euthyroidism she was refered to us for surgical management in view of her deteriorating exophthalmos and suspicion of malignancy. She underwent total thyroidectomy. Cut-section showed a colloid filled cyst in left lobe which was reported as colloid nodule and a single grayish white area measuring 0.5 cm in right lobe which was reported as papillary microcarcinoma. The patient was put on moderate TSH suppression and her follow-up Tg levels (both stimulated and unstimulated) are within normal limits (< 4 ng/ml).

QUESTIONS

How do you define papillary microcarcinoma?

Papillary thyroid carcinoma < 1 cm are termed papillary microcarcinoma (PMC) according to WHO. They account for upto 30% of all PTC.

How are the papillary microcarcinoma detected?

Patients with PMC can present as:

1. Visible or palpable nodule and are diagnosed on FNAC
2. PMC can also be found incidentally during postoperative histopathlogical examination of thyroidectomy specimen resected for benign thyroid diseases such as Graves' disease or multinodular goiter. This is known as incidental papillary macrocarcinoma or IPC.
3. PMC can also be diagnosed on guided FNAC done on thyroid nodules < 1 cm detected incidentally during a neck ultrasound

What is the appropriate surgical management of these cases?

The appropriate surgical treatment of PMC is debatable. On one hand, they exhibit a benign behavior without progression over a period of time. On the other hand, PMC can behave aggressively, presenting with lymph node metastates, distant metastases and can even result in cause specific mortality. Thus, prognostic factors for PMC are not so well-defined as for the typical PTC. The two management options are:

a. ***Observation:*** Few studies have also reported approx 4 year follow-up in patients with PMC without having any surgical treatment. No change in cancer focus was observed in > 70% cases and only < 1% cases developed lymph node metastases. In another study it was observed that tumors equal to or > 7 mm or those located in upper pole are more likely to show lateral LN metastases as compared to smaller tumors and should be observed more closely.
b. ***Surgical treatment:*** This could be either total thyroidectomy or hemithyroidectomy. Though recurrence rate in thyroid remnant following hemithyroidectomy is < 1.5%, overall consensus is for total thyroidectomy as it permits use of Tg measurement to follow-up these patients.

Do these patients require radioiodine therapy?

Radioiodine therapy for remnant ablation can be given if one or more of the following features are present—tumor multicentricity, positive lateral lymph nodes or caspsular/vascular invasion on histopathology.

Is there any difference between IPC or overt PMC?

It has been observed that multiple foci and LN metastases are more frequent with PMC that is identified pre-operatively as compared to the incidentally detected PMC

Is completion thyroidectomy required in patients with benign disease in whom PMC is incidentally detected on the lobectomy specimen?

It has been observed that recurrence in remnant following subtotal or hemithyroidectomy is very low. There are conflicting reports about the aggressiveness of PMC associated with Graves' disease and the effect of TSH receptor stimulating Antibody on the cancer focus is also debatable.

How should you monitor these patients?

In patients where the initial stimulated Tg is undetectable minimal monitoring is required.

What is the overall prognosis of PMC?

PMC have an excellent prognosis. However, it is important to make a distinction between IPC and overt PMC.

Chapter 23

Occult Papillary Carcinoma Presenting as Cervical Lymph Node Enlargement

CASE STUDY

A 32-year-old male presented with complaints of swelling on the left side of neck for 3 months. There was no history of pain or increase in size of swelling and no compressive features. On examination, the palpable swelling corresponded to a left jugulodigastric lymph node. However, there was no nodule in the thyroid. He underwent following investigations

- *FNAC:* from the lymph node: suspicious of papillary carcinoma
- ***Use thyroid:*** multiple nodules in thyroid, all less than 2 cm along with a large cystic lymph node at the level of carotid bifurcation with another lymph node in the jugular chain.
- *TFT:* within normal limit

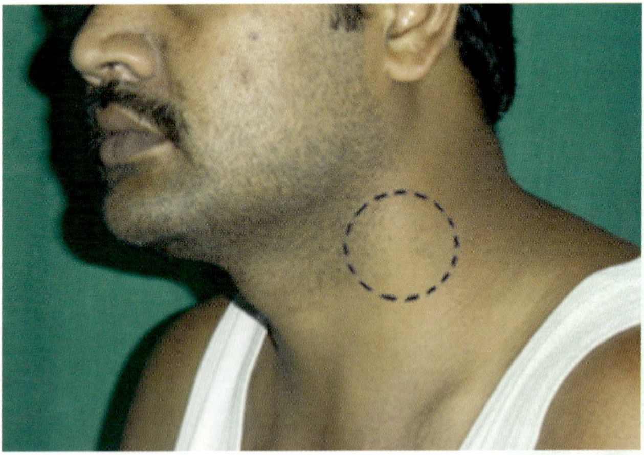

Fig. 23.1: Occult PTC presenting only as left deep cervical lymphadenopathy with normal thyroid gland

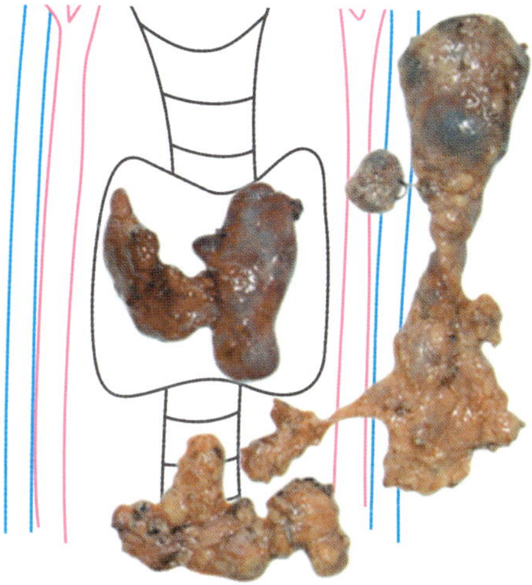

Fig. 23.2: Specimen of total thyroidectomy with left modified neck dissection and CCND

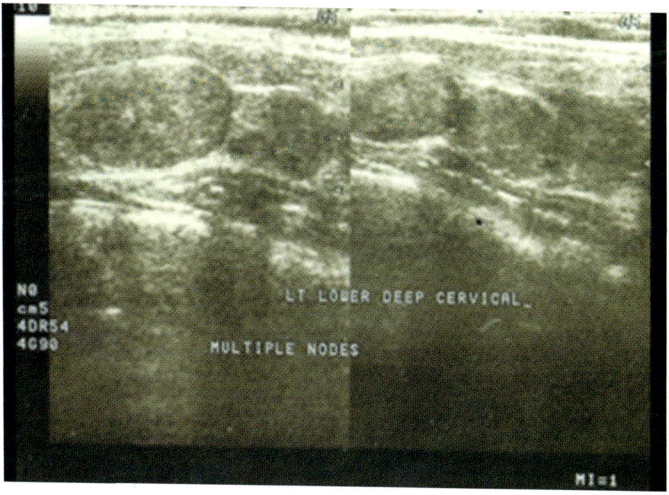

Fig. 23.3: Microcalcification in lateral lymph node

- *US-guided FNAC:* from the thyroid nodule suggestive of papillary carcinoma.
- The clinical impression was a occult papillary carcinoma thyroid metastatic to deep cervical lymph node.
- *CT scan:* of the neck and thorax was also ordered to rule out mediastinal lymph nodes.

Patient underwent total thyroidectomy with central compartmental lymph node dissection and left sided modified neck dissection. Postoperatively he developed thoracic duct fistula which did not close on conservative management for 12 days and he was then reoperated during which the cut end of the thoracic duct was identified and ligated. Subsequently he was discharged without any problems. Cut-section of the gross revealed a nodule in the left lobe (1.8 cm).The histopathology was papillary carcinoma thyroid with metastases to deep cervical lymph node (1/18); central compartmental nodes were free of tumor (0/6).

QUESTIONS

How does a cervical lymph node metastasis of papillary carcinoma look like on USG?

Ultrasonography is the most sensitive method for detection of metastatic lymph nodes from papillary carcinoma of the thyroid. Following ultrasonographic characteristics help in detecting metastatic lymph nodes from papillary carcinoma.

- ***Size and location:*** If a level II lymph node is more than 7 mm it is likely to be metastatic.
- ***Shape:*** a rounded lymph node (S/L ratio > 0.5) is likely to be metastatic.

- *Echogenecity:* a metastatic lymph node is more likely to be hyperechogenic as compared to adjacent muscle
- *Cystic necrosis:* is commonly seen in papillary carcinoma and this liquefactive necrosis is usually imaged as an anechoic area and if large it can sometimes be misinterpreted as a branchial cyst.
- *Hilum:* In a metastatic lymph node the normal echogenic hilum may be completely absent.
- *Intralesional calcification:* The presence of microcalcifications in lymph nodes which appear as bright echogenic flecks are frequent characteristics of lymph nodes affected by papillary carcinoma.
- *Margins:* Metastatic lymph node has well-defined borders.

Criteria most predictive of metastatic lymph node involvement are absent hilar echoes, and increase in short axis length (S/L ratio).

What further Investigations would you like to do?

US guided FNAC of the metastatic lymph node is an useful adjunct in arriving at a definite diagnosis especially because in papillary carcinoma metastatic lymph nodes may have cystic degeneration that can result in a false-negative FNAC if done without ultrasound guidance. US-guided FNAC has a sensitivity of 89-98%, specificity of 95-98% and accuracy of 95-97%.

Also an ultrasound of the thyroid in such a case would reveal one or more hypoechoic nodules in one or both lobes. The next step would be to get a US-guided FNAC from the thyroid nodules which would give a definite diagnosis of papillary carcinoma.

What is lateral aberrant thyroid?

Lateral aberrant thyroid is an old term used to define any thyroid tissue lateral to the carotid sheath and the jugular vein. However, over the years it is now established that such thyroid tissue was infact metastasis of thyroid carcinoma (mostly papillary carcinoma) to the lateral cervical lymph nodes and this has now become a surgical dictum.

How do you manage a thoracic duct fistula following neck dissection?

a. If the thoracic duct injury is recognized intra-operatively, it should be ligated.
b. If leakage of the duct is recognized post-operatively, as evident by excessive production of milky fluid from the drain conservative treatment should be tried (especially in low output leaks) which involves restriction of long and medium chain fatty acids or total parenteral nutrition, pressure dressings and closed drainage for at least two weeks. If conservative treatment fails (especially in high-output leaks, more than 500 ml in 24 hrs), the neck should be re-explored and an attempt is made to identify the cut end of the thoracic duct which is then ligated. Identification is made easy by giving the patient high fat diet prior to taking up for surgery which results in flow of milky fluid from the cut end of the duct during surgery. However, identification of the duct is not always possible; in such a case suturing the surrounding deep cervical fascia over the point of entry of duct into the internal jugular vein often controls the fistula. Fibrosis at the leak site can be accelerated by use of doxytetracycline soaked pledgets.

Chapter 24

Locally Invasive Papillary Carcinoma

CASE STUDY

A 35-year-old male presented to us with a neck swelling for last one year which has rapidly increased in size in last 2 months. He also complained of coughing out blood-stained sputum for last 2 months. There were no other compressive symptoms like pain, dyspnea, dysphagia or change in voice. On examination he was found to be having grade 2 goiter which was hard, approximate 8 × 6 cm, nodular with restricted mobility; the lower border was palpable and trachea was grossly shifted to opposite side. There was no cervical lymph node enlargement. He carried a FNAC report which was suggestive of adenomatoid nodular hyperplasia and CT of neck which revealed an enhancing space occupying lesion in left lobe of thyroid. However, in view of history of hemoptysis and a rapidly growing hard goiter, suspicion of malignancy was kept. A repeat FNAC was ordered which revealed follicular neoplasm. CECT was also repeated which revealed large, lobulated heterogeneously

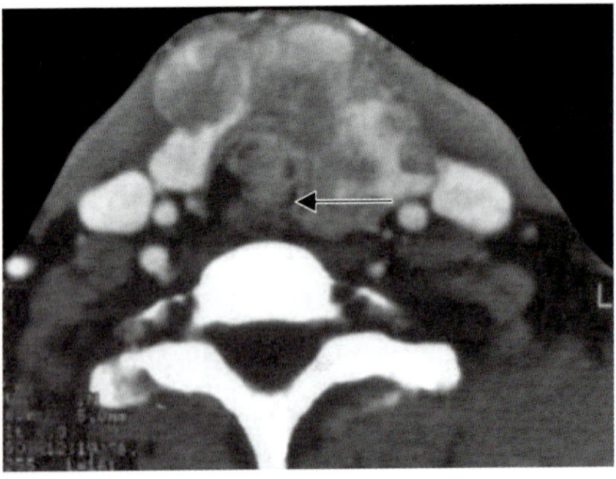

Fig. 24.1: CT scan of the patient with intraluminal extension into trachea (arrow)

attenuating mass in anterior part of left lobe of thyroid involving the isthmus; mass was seen to extend into the lumen of trachea, suggestive of tracheal invasion. Anticipating difficulty in intubation because of intraluminal tumor growth, a femoral-femoral bypass was planned but on the operating table intubation could be successfully done with a smaller caliber ET tube. Subsequently total thyroidectomy with central lymph node dissection was performed. The left sided strap muscles were found to be involved with the tumor mass and hence were excised en-bloc with the thyroid specimen. The left RLN was also found to be going through the tumor mass but since it was a functioning nerve as shown on preoperative I/L examination, every attempt was made to successfully save and dissect out the nerve. The tumor was found to be invading the cartilages between 2-4th ring and reaching the lumen. A window-resection of the trachea was performed and the opening closed primarily. A tracheotomy was done just below the excised portion of trachea. Postoperative period was uneventful and the patient could be successfully decannulated on the 10th postoperative day. The histopathology revealed papillary carcinoma with poorly-differentiated areas with central lymph node metastases (5/5). The excised portion of trachea at the site of invasion along with intratumoral invasion revealed tracheal wall infiltration. Whole body RAI scan done after 4 weeks revealed remnant thyroid tissue in the neck only while Tg values were grossly elevated (> 500 ng/ml). 125 mCi RAI was administered and post-therapy scan showed remnant thyroid tissue in the neck only. Subsequently he was again administered 150 mCi RAI and post therapy scan revealed remnant/metastatic thyroid tissue in the neck and superior mediastinum. He is since then in regular follow-up.

QUESTIONS

What are the presenting symptoms which should arouse suspicion of local invasion in DTC?

Patients may present as:

- Asymptomatic goiter
- Dysphagia
- Dyspnea
- Hemoptysis
- Stridor
- Hoarseness
- Cough with expectoration

What are the routes of local invasion in DTC?

Direct extension from either the primary tumor into the larynx (through the erosion of thyroid cartilage), trachea or esophagus, or

Direct extension from the metastatic paratracheal node into the RLN, trachea or esophagus.

Indirect extension into the larynx by extension posteriorly around the thyroid cartilage.

What are the contentious issues in the management of locally advanced DTC?

Though local invasion occurs rarely in DTC, once it occurs, it becomes the most common cause of mortality in patients of DTC who eventually die of thyroid cancer. The contentious issues in the management are:

i. What imaging modalities can be used to diagnose local invasion preoperatively?

ii. In cases of limited involvement of larynx, trachea or esophagus, what is the best option—shave excision or complete resection?
iii. What is the most appropriate/adequate procedure of excision and reconstruction in patients with intra-luminal involvement?
iv. What is the role of adjuvant therapy, particularly EBRT in such cases?
v. What is the optimal strategy in cases of local invasion of RLN?

What are management options in cases of limited involvement of larynx and trachea?

i. *Conservative management:* This involves shaving off the tumor from the larynx and trachea leaving behind only microscopic disease. This is also known as laminar ablation. However, the results are unpredictable and the local recurrence rates are likely to be high.
ii. *Aggressive management:* This involves full-thickness resection of a portion of aero digestive tract with the goal of removing all gross and microscopic disease (as shown by a negative margin on frozen section). Proponents of this aggressive management recommend this option not only in cases of frank cartilage invasion or intra-luminal involvement but also for cases with limited involvement.

In cases of tracheal invasion, what are the various options/extent of tracheal resection?

Various options are:

- Partial tracheal resection

- Circumferential tracheal resection with end-to-end anastomosis
- Palliative tracheostomy

Window resection or partial/wedge resection

When there is limited tracheal involvement requiring resection less than half of circumference of 1-2 tracheal rings, the defect can be managed either by putting a temporary tracheostomy through the defect (in cases of small anterior defects) or by rotation flaps (in larger defects) such as sternocleidomastoid myoperiosteal flap or pectoral myofascial flaps. Other options include permanent tracheostomy or delayed reconstruction using auricular cartilage. The disadvantages of these partial or continuity resections is that they may result in inadequate tumor removal because once the tumor has invaded the cartilage, it can grow transmurally and also spread circumferentially in the submucosal plane so much so that the latter spread may be more than the obvious outer adventitial invasion.

Circumferential resection

It is also known as sleeve resection. This becomes essential in patients with more extensive tracheal cartilage involvement. However, these advanced resection procedures are possible only in specialized units as they require multi-disciplinary care. Upto 6-7 tracheal rings can be resected using a primary end to end ansastomosis. In such resection the site of tumor invasion into the trachea is important when one has to select the level of resection and the operative technique which can be:

i. Primary closure by end-to-end anastomosis is feasible for defects < 2.5 cm

ii. For larger defects, additional tracheal releasing procedures are required
   a. *Suprahyoid release:* (level I resection)—this is accomplished by transecting the suprahyoid muscles (mylohyoid, genioglossus and geniohyoid) off the superior surface of hyoid bone
   b. *Combined cervical and mediastinal release (level II resection):* this is accomplished by median sternotomy. Sharp dissection is performed around the trachea, down to the carina and along the proximal major bronchi

iii. *Laryngotracheal step resection:* This is feasible in patients with unilateral laryngotracheal invasion usually at the laryngeal entry of one RLN. In such cases parital full thickness laryngectomy is performed and ipsilateral tracheal wall below the excised tumor is resected by an incision in the shape of a step. Reconstruction is accomplished by an oblique laryngotracheal anastomosis (by sliding the obliquely cut trachea up to fill the defect).

The cervical anastomosis is always covered by muscle flaps such as SCM flaps. While mobilizing the trachea for end-to-end anastomosis, blood supply of the trachea should be preserved. This can be achieved by keeping the plane of dissection along the anterior tracheal wall to avoid RLN injury and to avoid devascularization of trachea. Dissection of the posterolateral paratracheal tissue which contains the small vessels should be avoided.

One major advantage of tracheal resection is the immediate and sustained relief of tracheal bleeding and obstruction. Thus, aggressive resections may be indicated even in patients with distant metastases to prevent these local complications.

How do you manage the invasion of esophagus?

Invasion of esophagus is usually limited to the outer muscle layer which can be treated by excision and simple closure

What is the role of external beam radiotherapy (EBRT) in cases of locally invasive DTC?

The indications of EBRT in DTC would be:

- Gross residual disease after surgical excision
- In selected patients who have undergone presumed complete resection
  - Microscopic residual disease
  - Extensive extra-thyroidal extension
  - No RAI uptake

How do you manage the RLN invasion?

RLN is very commonly involved in locally advanced DTC, either directly from primary tumor (usually at the point of laryngeal entry) or more commonly by direct infiltration from a metastatic paratracheal node.

i. If the nerve is functioning (as shown by mobile VC on laryngoscopy) every attempt should be made to preserve it even if it entails leaving behind microscopic disease on the nerve which can be ablated later by RAI therapy
ii. However, if the RLN is already paralysed, no attempt should be made to preserve it in order to facilitate complete tumor removal.

Chapter 25

Differentiated Thyroid Carcinoma with Lung Metastases

CASE STUDY

A 23-year-old girl presented with right thyroid nodule along with right level 2 jugular lymph node. FNAC from thyroid nodule confirmed a papillary thyroid carcinoma metastatic to lymph node. Ultrasound revealed another small nodule in left lobe along with multiple right jugular chain nodes. Thyroid function tests were normal. She underwent total thyroidectomy with left sided modified neck dissection. At exploration the right strap muscles were found to be adhered to the thyroid nodule and were excised along with the thyroid. There were multiple level II,III,IV,V,VI and VII nodes which were cleared along with central compartmental dissection. Postoperative hypocalcemia was managed with IV calcium followed by oral calcium and vitamin D which

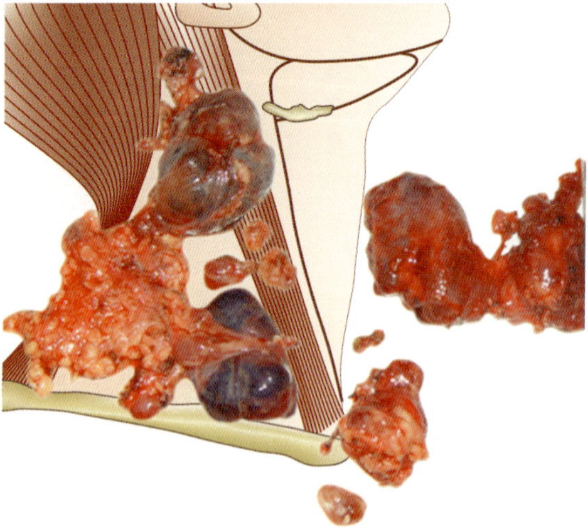

Fig. 25.1: Specimen of total thyroidectomy with right modified neck dissection

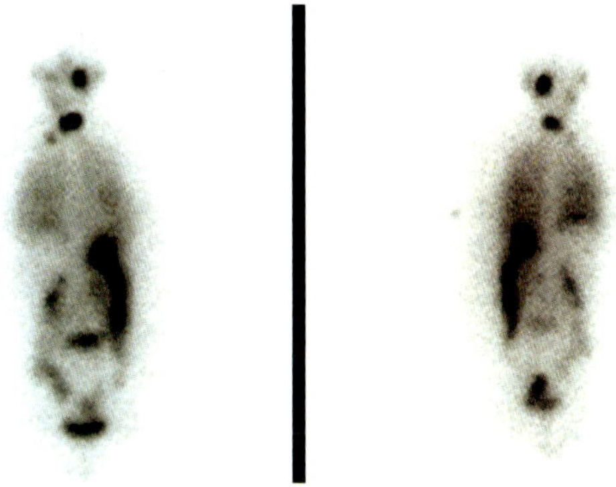

Fig. 25.2: RAI scan showing bilateral lung metastases and thyroid remnant

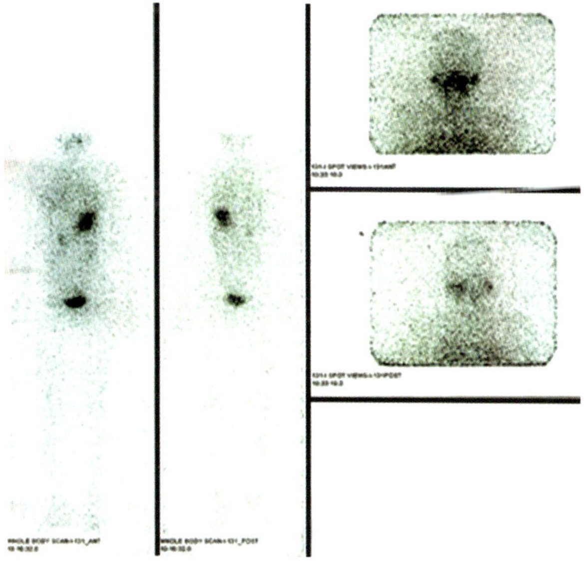

Fig. 25.3: Post-treatment scans of the same patient showing ablation of thyroid remnant and lung metastases

were gradually withdrawn over next 6 months. She underwent WBRAI scan after 4 weeks of total thyroidectomy which revealed thyroid remnant with bilateral pulmonary metastases. Serum Thyroglobulin levels at this time were 15 ng/ml. She was given 80 mCi' post-therapy scan did not reveal any other focus of uptake. She was again given 180 mCi 6 months later and post-therapy scan showed that pulmonary metastases disappeared. A repeat low-dose scan 6 months later showed only faint uptake in superior mediastinum and her Tg levels reduced to < 1 ng/ml.

QUESTIONS

How does the lung metastases present?

Lungs are the most common site of distant metastasis in DTC. 30% of patients have both lung and osseous metastases.

Pattern of lung involvement

Macronodular (>1 cm) nodules, or diffuse micronodular spread. The micronodular metastases are not detected by chest X-ray or by even CT thorax but are easily picked up on WBRAI scan.

Lung metastases are usually asymptomatic unless the pleura is involved.

What is the management?

Pulmonary metastases are almost always responsive to RAI therapy. Surgical treatment (enucleation or lobectomy) is required only in a minority of patients with a single macronodular metastases with or without mediastinal lymph node involvement, especially when these do not take up RAI

- *RAI therapy:* In adults the treatment dosage is usually 100-150 mCi repeated every 6-12 months.

How does management of children with lung metastases differ?

In children lower doses of RAI (empirically 1 mCi/kg body wt) should be used to avoid the risk of pulmonary insufficiency or chronic radiation-induced pulmonary fibrosis. This complication is particularly seen in extensive diffuse type of pulmonary metastases.

What is the long-term outcome?

Children, particulary with diffuse type of micronodular metastases do exceptionally well with RAI therapy.

FACTS AND FIGURES

RAI therapy is curative only in 10% of those lung metastases which are seen on X-ray film or CT whereas 70% of patients who have a normal X-ray and CT and whose lung metastases is detected only on the post-thyroidectomy WBRAI scan are likely to be completely cured with RAI therapy.

Chapter 26

Tall Cell Variant of Papillary Carcinoma (TCV)

CASE STUDY

A 67-year-old male patient presented with swelling in left side of neck for 3 months associated with URTI; got subsided with antibiotics but recurred again. No features of hypo/hyperthyroidism. No compressive symptoms. On examination thyroid was found to be normal but there was matted lymph node mass palpable in the upper deep cervical region 2 × 2 cm in size. Trachea was central. Other systemic and general examination was normal.

On investigations his thyroid function test was normal, FNAC from the lymph node mass was suggestive of metastatic papillary carcinoma and USG neck revealed a well-defined space occupying lesion in left lobe of thyroid with multiple deep cervical lymph nodes on the left side. subsequently a USG guided FNAC from thyroid was done which was also suggestive of papillary carcinoma. CT scan

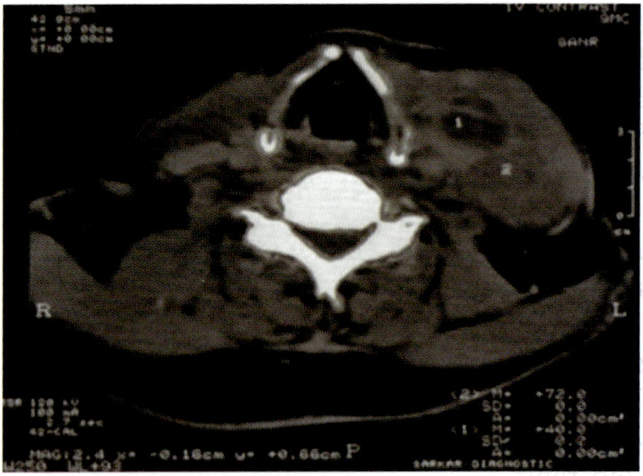

Fig. 26.1: CT scan showing large tumor arising from left lobe of thyroid and having necrotic areas

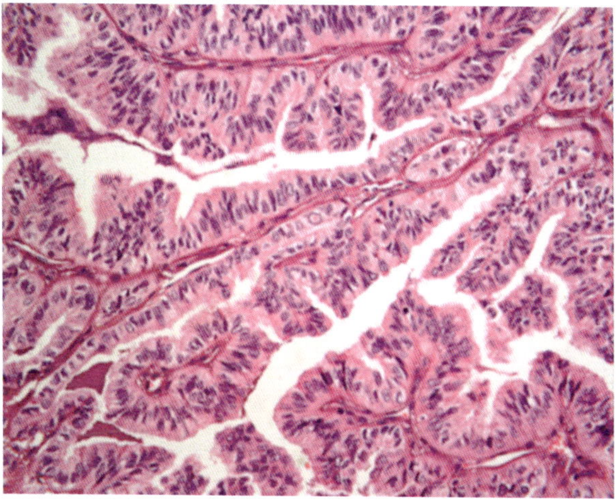

Fig. 26.2: Microphotograph showing papillae with fibrovascular core lined by tall cells with characteristic nuclear features of PTC (H and E)

was done which revealed a nodule in thyroid along with multiple jugular nodes on the left side. A diagnosis of papillary thyroid carcinoma was made and he was taken up for surgery. Total thyroidectomy with left radical neck dissection with left central compartmental dissection was done. Intraoperative findings were extrathyroidal invasion of tumor in strap muscles along with lymph nodes in level 2, 3 and 4, largest measuring 3.5 × 2cm which were adherent to IJV; hence left IJV and SCM was sacrificed. Cut section of the specimen showed 2 cm nodule present in upper pole of left lobe of thyroid. Postoperative recovery was normal. He was given high dose RAI therapy in view of significant thyroid remnant. Four months later he presented with recurrent lymph node in the neck which was confirmed on USG neck and FNAC. CT neck and thorax showed multiple neck nodes, mediastinal nodes and e/o lung metastasis. Excision of LN mass 3 × 2 cm was done and he was again given high dose RAI therapy. However, though his post-therapy scan did not reveal any uptake in the neck or lungs his Tg was still high and PET CT was suggestive of pulmonary metastases. Subsequently he developed malignant pleural effusion and later succumbed to his disease.

QUESTIONS

How do you define TCV and what is the incidence?

The common adopted histopathological definition of TCV is a papillary cancer of the thyroid in which a minimum of 30% (but according to some it should be 50-70%) of cells have a height at least twice their width, indicating a more aggressive pattern of growth. It constitutes upto 10% of all papillary thyroid cancers.

What are its clinical characteristics?

- Mean age of presentation: slightly higher than the usual variety of PTC
- Slight higher male preponderance
- Larger size of the tumor

Can the diagnosis of TCV made on FNAC?

If TCV is recognized in FNAC it can help in planning the extent of thyroidectomy. Features which can be helpful in distinguishing TCV from typical PTC are:

a. Larger cell size
b. More abundant granular cytoplasm

c. Increased nuclear pleomorphism and chromatin granules
d. Increased number of nuclear pseudoinclusions

What are unique biological characteristics of TCV?

TCV more commonly exhibits:
- extrathyroidal invasion
- greater incidence of invasion
- greater incidence of recurrence
- greater incidene of distant metastases
- higher cause-specific mortality

Thus, it follows a more aggressive course and can have a worse prognosis as compared to usual variety of PTC

Does the management of TCV differ from ususal variety of PTC?

- The recommend surgical treatment of choice is total thyroidectomy as well as enbloc resection of involved structures (e.g. strap muscles) as well as central compartmental dissection and modified or radical neck dissection depending upon LN involvement.
- All patients should undergo RAI WBS and if there is uptake RAI therapy should be given. Frequently in TCV no uptake can be demonstrated as compared to usual variety of PTC.
- Thyroxine suppression.
- EBRT may be more frequently required in TCV as compared to usual variety of PTC especially in cases of extrathyroidal invasion and where the tumor fails to take up RAI.

Chapter 27

Follicular Variant of Papillary Carcinoma

CASE STUDY

A 32-year-old lady presented with a neck swelling which was gradually increasing in size for last 6 years. There were no symptoms of hyper- or hypothyroidism and there were no compressive features. On examination there was a solitary thyroid nodule approx. 10 × 10 cm, mobile, firm in consistency, with a palpable lower border and without any cervical lymphadenopathy. Thyroid function tests were within normal limits, USG did not show any microcalcification. FNAC was suggestive of a colloid nodule. Patient was taken up for surgery where the right lobe was found to be normal while the left lobe was replaced by a single nodule; there was no extrathyroidal invasion and no lymphadenopathy. A hemithyroidectomy was performed and 8 × 8 × 4 cm nodule was removed, weighing 140 gm. The

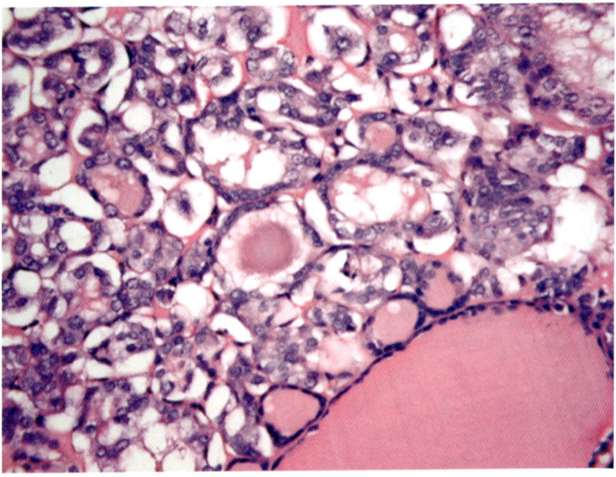

Fig. 27.1: Follicular variant of PTC showing closely packed follicles with characteristic nuclear features of PTC

histopathology was suggestive of follicular variant of papillary carcinoma. In view of this patient was taken up for completion thyroidectomy. Following total thyroidectomy, patient was given RAI ablation therapy and kept on thyroxine suppression. The histopathology revealed a circumscribed nodule which was composed of variably sized follicles. However, the epithelial cells display round to oval nucleus with chromatin clearing, nuclear overlapping and prominent nuclear grooves. Follicles display deep staining colloid with scalloping at places. Few display intraluminal papillary infoldings.

QUESTIONS

How do you describe this entity?

Follicular variant of papillary carcinoma (FVPTC) is the most common variant of PTC and constitutes approximate 9-16% of the papillary carcinomas. It is a well-differentiated thyroid carcinoma in which, though the nuclear features are of the usual PTC, the architectural pattern is predominantly follicular.

Why is the cytological diagnosis of FVPTC difficult?

The cytological diagnosis of FVPTC can be difficult for two reasons. Firstly, it has overlapping cytomorphological features with benign and follicular lesions owing to the presence of abundant thin colloid and monolayer sheets of follicular cells. Secondly, FVPTC contains very few of the nuclear features characteristic of PTC. Psammoma bodies are uncommon in FVPTC, which may be because of the relative paucity of fibrovascular structures. These two features contribute to the false-negative diagnosis of FVPTC on FNAC and Frozen Section.

What is the concern in cytological diagnosis of FVPTC?

FVPTC may be misdiagnosed as follicular neoplasm and an inadequate operation such as hemithyroidectomy may be perfomed. Also, FNAC may misdiagnose it as an adenomatous nodule and the patient may be wrongly offered conservative management.

When should you suspect the diagnosis of FVPTC on cytology?

When a specimen on cytological examination is highly cellular and contains monolayer sheets, eosinophilic cells with nuclear enlargement on a background of abundant watery and thick eosinophilic colloid, FVPTC should be included in the differential diagnosis. This should prompt a search of nuclear features of PTC such as chromatin clearing, nuclear grooves, and intranuclear inclusions that may be subtle and scarce in FVPTC. A diagnosis of FVPTC should be considered when FNAC is suggestive of papillary carcinoma based on nuclear characteristics but intra-operative FS suggests follicular neoplasm.

How can you increase the sensitivity of intraoperative diagnosis?

Intraoperative FS evaluation has poor sensitivity for FVPTC because of the loss of nuclear morphological details caused by freezing the tissue and the frequent appearance of tumor encapsulation resembling follicular adenoma. The use of touch preparations or smears from the cut surface of the nodule may increase the sensitivity of diagnosis of FVPTC because the cellular and nuclear details are preserved.

How does it differ from the usual variety of PTC?

In general, FVPTC tends to be smaller than PTC and is more likely to be encapsulated. Cervical metastases are less common in patients with FVPTC than in usual PTC. There is no evidence at present that early distant metastases, including pulmonary metastases, is increased in FVPTC.

Chapter 28

Completion Thyroidectomy

CASE STUDY

A 47-year-old lady was referred after undergoing an excision of thyroid nodule in a private hospital. The histopathology was reported as follicular neoplasm. On examination she was found to be having a hypertrophic scar but without any palpable neck swelling. She was not carrying any proper notes of previous operation. She was investigated by an USG neck which revealed intact right lobe of thyroid with fibrotic changes in the remnant of left lobe; Tc-99m-pertechnetate thyroid scan revealed intact right lobe and a significant remnant of left lobe. Review of slides of previous surgical specimen at our center was reported as papillary thyroid carcinoma. Subsequently CT scan was done which confirmed these findings and also ruled out any cervical or mediastinal lymphadenopathy. She was taken up for surgery. The previous scar was excised and the right lobe of

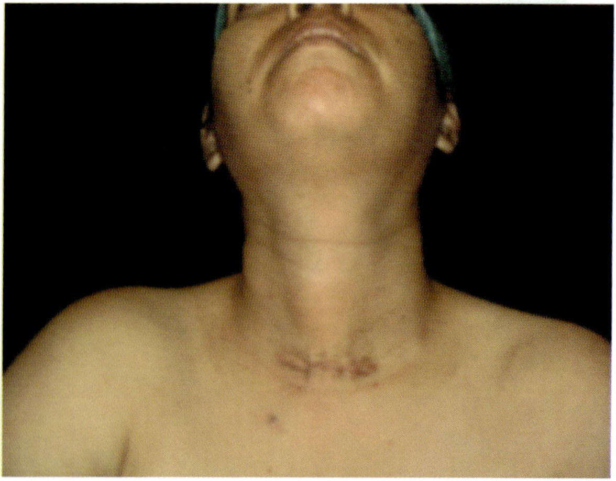

Fig. 28.1: Scar of previous surgery

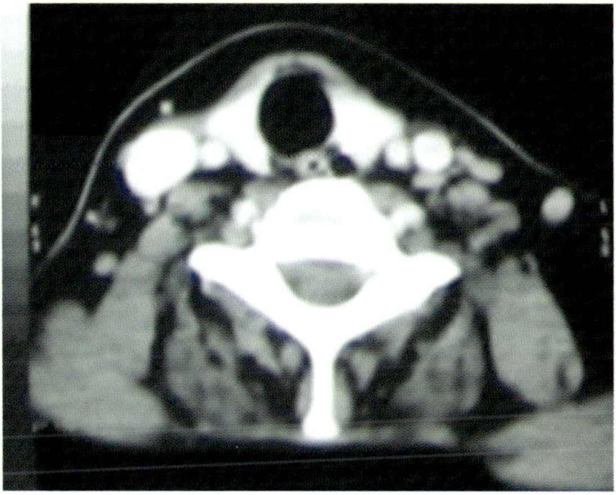

Fig. 28.2: CT scan showing both lobes of thyroid being present

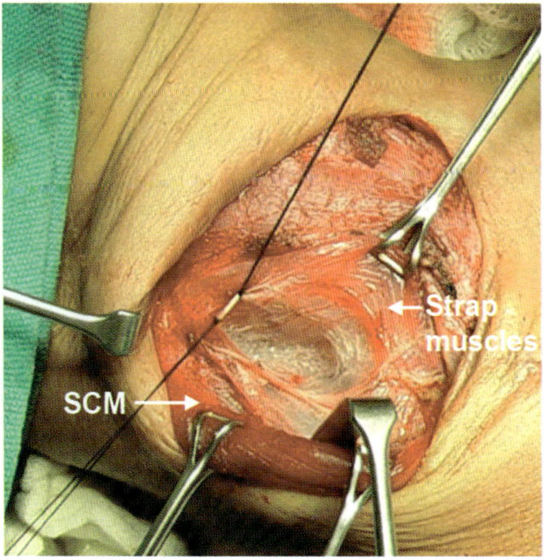

Fig. 28.3: Intraoperative photograph showing lateral approach between strap muscles and SCM

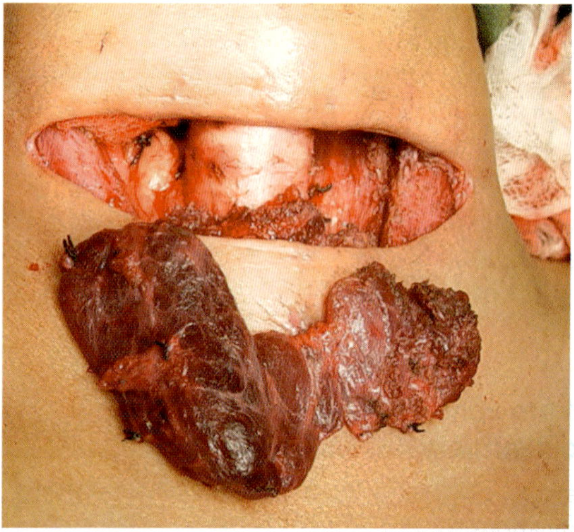

Fig. 28.4: Operative specimen showing intact right lobe and significant left lobe

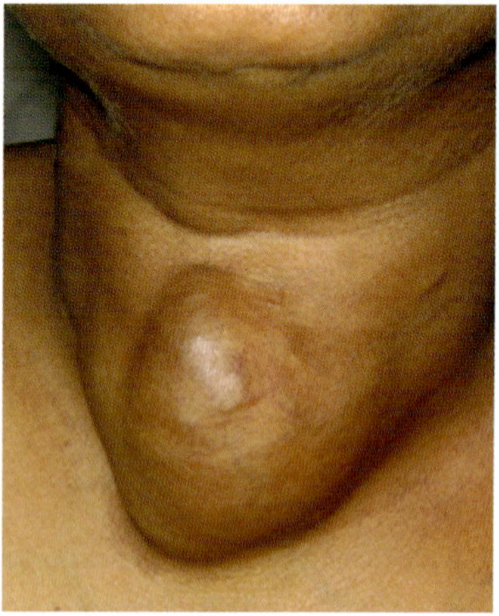

Fig. 28.5: Recurrent carcinoma in thyroid remnant of another patient

thyroid was approached through the lateral route. Right hemithyroidectomy along with excision of left remnant was performed. Both RLN and all 4 parathyroid glands were saved. The postoperative period was uneventful and the histopathology did not reveal any malignant focus in the specimen. A whole body RAI scan was performed 4 weeks later which revealed significant thyroid remnant which was ablated with 100 mCi of RAI.

QUESTIONS

What are controversial issues in re-operative thyroid surgery?

These are
- Indications
- Timing
- Operative approach

The indications of reoperative thyroidectomy are:

a. Completion total thyroidectomy because of presence of malignancy in the initial surgical specimen. Most common situation is when patient undergoes hemithyroidectomy for a thyroid nodule which is reported as follicular neoplasm on FNAC but the paraffin section report comes as follicular carcinoma.
b. Recurrent thyroid cancer
c. Development of thyroid carcinoma in the thyroid remnant after operation for benign thyroid diseases
d. Recurrent multinodular goiter
e. Recurrent thyrotoxicosis (if initial surgery is less than total thyroidectomy).

Timing

This is highly debatable. Usual recommendation is to operate either within one week of initial surgery in the same hospital admission or after 3 months to avoid inflammatory response and ensuing fibrosis. However, most studies have now shown that the technical difficulty of completion thyroidectomy does not change with time interval after initial surgery.

Operative approach

The lateral approach is extremely useful if one is forced to go on the side of initial surgery (either because less than a lobectomy has been performed or a large thyroid remnant is left behind which needs to be removed).

How do you define completion thyroidectomy?

It is defined as the removal of contralateral lobe along with the isthmus (if left behind) and pyramidal lobe of the thyroid after initial hemithyroidectomy or lobectomy.

Do thyroid cancer patients who belong to low-risk category require completion thyroidectomy?

The benefit of completion thyroidectomy in low-risk patients (< 45 years, LN negative and T1 tumors) has been debated. However, even low-risk patients carry a significant risk (approximately 40%) of harboring contralateral disease; further, it is very difficult to establish the presence or absence of contralateral disease. Hence, completion thyroidectomy can be considered even in low-risk patients, provided completion thyroidectomy is being performed by an experienced thyroid surgeon.

One of the strongest predictor of contralateral disease is multifocality in the initial hemithyroidectomy specimen. Thus, patients who have undergone hemithyroidectomy should undergo a completion total thyroidectomy if a multifocal carcinoma is detected in the first surgery. This is regardless of the risk category of the patient.

What kind of work-up is required before reoperative thyroid surgery?

a. Detailed study of operative notes of previous surgery, especially with reference to RLN, parathyroid glands and the extent of surgery. It should be noted whether the opposite lobe was palpated and whether this was done after mobilizing the contralateral strap muscles.
b. Vocal cord examination and any voice change has to be recorded.
c. Blocks/slides of previous surgery must be reviewed again.
d. Need/indication for completion thyroidectomy should be clearly noted.
e. RAI scan to be done to look for thyroid remnant on the side of initial surgery.
f. USG of thyroid to look for thyroid remnant because in some cases thyroid may not be iodine avid.

What operative technique should be employed for safe reoperative thyroid surgery?

a. Previous scar should be excised
b. Strap muscles can be divided
c. The side of initial surgery may not need to be entered if scan and USG clearly show no/very little thyroid tissue on affected side.

d. One can utilize the lateral approach – avoiding the scarred midline and instead dissecting the virgin area between sternocleidomastoid and strap muscles after dividing the omohyoid muscle.
e. Operating loupes (2.5*x*) can be used to identify the RLN and parathyroid glands.
f. RLN injury can be avoided if the nerve is identified low in the neck before it becomes engulfed by the scar tissue of previous surgery.
g. Another way of avoiding the RLN injury is to identify the RLN very high at the point of entry into larynx. This is done by dividing the isthmus and dissecting the thyroid from trachea in a medial to lateral direction so that the nerve is encountered at the point where it enters the larynx. This maneuver allows one to avoid the scar tissue entirely.

Can normal intact thyroid lobe be ablated with RAI instead of doing completion thyroidectomy?

Doses of RAI required for ablating a normal thyroid lobe will be very high. Such high doses carry a risk of leukemia / lymphoma as well as development of parathyroid adenomas and bone marrow depression.

Chapter 29

Thyroid Cancer in Children

CASE STUDY

A 12-year-old boy was referred to us after having undergone partial thyroidectomy (nodulectomy) at a private hospital for a thyroid nodule which was present for last one year. The histopathology was reported as poorly differentiated thyroid carcinoma. On examination a well healed cervical scar was present but there was no thyroid swelling and no cervical lymphadenopathy. Review of blocks/slides revealed that it was infact a papillary thyroid carcinoma with insular and poorly differentiated areas. A Thyroid scan was asked for to assess the residual thyroid – scintigraphic findings revealed normally functioning left lobe with minimal uptake in the region of right lower pole of thyroid. These findings were corroborated on USG of neck. The child was taken up for completion thyroidectomy. Operative findings included normal left lobe and a small remnant of right lobe without any lymphadenopathy. Both recurrent laryngeal nerves and left parathyroid glands were saved. The postoperative period was uneventful and the child was discharged on 4th postoperative day with advice to undergo a WBS scan after 4 weeks. The histopathology of left lobe did not reveal any malignancy. WBS scan done with 5 mCi of I^{131} revealed remnant thyroid tissue which was ablated with 50 mCi of I^{131} and post-therapy scan was performed at the time of discharge which revealed remnant thyroid tissue in the neck only. However, before the next appointment for WBS the child was admitted with us with massive pleural effusion. Evaluation revealed extensive bilateral lung metastases on CT scan and a positive pleural fluid cytology for malignant cells. The child was put on supportive management but succumbed to respiratory failure.

QUESTIONS

What are the risk factors for development of PTC in children?

PTC accounts for > 90% of all thyroid cancers in children. The various risk factors are:

a. Exposure to low-dose radiation to head and neck area
b. Previous existence and treatment of benign thyroid disease such as congenital hypothyroidism (dyshormonogenesis, iodide-transport defects, hemiagenesis, thyroglossal cyst).

How is the clinical presentation of PTC in children different from that of adults?

a. *Presence of solitary thyroid nodule:* Presence of solitary thyroid nodule in a child should be considered malignant unless proved otherwise because 50% of all thyroid nodules in children prove to be malignant.
b. Deep cervical lymphadenopathy is more common in children.
c. Pulmonary metastases are more common in children.

What are the histopathological characteristics of PTC in children?

a. Follicular variant of PTC is very common in children (seen in > 25%).
b. The more aggressive variants like diffuse sclerosing variant affects older children—it has a very high incidence of nodal metastases and lung involvement.
c. Tall cell variant, columnar cell variant and poorly-differentiated variants are less common.

d. Pure FTC is also rare in children and if they are found, they are usually of the minimally invasive type

What preoperative evaluation should be performed?

a. *FNAC:* If it is non-diagnostic then US-guided FNAC should be performed.
b. USG of thyroid.
c. Chest X-ray and if suspicion of pulmonary metastasis is high, non-contrast CT scan should be performed.

What is the optimal extent of surgery in children?

General consensus is that total or near-total thyroidectomy should be performed by experienced thyroid surgeons to have minimal complications in this age group. The rationale for this is :

a. Multicentricity and bilaterality is very high in children not only because of intraglandular lymphatic spread but because multifocal tumors can also arise *de novo* especially in cases of RET/PTC rearrangements. For the same reason, a child with PTC who has had less than total or near total thyroidectomy should be offered completion thyroidectomy.
b. ***For palpable nodes:*** Modified neck dissection should be done. There is no rationale for berry picking and Radical neck dissection is seldom required.
c. Total thyroidectomy allows the use of I^{131} therapy for remnant ablation as well as for distant metastases, the incidence of which is higher (15%) in children as compared to adults (2%).

What is the further management in a child with PTC who has undergone total thyroidectomy?

Thyroid remnant ablation should be routinely performed in all children even if they belong to the low-risk group. Remnant ablation should be performed 6 weeks after surgery; Diagnostic WBS is performed with 0.5 to 2.0 mCi of I^{131} (while in adults WBS is done with 5 mCi I^{131}). Thyroid remnant ablation is done with 30 mCi. A post ablation or post-therapy scan is done 5-7 days later to look for pulmonary metastases or a non-contrast CT can be done to look for pulmonary metastases (micronodular/interstitial metastasis). Most children may not require additional doses unless they have distant metastases. Some clinicians prefer to give fixed empirical doses of RAI (approx. 150 mCi). Following thyroid remnant ablation, next follow-up is scheduled at 3-6 months when following investigations are done following 4 weeks of thyroxine withdrawl (or only 2 weeks of withdrawal if LT3 is available) – WBS, Tg, neck USG and chest X-ray.

Subsequently cure is defined by a negative WBS, negative USG and a Tg level < 8.0 ng.ml (on hormone withdrawal). Once cure is achieved, annual FUP is done with Tg, neck USG, physical examination, serum TSH and chest X-ray. Only when Tg starts rising, should WBS be done.

Chapter 30

Follicular Neoplasm

CASE STUDY

A 28-year-old woman presented to us with gradually increasing swelling for last 4 months. She did not have any associated complaints. On examination she was found to be having a solitary thyroid nodule arising from right lobe of thyroid. There were no neck nodes. USG revealed a homogeneous well-defined solitary thyroid nodule without any microcalcification but with a central hypoechoic area. FNAC was suggestive of follicular neoplasm. She underwent right hemithyroidectomy and Frozen section done intraoperatively was that of a benign lesion which was later confirmed on permanent paraffin section.

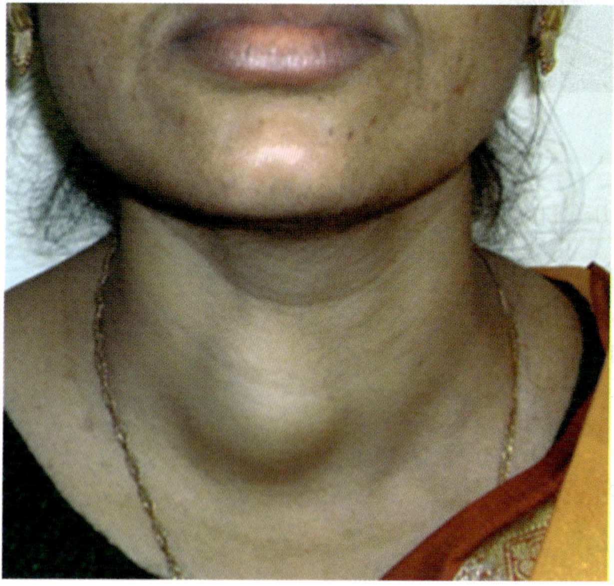

Fig. 30.1: Solitary thyroid nodule

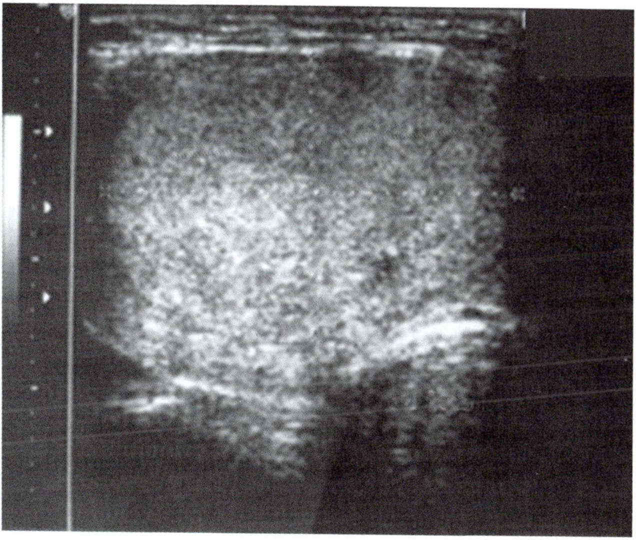

Fig. 30.2: Ultrasound showing a solid lesion without microcalcification

QUESTIONS

What is a cytologically indeterminate lesion?

Cytologically indeterminate category include four lesions: Follicular neoplasm, atypical lesions, benign follicular lesion, cellular follicular lesion.

Indeterminate follicular thyroid lesions comprise 10-30% of cytopathological diagnosis. Prevalence of cancer in indeterminate lesions varies widely between 3-31%.

What is a follicular neoplasm?

The term follicular neoplasm is a cytopathological term broadly applied to a heterogeneous group of thyroid tumors characterized by a proliferation of thyroid epithelial cells growing in a follicular pattern. Follicular neoplasm in turn include heterogeneous lesions like pure follicular neoplasms, Hurthle cell neoplasms and many neoplasms that ultimately prove to be FVPTC. FNAC cannot distinguish between follicular adenoma and follicular carcinoma. The probability of malignancy in a thyroid lesion demonstrated by FNAC to be a follicular neoplasm is 20%.

Can frozen section evaluation help in the diagnosis of follicular carcinoma?

The intraoperative FS evaluation cannot reliably distinguish benign from malignant lesions. The focal nature of tumor invasion may elude detection because of the limited sampling inherent to FS evaluation. Moreover, the artifact and cellular distortion induced by tissue freezing may mask the subtle morphologic atypia that characterizes the follicular variant of PTC.

What is the optimal management of a thyroid nodule with a FNAC diagnosis of follicular neoplasm?

All such patients should undergo at least a lobectomy + isthmusectomy. Also, the surgeon should look for certain intraoperative findings which would be a pointer towards presence of a carcinoma. These are presence of any nodule in the contralateral lobe, regional lymph nodes, extrathyroidal invasion and gross examination of specimen. In case of a highly suspicious finding, if facilities exist, a directed FS evaluation can be asked for. Further management is based on the permanent histological examination. If the diagnosis of follicular carcinoma most patients would require a completion total thyroidectomy.

Chapter 31

Hurthle Cell Neoplasm/ Carcinoma

CASE STUDY

A 40-year-old lady noticed a neck swelling following an upper respiratory tract infection. On examination it was found to be a right sided solitary thyroid nodule, 4 × 4 cm with no cervical lymphadenopathy. Subsequent investigations were as follows: FNAC: Hurthle cell neoplasm; USG: revealed 3 × 3 cm large nodule in right lobe with large dystrophic calcification and another small nodule in left lobe measuring 0.5 × 0.5 cm. There was no cervical lymphadenopathy. Thyroid function tests were within normal limits. In view of multifocality she was planned for total thyroidectomy. During surgery, strap muscles were found to be adherent to the thyroid and were excised along with

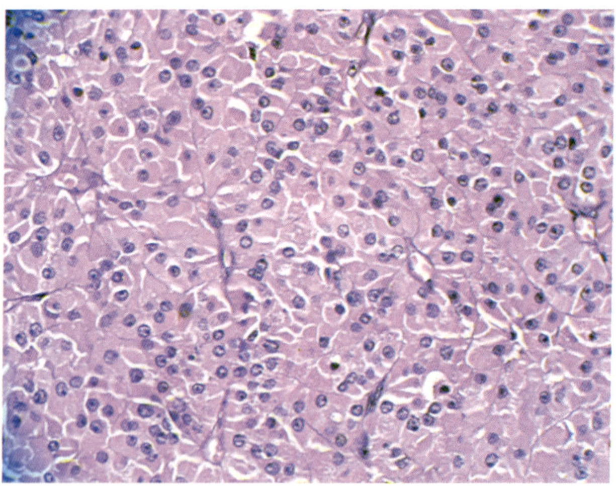

Fig. 31.1: Sheets and trabeculae of tumor cells with round nuclei and abundant eosinophilic cytoplasm from a case of Hurthle cell neoplasm (H&E stain)

total thyroidectomy. There was no other evidence of extra-thyroidal invasion. Postoperative period was uneventful and she underwent WBRAI scan after 4 weeks which revealed uptake in the thyroid bed which was ablated with 100 mCi RAI and scan done 6 months later showed no further uptake in the thyroid bed or elsewhere.

QUESTIONS

How are the Hurthle cell neoplasm classified?

Hurthle cells, like papillary and follicular tumors arise from follicular cell. Hurthle cell tumors (adenomas and carcinomas) are also known as oxyphilic tumors, oncocytomas or Askanazy cell tumors. It has also been classified as oxyphilic variant of follicular carcinoma. FNAC cannot distinguish between Hurthle cell adenoma or Hurthle cell carcinoma (HCC).

What are the clinical and histological characteristics?

i. Hurthle cell tumors are uncommon in children; peak incidence is in 5th-6th decade of life.
ii. Though Hurthle cell tumors are more common in women, men have proportionately more malignant tumors.
iii. They have a higher incidence of lymph node metastases (10-25%) as compared to FTC (5%).
iv. Hurthle cells are large, polygonal cells with fine granular, acidophilic cytoplasm representing an abundance of mitochondria.

v. To be considered a Hurthle cell tumor, more than 75% of cells must be Hurthle cells and they should be encapsulated because few, nonencapsulated Hurthle cells can also be seen in inflammatory conditions of thyroid as well in Graves' disease. The criteria used to diagnose HCC are capsular or vascular invasion, invasion of adjacent structures, lymph node metastases, and distant metastases.

What is the optimal management of a patient presenting with a solitary thyroid nodule with a FNAC of Hurthle cell neoplasm?

25-60% of such lesions ultimately prove to be HCC; hence all these patients require surgery. The extent of surgery is debatable. One option is to do a hemithyroidectomy and if the final histopathology is HCC, completion thyroidectomy can be performed in the same admission. The other option, and the one which I practice, is to do one-stage total thyroidectomy, especially if the size is more than 5 cm, if there is evidence of multifocality, lymph node or distant metastates or extra-thyroidal invasion, or if there is an aneuploid DNA pattern on FNA. A prophylactic central dissection is also recommended.

What is the postoperative management of such a patient?

Although less than 10% of HCC take up RAI, it can still be used to ablate any remaining normal tissue. This allows serum Tg level to be used as a marker of tumor recurrence as HCC and its metastases do secrete Tg. Subsequent follow-up and management is like that of follicular thyroid carcinoma. The role of external radiotherapy is limited and should be used only in patients with unresectable local invasion when there is no uptake of I^{131}.

How do HCC differ from FTC?

i. HCC are more likely to be multifocal within the thyroid gland.
ii. HCC have more lymph node metastases.
iii. HCC have more distant metastases.
iv. HCC are less likely to take up RAI after total thyroidectomy.
v. HCC have a high chance (50%) of a concomitant papillary thyroid carcinoma.
vi. Patients of HCC are more likely to give history of exposure to low-dose therapeutic radiation.

What are the prognostic factors and what is the prognosis?

HCC are more aggressive than follicular carcinomas The 10-year survival of HCC in only 65% compared to that of 85% for FCC. Important prognostic factor are extra-thyroidal invasion, nodal metastases and distant metastases.

Chapter 32

Follicular Carcinoma Presenting with Bone Metastases

CASE STUDY

A 47-year-old female was referred from the department of Neurosurgery as a case of carcinoma thyroid with spine metastases. Patient had presented to the department of Neurosurgery with complaints of progressively increasing pain in back and lower limbs for 1-2 years. Evaluation revealed destruction of L2 vertebra on plain X-ray while MRI was suggestive of metastasis in L2 vertebra. In view of severe radiculopathy she was taken up for surgery and laminectomy was done. The postoperative period was uneventful but the histopathology revealed metastatic follicular carcinoma of thyroid and she was subsequently referred to us. On examination she was found to be having a solitary thyroid nodule, 6 × 6 cm arising from the right lobe along with a globular bony swelling arising from the medial end of the clavicle. FNAC from the solitary thyroid nodule was suggestive of follicular neoplasm while that from the clavicular swelling was suggestive of metastatic follicular carcinoma. She was taken up for surgery and total thyroidectomy along with excision of the clavicular metastatic mass was successfully done. The histopathology was widely invasive follicular carcinoma with bony metastasis. The postoperative period was uneventful but she continued to have incapacitating pain in lower limbs. She was then referred to the department of Nuclear Medicine for WBRAI scanning and therapy. WBS revealed thyroid remnant and metastases to lumbar vertebra and pelvis. Serum thyroglobulin was significantly elevated (> 320 ng/ml). She was treated by RAI therapy in multiple sittings with a cumulative dose of 605 mCi over 3 years. Her last WBS revealed no tracer uptake and her serum thyroglobulin levels decreased (145 ng/ml). There was marked improvement in her pain and she could resume her daily activities.

QUESTIONS

How do patients of follicular carcinoma with bone metastases present?

i. Skeletal pain
ii. Soft tissue swelling.
iii. Pathological fracture
iv. Spine metastases with symptomatic spinal cord compression- paraperesis or paraplegia
v. Asymptomatic

Bone metastases usually occur in older patients and more in follicular cancer as compared to papillary cancer.

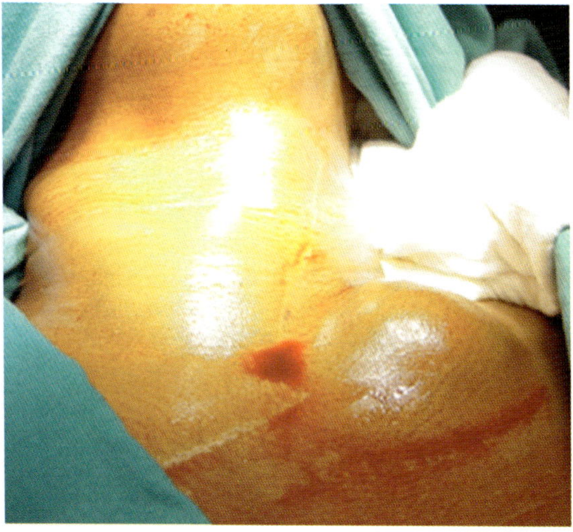

Fig. 32.1: Patient with goiter and a clavicular mass

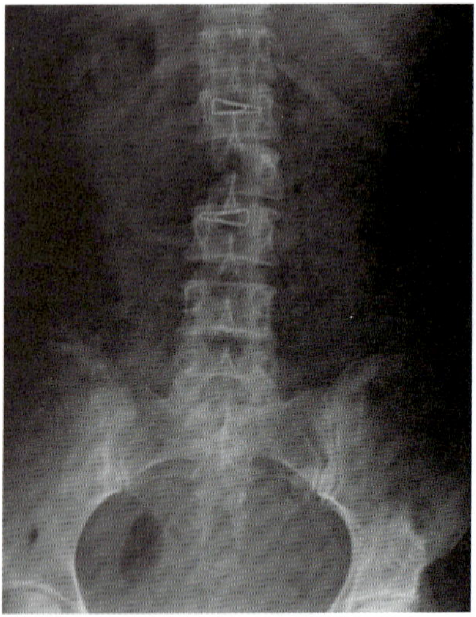

Fig. 32.2: Same patient with metastases to lumbar vertebrae

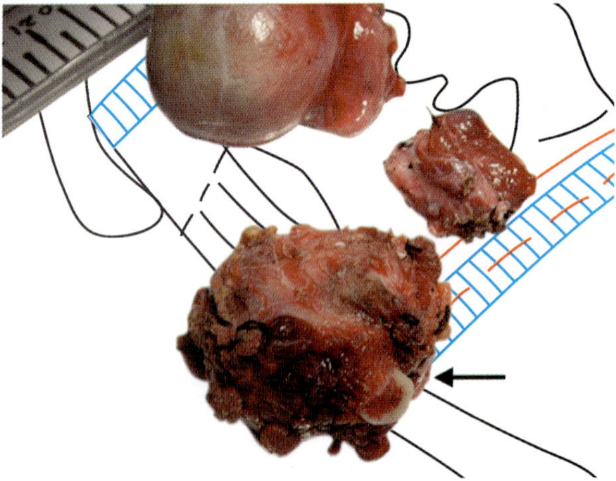

Fig. 32.3: Total thyroidectomy and partial claviculectomy (arrow) specimen

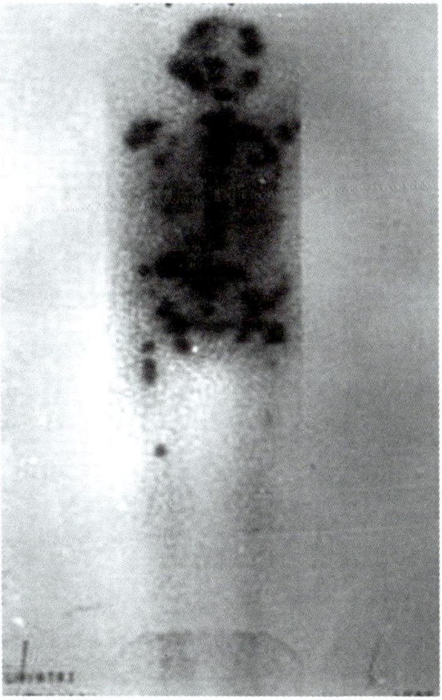

Fig. 32.4: WBS showing multiple bony metastases

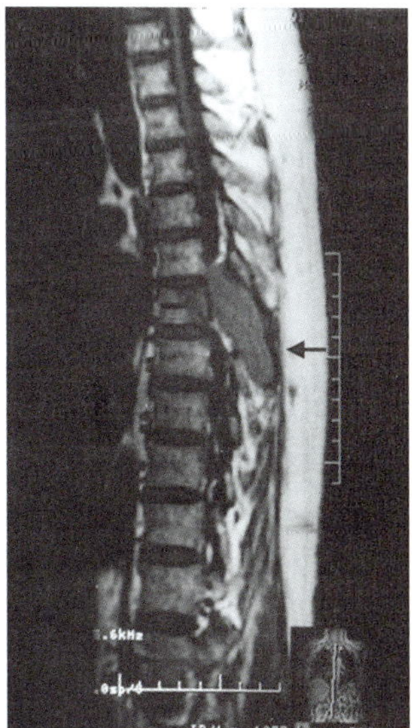

Fig. 32.5: MRI of spine showing both bony and soft tissue metastases to spine (arrow)

The commonest *sites of osseous metastases* in decreasing order of frequency are:

Vertebrae, pelvis, skull, long bones, sternum, and clavicle

What are the diagnostic procedures for detection of skeletal metastases?

Radiography

Radiography of selected/suspected site to assess the extent of osteolytic/osteoblastic activity (the latter is an index of respone to therapy). Major disadvantage is that total survey is difficult as radiation exposure is significant.

MDP bone scan

It has poor sensitivity and specificity because these metastases are generally osteolytic which result in a photopenic lesion on MDP scan which can be easily missed. With WBRAI it has a concordance of only 50% (especially in thorax and vertebrae).

WBRAI

Has highest sensitivity and specificity. WBS most of the times would reveal multiple bone metastases in a patient with an apparently solitary metastasis.

A combination of all the three techniques is required to evaluate the extent of bone involvement.

What is the therapeutic approach to such a patient?

Despite distant metastases one should not deter from offering total thyroidectomy followed by radio-active iodine therapy and thyroxine suppressive therapy as well as surgical metastectomy as and when indicated.

RAI therapy

Bony metastases concentrate RAI avidly but require several I ^{131} therapies. Individual dose varies from 250-300 mCi and total cumulative dosage may go upto 1-1.2 Ci. First dose is usually given within 4 weeks of total thyroidectomy and the second dose is given after 6 months and then at 9 and 12 months. Most patients require more than 4 sittings. Complete response is considered if there is clearance or ablation of the bone metastases as demonstrated by healing of the lesion on radiograph or if MDP bone scan or RAI scan is negative or the patient becomes asymptomatic with normal s-Tg levels.

It is considered as partial response if number of lesions decrease or the avidity of I^{131} is reduced or s-Tg levels decrease from initial high levels. The cure rate is very low, 4-8% because the lesions are usually large, heterogeneity of cancer cells with respect to I^{131}, loss of trapping function due to partial dedifferentiation or due to stunning effect after a non-lethal dose of I^{131}. Even though majority of patients have partial responses, quality of life improves considerably as seen by relief of pain, reduction in size of soft tissue swelling and reduction in pressure symptoms like paraperesis, radiculitis.

External beam therapy

Indicated if bone metastases are painful or if there is impending paraplegia. Usually administered after RAI therapy.

Surgical management (Metastatectomy)

Usually a solitary metastases in an accessible bone like clavicle or manubrium sterni can be excised. When the bone metastases are large or are not totally respectable, surgery may help reduce the tumor mass, making subsequent treatment with RAI theapy more effective.

How would you manage a patient with vertebral metastases?

Patients with impending paraplegia should be emergently operated. Such patients usually require laminectomy with excision of any associated soft tissue mass along with total thyroidectomy. Patients without paraperesis but with vertebral metastases should undergo total thyroidectomy as soon as possible followed by radio-iodine therapy. The period of hypothyroidism can be shortened by use of recombinant TSH.

What are the indications of surgical intervention?

Palliative intent

Palliative resection is indicated to improve quality of life for patients with symptomatic osseous lesions associated with pain, pathologic fractures (usually in long limbs, spine) or neurologic symptoms from spinal cord compression (verterbral metastases) or brain metastases. Palliative resection is also indicated for symptomatic disease that fails to concentrate RAI.

Curative intent

Potentially curative resection has been indicated for apparent solitary bone metastases as this may be associated with improved survival.

What are the side effects of RAI therapy?

Side effects are frequent but are mild and transient and include nausea, vomiting, GI symptoms, and acute sialoadenitis. Sialoadenitis may become chronic after several doses and can be avoided by maintaining hydration, oral hygiene and by giving low doses of steroids for 2-3 days after RAI administration.

What is the long-term prognosis of such patients?

Presence of metastases puts these patients of differentiated thyroid carcinoma in High Risk category. Despite the absence of curative capability of I^{131} it still remains one of the most important modalities of treatment for skeletal metastases in DTC. With RAI therapy there is considerable improvement of quality of life in patients with paraplegia An aggressive surgical approach to resectable solitary bone metastases is warranted on the basis of survival benefit associated with potentially curative resection.

What are newer modalities for treatment of bone metastases?

i. Preoperative embolization and cementoplasty as alternative therapies in cases of impossible complete surgery, for pain and for reducing hemorrhagic risk during surgery for metastases.
ii. Indium-111-labelled octreotide scintigraphy and therapy
iii. *Bisphosphonates:* Inhibit the function of osteoclasts. Effective in reducing the pain and morbidity of pathological fracture. They may also delay or prevent the development of skeletal metastases.

FACTS AND FIGURES

1. The incidence of distant metastases is approximate 12.5%.
2. Two thirds have lung metastases while one-third have bone metastases.
3. Curative treatment is possible only in less than 10% cases of bone metastases.
4. These patients have 30% 15 year survival compared to 90% 15-year survival of low risk patients.

Chapter 33

Sporadic MTC

CASE STUDY

A 30-year-old female patient was referred with complaints of gradually increasing neck swelling and increased frequency of stools for last 5 years. The neck swelling was not associated with any compressive symptoms. The frequency of loose stools was 6-10 times a day, it was watery in consistency without any foul smell and was not associated

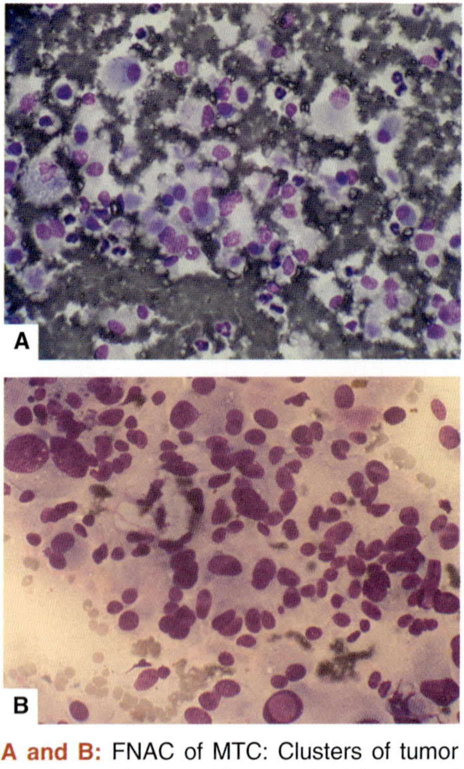

Figs 33.1A and B: FNAC of MTC: Clusters of tumor cells with moderate nuclear anisomorphism, central to eccentric nuclei, hemorrhagic background, formation of microfollicles and binucleate and multinucleate cells (MGG stain)

with any abdominal pain. Family history was not significant. On examination she was found to be normotensive. Local examination of the neck revealed solitary thyroid nodule of the left lobe, measuring approximately 4 cm and moving well with deglutination. She also had left sided multiple

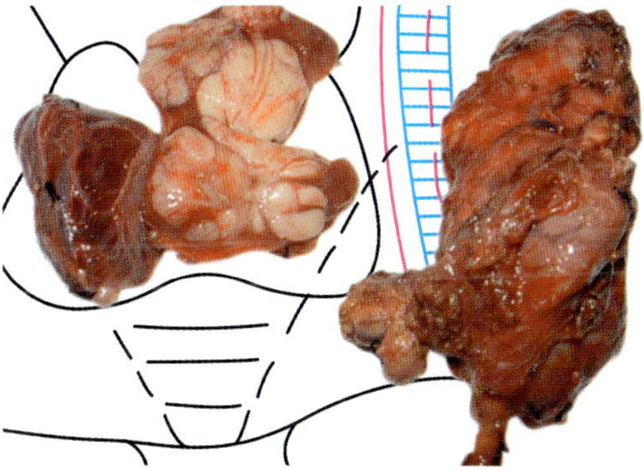

Fig. 33.2: Total thyroidectomy specimen with left MRND showing solitary tumor focus

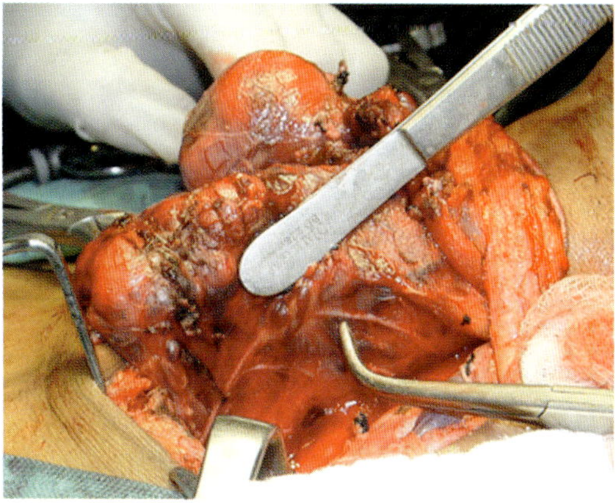

Fig. 33.3: Intraoperative photograph showing RLN lying lateral to the lymph node mass

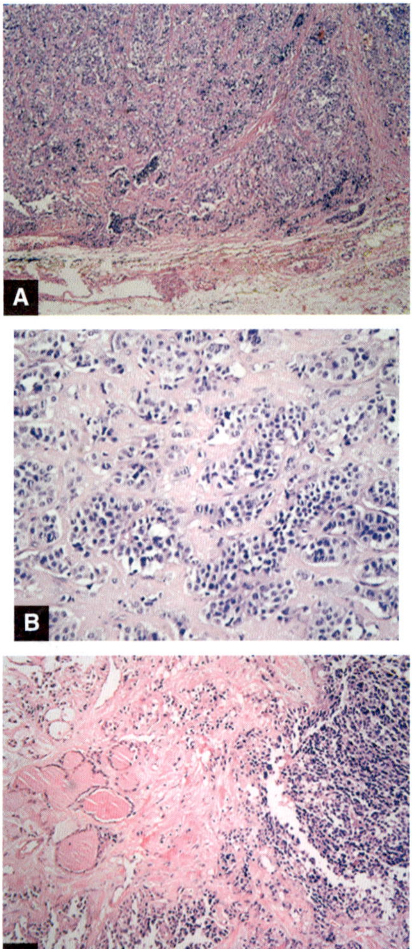

Figs 33.4A to C: Round, polygonal to spindle cells arranged in nests and cords, defined by sharply outlined fibrous bands, stippled nuclear chromatin, granular cytoplasm (H and E stain)

cervical lymph node enlargements. Her FNAC was suggestive of medullary thyroid carcinoma with metastases to lymph nodes. Subsequently serum calcitonin was estimated which was found to be significantly elevated (19764 pg/ml). After confirming the diagnosis of medullary

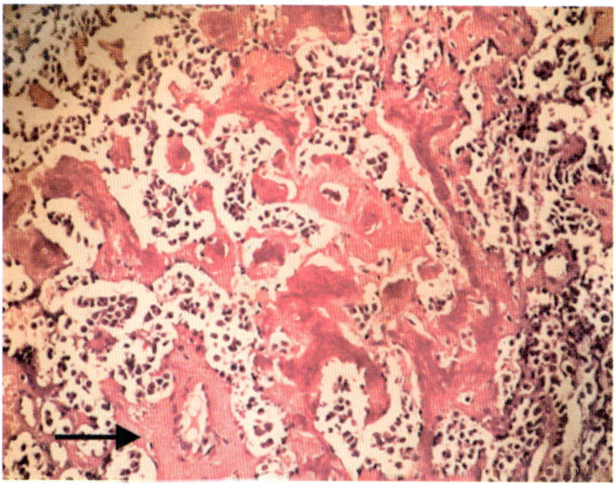

Fig. 33.5: Congo-red stained positivity for amyloid (arrow) in a case of MTC

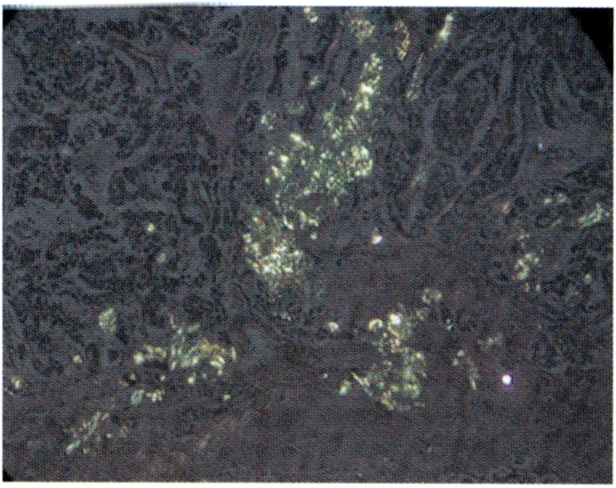

Fig. 33.6: Apple green bifringence of amyloid under polarized light in a case of MTC

thyroid carcinoma, metastatic work-up was done: Plain X-ray of chest and CT thorax and lungs did not show any mediastinal lymph node deposits or lung metastases; CT liver did not reveal any hepatic metastases and bone scan was negative for any skeletal metastases. She underwent total thyroidectomy with bilateral central compartmental dissection and left-sided modified radical neck dissection. The postoperative period was uneventful. The

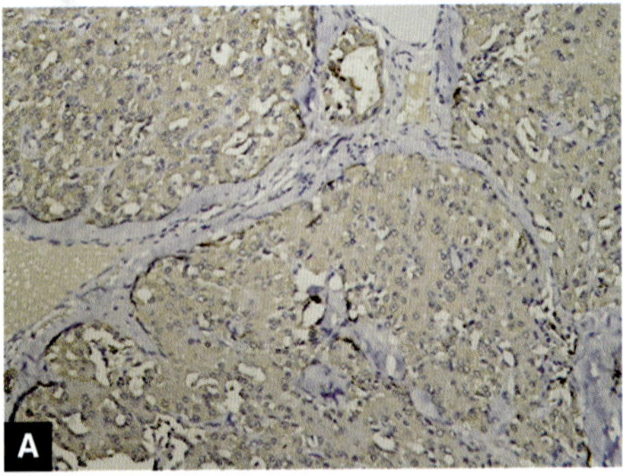

IHC: Calcitonin +ve

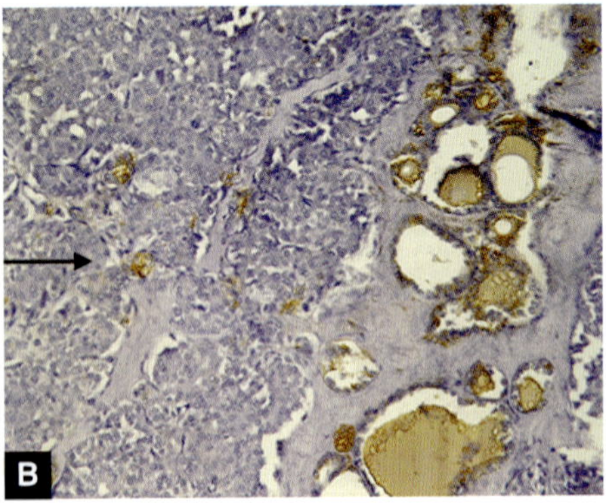

IHC: Thyroglobulin –ve (arrow)

histopathology confirmed medullary thyroid carcinoma with all lymph nodes of the lateral compartment showing tumor deposits; however, the lymph nodes of central compartment were free of tumor. Immunohistochemistry was positive for calcitonin but negative for thyroglobulin. The postoperative calcitonin was estimated at 8 weeks and was found to be within normal limits-7.40 pg/ml (normal :< 13 pg/ml).

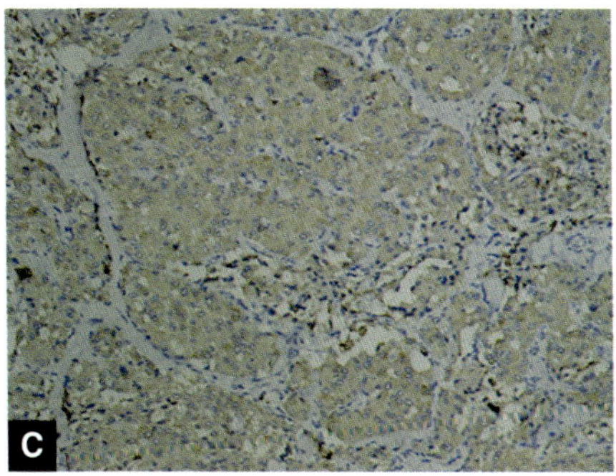

IHC: Chromgranin+ve

Figs 33.7A to C. Immunohistochemistry

QUESTIONS

What is the appropriate preoperative evaluation of such a case?

Majority of patients diagnosed with MTC present with a solitary thyroid nodule.

- Some features of thyroid nodule may prompt suspicion of MTC-location in the upper 1/3 of thyroid lobe, pain on palpation, history of diarrhea and flushing, presence of large, discrete rubbery lymph nodes along with thyroid nodule.

- Careful clinical examination should be done to seek signs of MEN2B (marfanoid habitus, mucosal neuromas) and family history suggestive of thyroid, parathyroid tumors and pheochromocytoma should be sought.
- Signs and symptoms of locally invasive tumor such as hoarseness, dysphagia, dyspnea, stridor or hemoptysis should be looked for.
- Examination findings with respect to size of the mass, fixation to surrounding structures, unifocal or bilateral lesion and presence of regional lymphadenopathy should be noted.
- The diagnosis is accurately established by FNAC of the nodule along with immunocytochemistry with calcitonin (if available)
- Measurement of basal and/or stimulated serum calcitonin
- USG would reveal a hypoechoic solid nodule with microcalcification and lymph node enlargement in the central and lateral compartments.
- All patients of MTC should be screened for pheochromocytoma with a 24-hour urinary metanephrine or VMA or free catecholamines.
- Blood sample should also be taken for genetic testing (RET proto-oncogene analysis) as approximately 25% of patients with presumed sporadic MTC have hereditary disease.
- High resolution cervical ultrasound should be done to assess the locoregional area—central, lateral and supraclavicular region for lymph node metastases. In large or locally advanced lesions spiral CT should be performed as it can assess the operability and the antero-superior mediastinum for presence of lymph nodes which would help in deciding the need for sternotomy.

- Metastatic survey for staging the disease should be performed which includes chest CT, MRI of the liver and radionuclide bone scan.

What is the site of origin of MTC?

MTC arises from the C-cells or parafollicular cells which are part of APUD system of neuroendorine cells. Within the thyroid gland, the highest concentration of C-cells is at the junction of upper one-third and lower two-third. The primary hormone secreted by MTC is the calcitonin. However, MTC can also secrete a variety of substances such as CEA, histamine, NSE, somatostatin, ACTH, chromogranin A, etc. These hormones and peptides may produce flushing, diarrhea, and even clinical syndromes like Cushings' syndrome

What is the clinical behavior of sporadic MTC?

Sporadic MTC exhibits a heterogeneous behavior. On one hand it may behave as a slow growing indolent disease and on the other hand it may behave as a very aggressive disease producing extensive local invasion as well as florid distant metastases. In MTC, unlike DTC, lymphatic spread to regional lymph nodes—central, lateral and mediastinal is very common. In the neck it may rapidly invade structures like IJV, strap muscles and trachea. RLN may be invaded by large metastatic perithyroidal and paratracheal nodes.

What is the gross and microscopic pathology of MTC?

Cut-surface of MTC is usually whitish or red. Microscopic features are sheets of cells-spindle shaped, round or polygonal, separated by fibrous stroma. Nuclei are usually uniform in shape and mitotic figures are rare. Cytoplasm is usually eosinophilic and characteristically granular. Amyloid deposits which show positive staining with Congo Red or apple green bifringence on polarized light, are seen interspersed between tumor cells in approximately 75% of cases. Most of the tumor cells show positive immunostaining for calcitonin and CEA but negative staining for thyroglobulin antibodies. Rare subtypes of MTC are medullo-follicular type which shows a combination of C-cell and follicular features.

What is the pattern of loco-regional and metastatic spread?

MTC commonly metastasizes to lymph nodes usually in a stepwise fashion and the frequency is related to the size of tumor

Tumor size	*Frequency of LN metastases*
< 1 cm	20-30%
1-4 cm	50%
> 4 cm	90%
Skip metastases	35%

Distant metastases

Common sites are liver, lungs and bone. Seen in 20% of cases. The distant metastases are usually small, multiple and diffuse. Distant metastases are responsible for cause-specific mortality in MTC. In 20-30% it is the initial presentation and multiple organs may be involved simultaneously. Lung metastases are usually diffuse while liver metastases are multiple, small and superficial. The treatment is directed towards relief of symptoms.

- *Diarrhea:* loperamide, octreotide
- *Isolated metastases:* of liver and lung can be surgically excised
- *Multiple liver metastases:* chemoembolization, chemotherapy, usually combination of 5-FU, streptozotocin and dacarbazine

There is no role of EBRT. Somatostatin analogues alone or in combination with interferon alpha-2b can be tried. Novel drugs such as inhibitors of tyrosine kinase are being tested as well as radio-immunotherapy with I^{131} antibodies are being tried.

What is the role of EBRT in management of MTC?

MTC is not radiosensitive but EBRT can be given if gross disease is left behind after palliative surgery. It is, of course, useful in the treatment of skeletal metastases.

If the patient has distant metastases at presentation, should he be offered surgery for local control?

In MTC even distant metastases is compatible with prolonged survival, hence palliative intervention is useful in the form of total thyroidectomy and central LN dissection as well as selective removal of bulky LN masses to provide symptomatic relief and to reduce the tumor burden, if this can be achieved with minimal morbidity and without sacrifice of vital structures.

What is the incidence of cure rate or normo-calcitoninemia?

a. Without lymph node involvement : 75-90%

b. With lymph node metastases : 20-30%
c. If involved LN are > 10 : 4%

What are other causes of elevated calcitonin (CT)?

a. *Other NET:* GI enteropancreatic endocrine tumors and others such as pheochromocytoma and paraganglionoma
b. Cell hyperplasia and consequently marginal elevation of Calcitonin can occur normally in children < 6 years of age and older people > 50 years.
c. Presence of anti-IgG antibodies in patients sera may cause spurious elevation of calcitonin in IRMA assays.

How do you stage the tumor?

UICC TNM Classification

Stage I	T1, N0, M0
Stage II	T2-T4, N0, M0
Stage III	Any T, N1, M0
Stage IV	Any T, any N, M1

T1 : Tumor < 1 cm, confined to thyroid gland
T2 : Tumor > 1 cm and < 4 cm, confined to thyroid gland
T3 : Tumor > 4 cm, confined to thyroid gland
T4 : Tumor of any size, infiltrating the thyroid capsule
N1a : Metastases to ipsilateral nodes
N1b : Metastases to bilateral, midline, contralateral or mediastinal nodes

What is the appropriate surgical management?

a. The main stay of primary treatment of MTC in both sporadic and hereditary forms is surgical, i.e. total thyroidectomy with prophylactic bilateral central compartmental dissection. The evidence for this comes in form of bilateral and diffuse distribution of C-cells, bilateral MTC can be present in one-third of even sporadic cases and 25% of presumed sporadic cases eventually turn out to be hereditary MTC.

b. The central compartment involvement is very high, approximately 75% (33% even in small, <1cm tumors) and these nodes cannot be reliably detected preoperatively (neither by clinical examination nor by USG). Thus, central neck clearance is required in all cases of MTC even in the absence of grossly evident central LN enlargement.
c. If the central group of LN are positive intraoperatively (on frozen examination), lateral compartments should be dissected.
d. There is enough evidence that compartment-oriented lymphadenectomy decreases the incidence of loco-regional recurrence and can achieve normal calcitonin postoperatively.
e. An aggressive approach is warranted in MTC unlike DTC—the rule of thumb is to treat one stage ahead of the existing stage. Thus
   i. In patients with MTC < 1 cm with central group of LN enlargement: Total thyroidectomy with central dissection (mediastinal dissection can be avoided).
   ii. ***In patients with palpable thyroid nodule which is positive on FNAC preoperatively:*** Total thyroidectomy with full central compartmental dissection (avoiding mediastinal dissection) with modified neck dissection on the side of lesion.
   iii. In patients with thyroid nodule with palpable lateral neck nodes or in cases of large nodule even in the absence of lateral neck nodes: total thyroidectomy with

full central compartmental dissection (including anterior-superior mediastinal nodes) with bilateral modified neck dissection.

How do you handle the parathyroid glands during surgery for MTC?

There are 3 ways to manage the parathyroid glands:

i. Preservation of all 4 parathyroid glands in situ.
ii. Preservation of superior parathyroid glands and autotransplanting inferior parathyroid glands: The inferior parathyroid glands are in close proximity to the LN of the central compartment and it can be very difficult to distinguish between the normal parathyroid gland and the lymph node. Attempting to preserve the parathyroid gland risks leaving behind positive lymph nodes and similarly extensive dissection may result in an avascular/ischemic parathyroid glands. Thus, one can autotransplant the two inferior glands after FS confirmation.
iii. Auto-transplantation of all 4 parathyroid glands. Before starting dissection of central compartment, all parathyroid glands can be dissected off and kept in cold saline to be autotransplanted later.

What is central compartmental dissection?

It entails removal of all fibro-fatty and lymphatic tissue in a space which is bound by hyoid bone superiorly, innominate vessels inferiorly and carotid arteries laterally. Careful attention should be paid during dissection to avoid injury to the RLN and the inferior parathyroids. To obtain exposure the strap muscles should be divided in the inferior portion. The cervical portion of thymus is also removed.

What are histopathological features of medullary thyroid carcinoma?

- *Patterns:* lobular, trabecular, insular and sheets
- *Cells:* round, polygonal, spindle shaped
- Coarse clumped or speckled chromatin, fine granular eosinophilic cytoplasm, binucleate and tumor giant cells, mitosis and necrosis are frequent in large tumors.
- Stromal amyloid deposits are seen in approximately 75% cases
- Tumors are positive for calcitonin, CEA and chromogranin antibodies but negative for thyroglobulin antibody.

What is the postoperative management of MTC?

- Thyroxine is given to maintain TSH concentration within normal range. There is no role of TSH suppression in MTC
- Calcitonin and CEA are measured usually at 6weeks to 3 months after surgery. If basal calcitonin is undetectable, stimulated (by calcium as pentagastrin is unavailable in India) should be done to establish cure
- Calcitonin and CEA are estimated at 6 monthly intervals for first 2 years and thereafter annually even if calcitonin normalizes.
- However, a detectable calcitonin is compatible with long-term survival. A rising calcitonin or CEA level indicates progressive disease.
- If the elevated postoperative calcitonin suddenly normalizes one must think of de-differentiation of tumor rather than cure.

What are prognostic markers in MTC?

Sporadic MTC is a heterogeneous disease as patients may survive several decades or die within few years of diagnosis. Amongst all the forms of MTC it has a better prognosis than only MEN2B. The various prognostic markers are:

a. ***Stage of disease:***

Stage	10-year survival
I	100%
II	93%
III	71%
IV	20%

b. *Age:* Older patients have poor outcome. Both age and stage of disease are independent prognostic factors.
c. ***Plasma calcitonin levels:*** High preoperative levels, especially if >10,000 pg/ml, is a bad prognostic indicator.
d. ***DNA aneuploidy:*** is a poor prognostic marker.
e. Positive immunostaining with calcitonin or somatostatin as well as presence of amyloid are associated with better outcome.
f. Elevated CEA level is a marker of disseminated disease
g. Presence of symptoms like diarrhea (which indirectly indicates high calcitonin levels) is associated with poor prognosis.

An important point to remember is that once MTC has become clinically manifest the prognosis of sporadic and familial cases is the same.

Chapter 34

Multiple Endocrine Neoplasia Type 2A (MEN 2A)

CASE STUDY

A 14-year-old girl presented with gradually increasing swelling in front of neck for last one year and increased frequency of watery stools for last 3 months. On examination she had a 4 × 4 cm firm swelling which was moving with deglutination and arising from right lobe of thyroid. Fine needle aspiration was suggestive of medullary thyroid cancer. She was worked up for MEN syndrome – 24 hour urinary metanephrine, serum calcium and PTH were within normal limits. However, family history revealed that her grandmother who was still alive had been operated for MTC 25 years back, her father died at the age of 34 from metastatic thyroid carcinoma and two of her siblings out of 4 were found to be having solitary thyroid nodule. Serum calcitonin was significantly elevated (4599 pg/ml). Genetic analysis of the index case was done and mutation was detected in

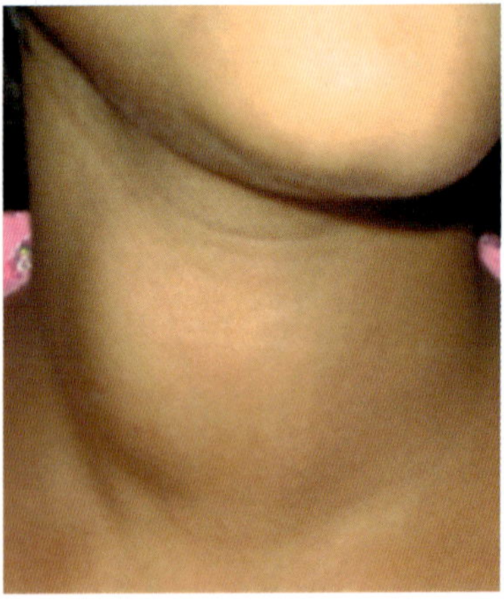

Fig. 34.1: Young girl of MTC presenting with solitary thyroid nodule

the RET proto-oncogene, Exon 11 codon 634, resulting in TGC conversion to CGC, substituting cystine to Arginine indicative of MEN2A. The patient was taken up for surgery. At exploration, the two inferior parathyroid glands were found to be enlarged-after confirmation by frozen section the two glands were excised. Total thyroidectomy with central compartmental dissection with 2 gland parathyroidectomy was thus performed. Cut section of the

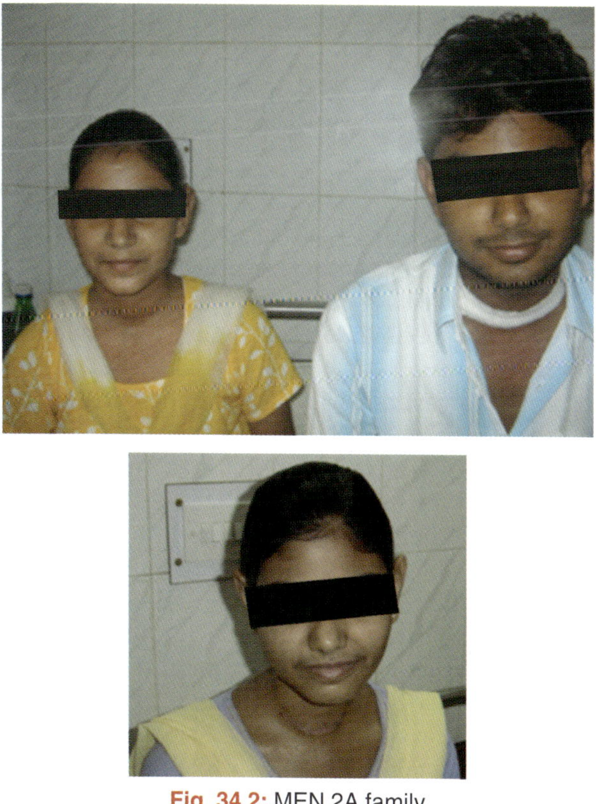

Fig. 34.2: MEN 2A family

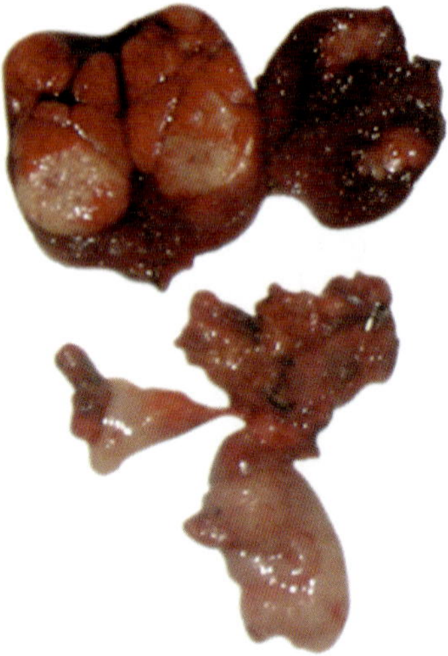

Fig. 34.3: Surgical specimen of the same patient showing bilateral tumor in hereditary MTC

thyroidectomy specimen revealed grayish white tumor in both lobes and histopathology confirmed medullary thyroid carcinoma; however, all 12 lymph nodes of the central compartment were free of tumor tissue. The inferior parathyroid glands weighed 100 mg and 56 mg and histopathology revealed reduced fat cells suggestive of parathyroid hyperplasia. The immunohistochemistry revealed that the tumor cells were positive for CEA, Calcitonin and chromogranin and negative for thyroglobulin. She was put on oral calcium and vitamin D3. Her 3 siblings were investigated by basal serum calcitonin which was found to be normal in all the 3 siblings. However, genetic analysis revealed that all the 3 siblings had positive mutation in codon 634 of the RET proto-oncogene. Two of her siblings, aged 18 and 16 years underwent total thyroidectomy and central compartmental dissection and histopathology was confirmatory of medullary thyroid carcinoma. Her 4th sibling who is 10 years old is awaiting surgery.

Test Results

Exon no.	*Codon*	*Presence of mutation*
Exon 10	602 / 603 / 606 / 609 / 611 / 615 / 620	Not detected
Exon 11	634	Detected
Exon 13	768 / 777 / 770 / 781 / 790 / 791	Not detected
Exon 14	804	Not detected
Exon 16	918 / 922	Not detected

Fig. 34.4: Mutation analysis of index case

QUESTIONS

What are the components of MEN 2A?

It is also known as Sipple syndrome. It is an autosomal dominant syndrome characterized by multiple tumors: Medullary thyroid cancer, parathyroid tumors and pheochromocytoma. Besides this it also includes some variants such as:

- Familial MTC (FMTC)
- MEN 2A with cutaneous lichen amyloidosis (CLA)
- MEN 2A and Hirschsprung's disease

What is the causative gene?

The causative gene is RET protoncogene which encodes a tyrosine-kinase receptor. The receptor has three domains, an extracellular domain, an intracellular tyrosine-kinase domain and a cysteine rich domain immediately external to cytoplasmic membrane.

RET protoncogene has 21 exons. Mutations associated with MEN 2A affect six exons in each two major domains. The commonest affected codon is 634 which is responsible for 80-90% of all MEN 2 mutations.

What is the frequency of different tumors in MEN 2A?

- MTC: 100%
- Pheochromocytoma: 45%
- Hyperparathyroidism: 35%

What are unique histological and clinical features of hereditary MTC?

- 95% are bilateral and multifocal
- associated with background C-cell hyperplasia
- Node involvement is more extensive in MEN 2A than in sporadic disease.

What are the characteristics of HPT in MEN 2A?

- It presents late, around the age of 40 years
- It is rarely the presenting feature of the syndrome and is not clinically significant as patients are normocalcemic.
- It is highly associated with a mutation of codon 634
- Though the underlying process is hyperplasia, only one or two glands may be enlarged.

What are the issues in genetic testing for MEN 2A?

i. Genetic testing of at-risk family members for mutated MEN 2A gene allows early or prophylactic thyroidectomy which could prevent development of metastatic disease and prevent mortality.

ii. ***Reproducibility and simplicity:*** Since the disease is inherited in an autosomal dominant fashion, 50% of at-risk first degree relatives will never develop disease and once they are found not to be having the mutated gene, they are spared the expense and inconvenience of routine/annual biochemical calcium/pentagastrin stimulated calcitonin testing which has to be done life-long. Genetic testing requires drawing of blood for extraction of lymphocyte DNA, and need be performed once in an at-risk individual's lifetime. Also, provocative calcitonin testing is unpleasant and uncomfortable and compliance is limited. However, genetic testing error can occur in 5-10% of cases, especially due to sample mix-up resulting from kindreds with similar first and last names in a family.

Is genetic testing required in patients with apparently sporadic MTC/HPT/Pheochromocytoma?

Almost 25% of persons with apparently sporadic MTC or pheochromocytoma have RET protoncogene mutation, hence genetic analysis should be performed in all patients with such tumors. Further, genetic testing is likely to be far more effective in identifying hereditary MTC than provocative tests of calcitonin in first-degree relatives. Thus, the current recommendation is to perform a germline genetic analysis of exons 10, 11, 13,14, 15,16 of RET to exclude hereditary disease with a probability of greater than 99%.

What is the role of preventive surgery for carriers of MEN 2A gene?

At risk family members who are found to have inherited a RET gene mutation will certainly develop MTC at some point in their lives, usually before the age of 30 and thus likely to benefit from a prophylactic thyroidectomy.

How can you utilize the genetic information for therapeutic purposes?

Genetic information can be utilized to stratify the RET mutations into risk categories and then performing codon based surgery. This is possible because RET mutations are associated with very aggressive clinical behavior.

i. ***Highest risk category:*** This includes mutations in codons 883,918,922. Total thyroidectomy with CCND should be performed during first few months of life (< 1 year of age).
ii. ***High risk category:*** This includes mutations in codon 634,611,618,620. Total thyroidectomy with or without CCND should be performed between 5-10 years. Trade off between age at surgery and extent of surgery – either earlier surgery without CCND or later surgery with CCND
iii. ***Intermediate or low risk category:*** This includes mutations in codons 609,768,791,804,891. MTC develops at a later age and the tumor grows slowly. No consensus on the treatment protocol. The options are either total thyroidectomy by the age of 5 years, or total thyroidectomy by the age of 10 years or continued stimulated calcitonin testing and whenever it is elevated a total thyroidectomy is performed.

What are the general guidelines for managing hyperparathyroidism in MEN 2A?

Patients with hyperparathyroidism and MEN 2A are most often asymptomatic or have only mild hypercalcemia. It is often detected either as a mild hyperparathyroidism (elevated or inappropriately elevated PTH) in a normocalcemic individual found before a thyroid operation for MTC or as one or more enlarged parathyroid glands found during the thyroid operation for MTC; or as hyperplastic enlarged parathyroid glands on histology of the central lymph node clearance done for MTC.

Parathyroid disease in MEN 2A is much less aggressive than in MEN1 patients. The general accepted operation, particularly in a normocalcemic individual, is routine identification of all 4 parathyroid glands and excision of only macroscopically enlarged glands. A cervical thymectomy and a careful search for supernumerary parathyroid glands should also be done. The rationale behind this approach is that the incidence of recurrent or persistent hyperparathyroidism in MEN 2A is not as common as seen in MEN1. Infact, the primary surgical concern in MEN 2A is to avoid hypocalcemia.

The other option, particularly in a hypercalcemic individual, is to perform either a subtotal parathyroidectomy or total parathyroidectomy with autotransplantation in nondominant forearm. The advantages of this approach felt by its proponents are: routine removal of parathyroid glands ensures adequate cervical lymph node clearance in MTC; if recurrence develops in central compartment and re-operation is required, parathyroid function will not be jeopardized; and the fact that patients with MEN 2A are always at risk for development of HPT later, when localization of hyperfunctioning tissue is simpler if all the parathyroid tissue is in the arm only.

How do you follow-up these patients?

The follow-up of hereditary MTC is life-long. It is advisable to follow these patients (who have undergone prophylactic/ therapeutic thyroidectomy) with stimulated plasma calcitonin levels every 1-2 years. They must also be followed for development of pheochromocytoma and hyper-parathyroidism.

Chapter 35

Persistent Hypercalcitoninemia

CASE STUDY

A 32-year-old male patient presented with complaints of alteration of voice-hoarseness and decrease in amplitude for one month. He had no other significant history. On examination he was found to be normotensive with no significant finding on general examination. On local examination he was found to be having a 2 × 2 cm nodule in the left lobe of thyroid which was firm, moving with deglutination and its lower border was palpable. There was no lateral neck lymphadenopathy. On evaluation, USG revealed 1.2 × 1.5 × 1.2 cm nodule in the midportion of thyroid. There was also evidence of multiple bilateral cervical lymph node enlargement. FNAC from the nodule was then performed and it was suggestive of Medullary thyroid carcinoma. Subsequently a serum calcitonin was collected and was found to be elevated (1505 pg/ml). Vocal cord examination revealed bilateral normal vocal cord movement. CECT was done to assess the neck and mediastinum and it confirmed the presence of thyroid nodule and only left sided cervical lymphadenopathy but no mediastinal lymph nodes. It also picked up lung and pleural lesions—a peripherally enhancing irregular mass, 3 × 2 cm having spiculation and associated pleural thickening was noted in the right lung. Bilateral upper and mid zones of the lung showed multiple soft, ill-defined nodules.

The patient was taken up for surgery. After raising the flaps, left midjugular (level III) lymph node was sampled and sent for frozen section examination. Meanwhile total thyroidectomy with central compartmental neck dissection was performed. Both superior parathyroid glands were preserved *in situ* with good vascular supply while both inferior parathyroid glands were removed prior to CCND and autotransplanted in the SCM. Left RLN was found to be adherent to the central compartmental (paratracheal LN) from which it could be dissected out only with great difficulty. Every attempt was made to preserve the RLN because it was a functioning nerve (as shown on I/L examination). On receiving the positive FS report Modified Radical Neck Dissection was performed on the left side. The post-operative period was uneventful and histopathology revealed a solitary focus of MTC in left lobe while 6 out of 21 LN in the central compartment were positive and 8 out of 12 lymph nodes of left lateral neck compartment were positive. On immunohistochemistry the specimen stained positive for calcitonin. Serum calcitonin was estimated 2 months after surgery and was found to be still elevated (1050 gp/ml) and CEA was also elevated (14.2 pg/ml). He was kept under surveillance and repeat values after 6 months were 927 and 9.3. Since he had persistent hypercalcitoninemia, further evaluation was done-DMSA penatavalent scan was found to be negative; CECT of abdomen did not reveal any liver metastases and USG neck did not reveal any loco-regional disease. He was then advised to undergo a PET scan which revealed multiple bilateral lung lesions while there was no increased uptake in the neck or elsewhere. He was then given EBRT of the mediastinal area. He is still in follow-up and the Calcitonin and CEA values though still elevated, are not rising.

QUESTIONS

What is the appropriate postoperative management of these patients?

After adequate initial surgery, all patients should receive life-long replacement therapy with thyroxine. The dose is adjusted by annual serum TSH levels. There is no need for TSH suppression and the serum TSH should be maintained within the normal range unlike in papillary thyroid carcinoma.

What is persistent or recurrent hypercalcitoninemia?

Presence of residual disease in MTC can be easily picked up by a persistently elevated basal or stimulated serum calcitonin level 6 months after initial operation. Though persistent hypercalcintoninemia is expected after incomplete/inadequate initial surgery, it is common even after an apparent complete/adequate surgery for MTC. Persistent hypercalcitoninemia is a perplexing and challenging problem because the localization of residual MTC responsible for elevated calcitonin level is difficult.

How to localize and manage occult MTC?

The foremost aim is to localize the site of metastatic or residual MTC. A number of methods may be used to localize residual or recurrent disease.

- Physical examination: A careful physical examination is extremely important to identify neck nodes or recurrent/ persistent thyroid tissue

- Imaging studies:
  - USG: High resolution USG along with guided FNAC of impalpable neck nodes is one of the most sensitive method for detecting residual/metastatic disease in the neck
  - CT thorax and abdomen
  - MRI is useful for detecting residual MTC in the mediastinum
  - Nuclear studies like MIBG, Tc 99m Pentavalent DMSA, anti-CEA monoclonal antibody imaging
  - PET has been used with great success
  - Invasive studies like selective venous catheterization are now being used less and less
  - Diagnostic laparoscopy can be utilized to detect superficial miliary liver metastases.

How will you manage loco-regional or metastatic MTC?

There are different views in approaching this problem and several authors have documented that both these approaches are valid. The *first* is an aggressive approach which recommends loco-regional reoperation involving meticulous microdissection. Though it rarely results in long-term biochemical cure, it may limit progression of MTC. However, microdissection does carry a higher rate of complications. An attempt can be made to identify patients who are more likely to benefit from this aggressive surgical approach-these are patients whose primary tumors do not have capsular invasion, extralymphatic spread or invasion of local structures. The *second* approach is the more conservative approach based on the fact that patients who had apparently curative surgical treatment with no identifiable MTC may have a long survival time 10-year survival rate being 85%. Thus, in a patient with persistent hypercalcitoninemia, the first step is to determine whether the initial surgery has been adequate or not. An adequate intial surgery for MTC is defined as total thyroidectomy with bilateral central compartmental dissection and in larger tumors or palpable lateral nodes, unilateral/bilateral neck dissection with or without mediastinal neck dissection has been perfomed.

a. If the initial surgery is adequate and no loco-regional or distant metastatic site can be identified by optimal imaging, then one should follow the policy of "observation".
b. If the initial surgery is adequate but loco-regional recurrent or persistent disease is identified either in the neck or more commonly in the mediastinum, a reoperation is advisable because the removal of residual disease may arrest the course of the disease and result in either normalization of calcitonin or at least some decrease in the calcitonin levels. Re-operation can range from formal lymph node dissections and mediastinal dissection (requiring even sternotomy) to micro-dissection. Microdissection involves a meticulous dissection of all lymph nodes and fatty tissue of cervical and lateral zones of the neck sometimes combined with mediastinal clearance. However, reoperation, particularly microdissection may result in significant morbidity in the form of permanent hypoparathyroidism and recurrent laryngeal palsy, hence reoperations should be performed by experienced endocrine/thyroid surgeons.
c. If the initial surgery is inadequate (either less than total thyroidectomy or without a central compartmental clearance) and the residual disease is localized in the neck, reoperation is advisable.

Chapter 36

Anaplastic Carcinoma: Diagnostic and Therapeutic Challenge

CASE STUDY

A 45-year-old lady presented with rapidly increasing thyroid swelling for last 1 month. She gave history of cervical pain, hoarseness of voice, difficulty in swallowing, occasional difficulty in breathing, loss of appetite and loss of weight. She gave history of goiter of 8 months duration. Examination revealed a large thyroid mass with ill-defined borders, hard consistency and severely restricted mobility. There was no cervical lymph node enlargement. Vocal cord examination revealed left vocal cord palsy and FNAC was suggestive of anaplastic thyroid carcinoma. CT showed a large heterogeneous mass arising from thyroid. She was put on hyperfractionated radiotherapy along with cisplatin chemotherapy. There was 50% reduction in size and relief in pain and swallowing.

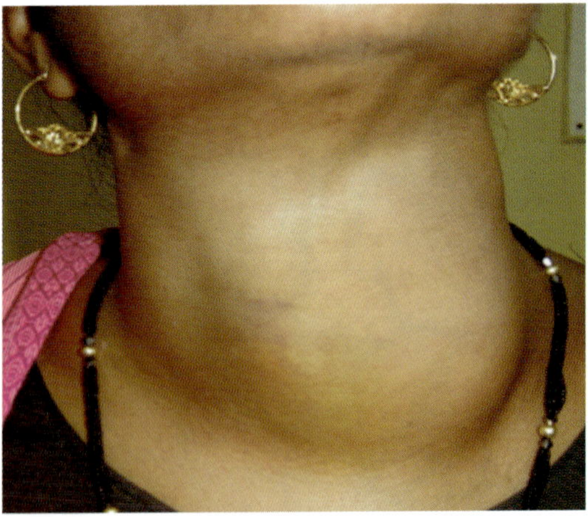

Fig. 36.1: Patient presenting with large, fixed mass

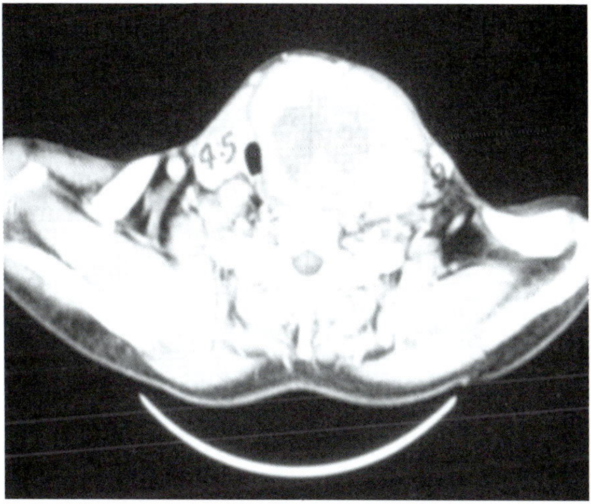

Fig. 36.2: CT scan showing large thyroid mass with necrotic areas and involvement of IJV

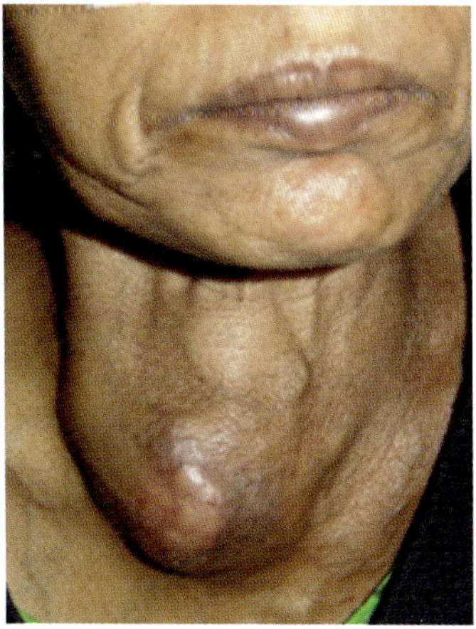

Fig. 36.3: Large thyroid mass with impending rupture

QUESTIONS

What is the common clinical presentation?

Anaplastic thyroid carcinoma (ATC) can present in two different ways:

Commonly it presents as a rapidly growing large thyroid mass associated with signs and symptoms arising due to expansion and infiltration of the tumor in the neck, such as dyspnea, dysphagia and hoarseness and neck pain. The other presentation is more insidious and may be in the form of long-standing goiter or pre-existing papillary carcinoma transforming itself into anaplastic thyroid carcinoma.

How do you diagnose ATC?

The typical case of ATC strongly suspected on clinical grounds is easily confirmed in majority of cases by fine needle aspiration cytology. FNAC is an effective method because the tumor is widely disseminated throughout the thyroid gland rather than being localized to a single focus.

However, there are certain pitfalls:

a. Sometimes the aspiration may be paucicellular in which case it may be misdiagnosed as Riedel's struma. In such a situation, tru-cut needle or open biopsy is advisable.
b. ATC in 90% of cases has co-existing areas of differentiated thyroid carcinoma (papillary or follicular). Therefore, cytological diagnosis of papillary or follicular carcinoma in a clinical setting that is highly suspicious of anaplastic carcinoma, does not exclude the presence of anaplastic carcinoma.
c. Spindle cell predominant ATC can be confused with sarcoma.
d. Multinucleated tumor giant cells can mimic metastatic breast carcinoma.

e. Squamoid predominant ATC can be falsely reported as upper aero-digestive squamous carcinomas that have locally invaded the thyroid gland and cervical soft tissues.
f. May also be confused with lymphoma and medullary thyroid cancer.

What is the role of immunohistochemistry?

The differential diagnosis of ATC includes the following:

a. ***Lymphoma:*** Historically lymphomas (small and large cell) were frequently misdiagnosed as ATC. With the wide availability of T-cell and B-cell immnunochemical markers lymphoma can be readily distinguished from ATC.
b. ***Medullary thyroid cancer:*** They express calcitonin and carcinoembryonic antigen (CEA) and thus can be easily distinguished from ATC.
c. Primary or secondary squamous carcinoma: IHC cannot reliably distinguish ATC from these.
d. ***Poorly differentiated follicular carcinoma (Insular carcinoma):*** Thyroglobulin and TTF-1 are rarely expressed by the ATC and also Insular carcinoma has a distinctive histology.
e. ***Sarcomas and melanomas:*** ATC express keratin and this is the single most useful epithelial marker in distinguishing from sarcomas and melanomas.

What is the role of local disease control?

The different surgical strategies for local control of disease are as follows:

a. ***Total thyroidectomy:*** Since the disease presents as advanced disease, only rarely is total thryoidectomy possible,except in those patients in whom papillary carcinomas has transformed into anaplastic carcinoma.

b. Extensive resection: involving aero-digestive tract or major vessels are not justified in view of short survival
c. Debulking: though possible, does not add to survival.
d. ***Therapeutic tracheostomy:*** this is required when tumor obstructs the airway and patients presents with stridor. However, its utility in the overall management is doubtful
e. ***Prophylactic tracheostomy:*** Again the value of prophylactic tracheostomy for prevention of respiratory obstruction is doubtful. Many patients with tracheostomies can have local wound healing complications which would prevent or delay postoperative external beam radiotherapy.

What is the role of hyperfractionated radiotherapy?

Even though ATC is a radio-resistant tumor, EBRT can aid in local disease control, especially by the use of hyperfractionated RT along with doxorubicin radiosensitization.

Hyperfractionation of RT permits administration of higher total radiation doses with less toxicity. The results are conflicting and overall consensus is that even after using doxorubicin radiosensitization with hyperfractionated RT, local disease control as well as survival have not improved.

What is the role of chemotherapy?

Various chemotherapeutic agents have been used but with disappointing results. Almost all regimes include doxorubicin. Recently paclitaxel has been tried and is said to have equal or more potency.

What is the treatment with combined modalites?

Since local disease control can prevent suffocation and patients die of metastatic disease which is there even prior to the discovery of primary tumor it makes sense to combine all the three modalities. Various protocols of hyperfractionated radiotherapy in combination with doxorubicin and surgery when feasible have been evolved. These have resulted in a slightly better survival.

What is the prognosis?

It is the most lethal endocrine malignancy. Survival is measured in months and death is commonly due to suffocation as a result of tumor causing obstruction of the thoracic inlet. Tumor volume can double over a week of observation.

FACTS AND FIGURES

1. Only 2-5% of thyroid carcinomas are anaplastic, but account for 50% of deaths from thyroid carcinoma
2. Average survival is only 3-6 months; only 10% survive more than one year
3. Usually occurs in elderly, 7-8th decade
4. Mean size at presentation is 5-6 cm
5. 33% present with one or more compressive symptoms—dyspnea, dysphagia, hoarseness
6. 50% present with distant metastases—90% in lungs
7. 40% have lymph node involvement which may not be separately palpable from the thyroid mass
8. All anaplastic thyroid carcinoma are classified as Stage IV regardless of tumor size, lymph nodes or distant metastases
9. 80% of ATC express keratin and this helps in distinguishing from malignancies of non-thyroidal origin like sarcomas, lymphomas and melanoma.

Chapter 37

Thyroid Lymphoma

CASE STUDY

A 65-year-old lady was referred with complaints of increasing breathlessness for last 2 months. She has been unable to take anything orally for last 7 days. On examination she was found to be having severe stridor

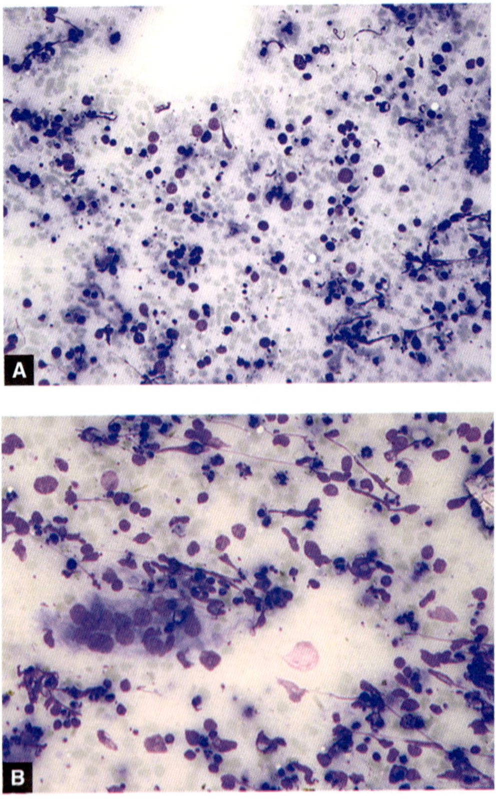

Figs 37.1A and B: FNA of thyroid lesion positive for atypical lymphoid cells (non-Hodgkin's lymphoma) (MGG stain)

resulting from large fixed thyroid. She also had bilateral bulky cervical lymph nodes. The thyroid was not moving on deglutination. She was immediately put on resuscitative measures and FNAC was ordered which revealed high grade lymphoma. The option of tracheal stenting followed by chemoradiation was explored; however, she expired due to respiratory failure.

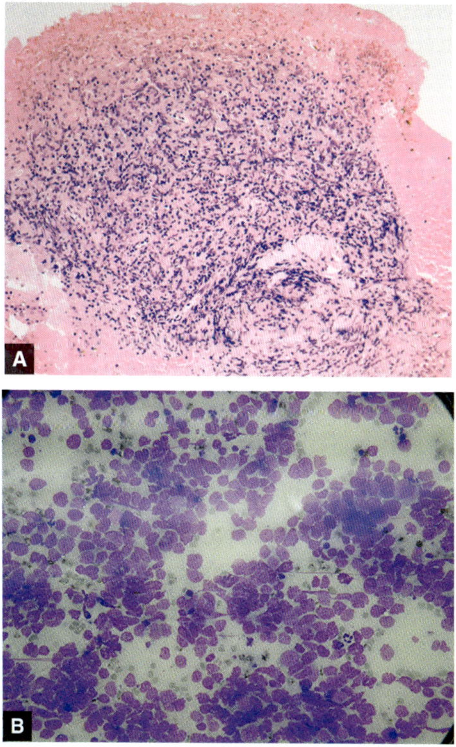

Figs 37.2A and B: (A) Tru-cut biopsy showing small to intermediate sized atypical lymphoid cells along with follicular cells from a case of low grade (marginal zone lymphoma of thyroid (H and E); (B) Cytology of same case showing atypical lymphoid cells (MGG stain)

QUESTIONS

What is the incidence and clinical presentation of thyroid lymphoma?

1-5% of all thyroid carcinoma are primary thyroid lymphoma. Amongst all extra-nodal lymphoma only 2% are thyroid lymphoma. They have a female preponderance (3:1) and usually present with a rapidly enlarging neck mass along with compressive features like stridor, dysphagia and hoarseness of voice.

What are various sub-types of lymphoma?

Almost all of the primary lymphoma of thyroid are Hodgkin's lymphoma of B-cell origin and can be further classified into 4 sub-types:

a. Diffuse large B-cell without marginal zone B-cell hyperplasia
b. Diffuse large B-cell lymphoma with marginal zone B-cell hyperplasia
c. Marginal zone B-cell lymphoma of mucosa associated lymphoid tissue (MALT)
d. Follicular lymphoma.

How do you make a pathological diagnosis of lymphoma?

FNAC is virtually diagnostic in large cell lymphoma but can be difficult in MALT lymphomas because of 3 reasons: Firstly, because MALT lymphoma has a more heterogeneous appearance, secondly, the cytological picture is quite similar to that of Hashimoto's thyroiditis and thirdly in most cases, MALT lymphoma arises on a background of Hashimoto's thyroiditis and thus may result in false negative sampling

When should the patient be subjected to open/trucut biopsy?

Since the prognosis of primary thyroid lymphoma is directly related to the pathological subtype of lymphoma it is imperative to classify into a distinct clinico-pathological subtype. Though immunophenotyping increases the sensitivity of FNAC, sometimes it may not be helpful or may simply be unavailable. In such a situation, one should resort to trucut or even open surgical biopsy.

What is the role of thyroidectomy in lymphoma of thyroid?

The only situation where surgery or even radiation alone can be indicated is MALT lymphoma in early stage, i.e. confined to thyroid gland (Stage 1E).

What is the role of palliative surgery?

The role of palliative surgery alone is controversial. Immediate tracheostomy or tracheal stenting seem logical but can result in complications especially in bulky lymphomas.

What is the best modality of treatment for primary lymphoma of thyroid?

Combined chemoradiation is thought to be the best modality of treatment. The overall relapase rates of chemoradiation has been 7.7% compared to radiation alone (37.1%) and chemotherapy alone (43%). The most commonly used regimen is CHOP (Cyclophosphamide, Doxorubicin, Vincristine and Prednisone).

Section 2

PARATHYROID DISORDERS

Chapter 38

Primary Hyperparathyroidism

CASE STUDY

A 28-year-old male was seen with history of fractures in both upper arms sustained 2 years back from trivial trauma and managed by intramedullary nailing and iliac graft. Subsequently he also sustained fracture of left femur, also from trivial trauma, which was managed by nailing again. He gave history of bone pains, difficulty in getting up from squatting position and climbing stairs. There was no history of renal colic and stones. He gave history of dyspepsia and upper abdominal pain. Biochemistry revealed elevated serum calcium (10.2 and 10.4 mg/dl), low phosphorous (2.3 and 2.4 mg/dl), high alkaline phosphatase (440 IU/L), elevated PTH (779 pg/ml), low vitamin D (3.94 ng/ml). A diagnosis of primary hyperparathyroidism was made. Skeletal survey revealed subperiosteal resorption, brown tumors, non formation of callus at fracture site. BMD was significantly reduced. Localization was done by USG which revealed right inferior parathyroid adenoma which was confirmed on MIBI scan. He was taken up for focused parathyroidectomy and a 2 gm right inferior parathyroid adenoma was removed by 2.5 cm incision. Postoperatively he developed symptomatic hypocalcemia which was managed by intravenous calcium infusion and oral vitamin D and calcium. The histopathology revealed well circumscribed tumor disposed in nests and solid sheets traversed by thin fibrovascular septae. The tumor cells were uniform in appearance with round centrally placed mildly anisomorphic nuclei, small nucleoli discernible in places, and moderate amount of pale eosinophilic to clear cytoplasm. At the periphery normal compressed parathyroid gland was. The final impression was parathyroid adenoma.

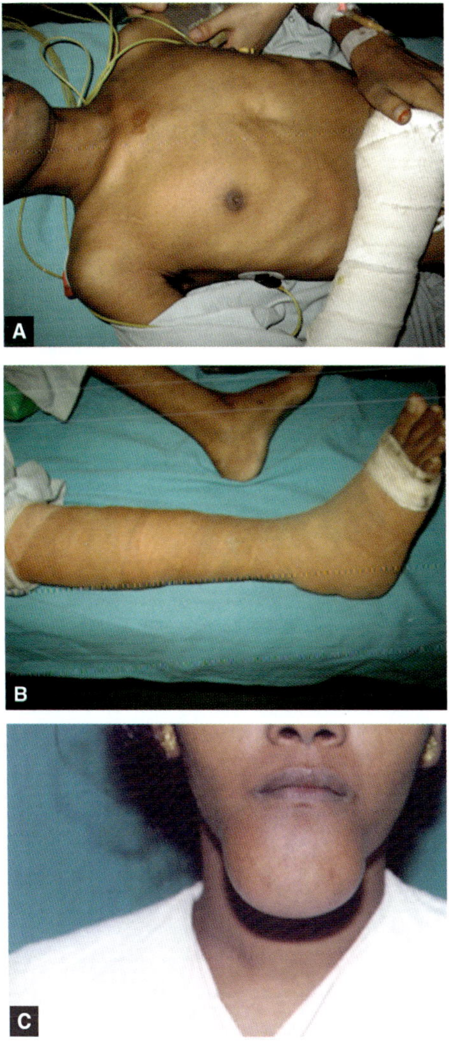

Figs 38.1A to C: Clinical presentation of patients of PHPT

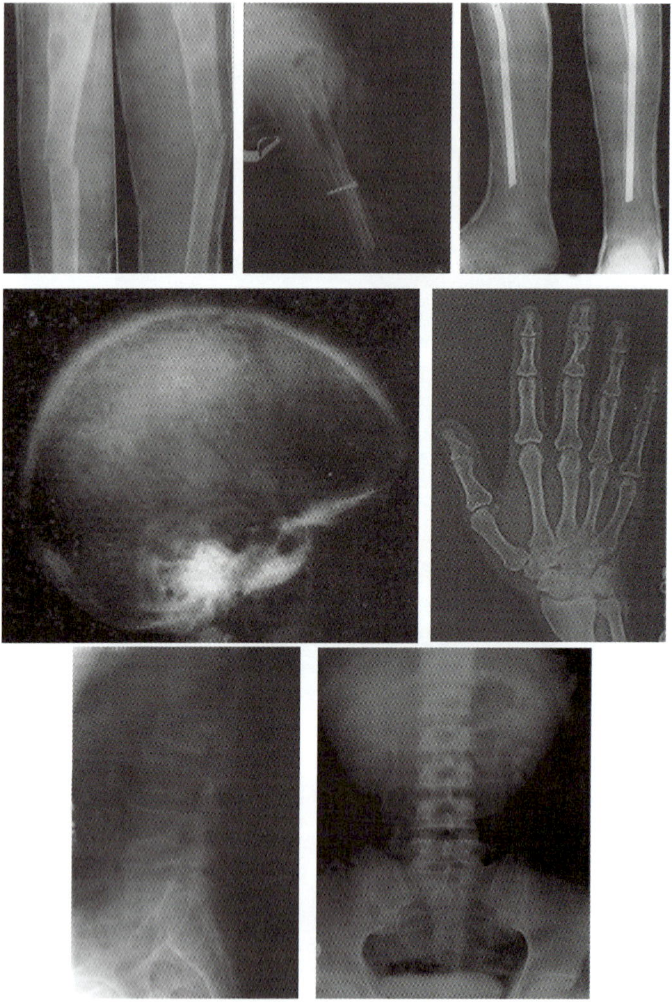

Fig. 38.2: Skeletal survey of PHPT patients showing brown tumors in long bones, subperiosteal resorption, nephrocalcinosis and rugger jersey spine

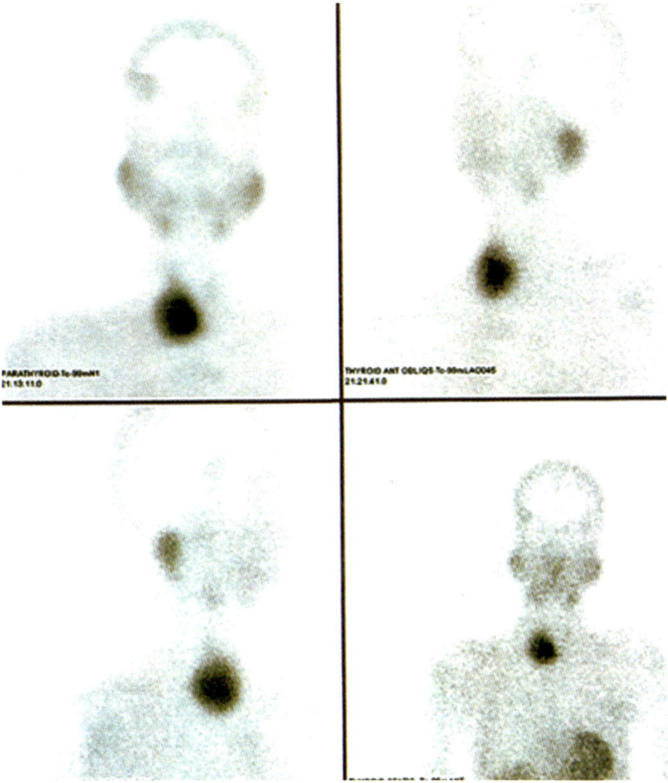

Fig. 38.3: MIBI scan showing single, intense focus of retained tracer in parathyroid adenoma

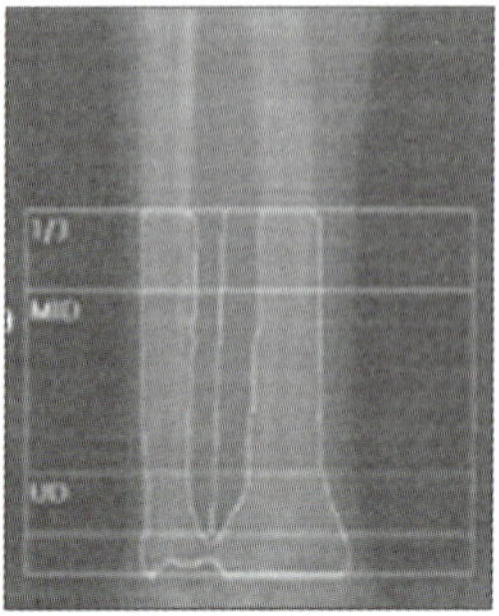

Image not for diagnostic use
228 × 91

Scan Information:
Scan Date: January 15, 2007 ID: S0115070D
Scan Type: a R.Forearm
Analysis: January 15, 2007 12:30 Version 12.4
Right Forearm
Operator: RKS
Model: Discovery A (S/N 45227)
Comment:

OXA Result Summary:

Radius+ Ulna	Area (cm^2)	BMC (g)	BMD (g/cm^2)	T - Score	Z - Score
1/3	5.31	2.90	0.516	-4.9	-4.7
MID	11.49	5.81	0.506	-3.4	-3.4
UD	5.06	2.55	0.504	-0.1	0.1
Total	**21.86**	**11.26**	**0.515**	**-3.0**	**-2.9**

Total BMD CV 1.0%
WHO Classification: Osteoporosis
Fracture Risk: High

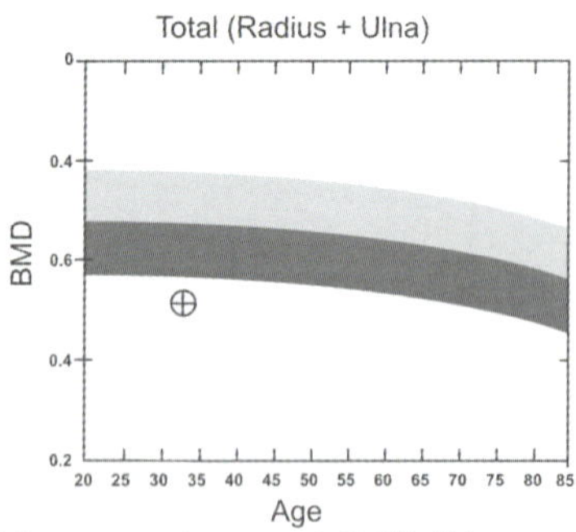

Physician's comment:

Reference curve and scores matached to White Male

Source: Hologic

Fig. 38.4A

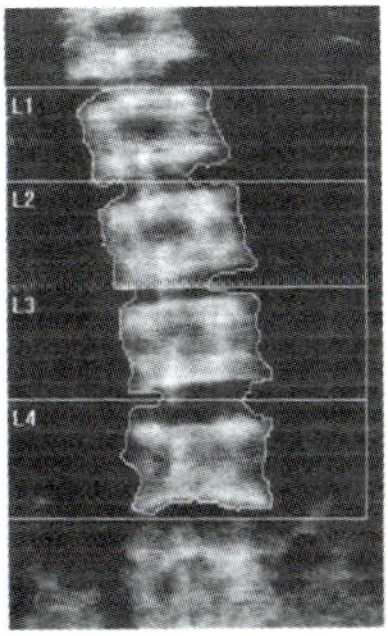

Image not for diagnostic use
121 × 139

Scan Information:
Scan Date: January 15, 2007 ID: S0115070D
Scan Type: f Lumbar Spine
Analysis: January 15, 2007 12:25 Version 12.4
Lumbar Spine
Operator: RKS
Model: Discovery A (S/N 45227)
Comment:

OXA Result Summary:

Region	Area (cm^2)	BMC (g)	BMD (g/cm^2)	T - Score	Z - Score
L1	12.81	11.61	0.907	-0.9	-0.9
L2	15.17	13.96	0.920	-1.6	1.6
L3	15.86	13.82	0.871	-2.1	-2.1
L4	15.57	12.62	0.811	-3.0	-3.0
Total	**59.42**	**52.02**	**0.875**	**-2.0**	**-2.0**

Total BMD CV 1.0%
WHO Classification: Osteopenia
Fracture Risk: Increased

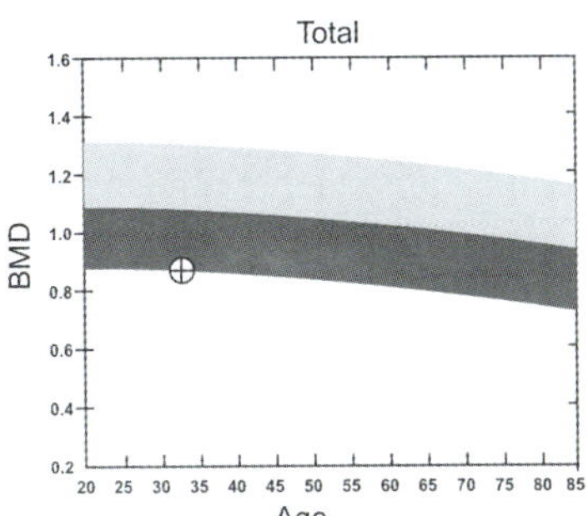

Reference curve and scores matached to White Male

Physician's comment:

Source: Hologic

Fig. 38.4B: BMD showing reduced bone density

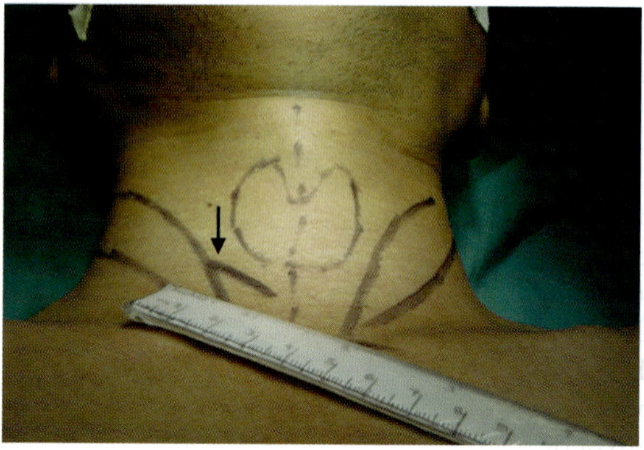

Fig. 38.5: Incision marking (→) for focused parathyroidectomy

QUESTIONS

What are the clinical features of Primary Hyperparathyroidism?

They can be divided into two broad categories:

- ***Classical symptoms:*** Patients present with advanced symptoms related to end-organ damage. Though only 20% of Caucasian patients present with classical disease, majority of Indian patients and those of other developing nations still present with the advanced symptomatology such as:
  - *Kidney:* Renal lithiasis, Nephrocalcinosis
  - *Skeletal system:* Hallmark is osteitis fibrosa cystica (OFC) due to extensive bone resorption resulting in bone pain, sub-peristeal resorption, brown tumors and pathological fractures.
  - *Neuromuscular system:* Severe proximal muscle weakness and extreme fatiguability

  - *GI system:* Dyspepsia, peptic ulcer disease and pancreatitis
  - *Neuro-psychiatric:* Mental state changes—irritability, mood swings, depression
  - Hypercalcemic crisis.
- ***Modern presentation:*** Most of the patients of the developing nations now are diagnosed when either they are minimally symptomatic or when elevated serum calcium is found on routine biochemical evaluation of otherwise healthy individual. Such patients are usually not truly asymptomatic because they do have vague neurocognitive symptoms like depression, easy fatiguability and lethargy. Further, target end-organ damage can be detected in the form of asymptomatic renal lithiasis (on USG) or low bone mineral density (on BMD).

How would you establish the biochemical diagnosis of PHPT?

- The biochemical hallmark is the presence of an increased serum calcium level along with inappropriately elevated intact PTH. Serum calcium is usually >2.55 mmol/L or 10.2 mg/dl (1 mg/dl = 0.25 mmol/L).
- Other biochemical features include
  - Hypophosphatemia
  - Hypercalciuria
  - Elevated alkaline phosphatase
  - Low serum 25-OH vitamin D
  - Mild hyperchloremia

What is the differential diagnosis of hypercalcemia?

- *Those with elevated PTH*
  - PHPT

  - Lithium toxicity
  - Thiazide diuretics
  - FIHH
  - Non parathyroid endocrine disorders: thyrotoxicosis, pheochromocytoma, islet-cell tumors
- *Those with suppressed PTH*
  - Vitamin D intoxication
  - Vitamin A intoxication
  - Prolonged immobilization
  - Milk-alkali syndrome
  - Parenteral nutrition

How will you assess the end-organ damage?

Bone mineral density

This is best assessed by measuring density at three sites by the dual energy X-ray absorptiometry (DEXA) scan. Bone mineral density provides accurate information about the actual state of bone mineral content even when the PHPT patients are asymptomatic and do not have obvious radiological features of PHPT. It is now well established that PTH is catabolic on cortical bone and anabolic on cancellous bone. Since distal third of radius contains cortical bone, in PHPT bone density at distal third is diminished. Similarly lumbar spine is predominantly cancellous bone and least affected in PHPT. The hip region shows bone density which is intermediate between cortical and cancellous sites as it contains almost equal mixture of cortical and cancellous bone.

BMD results are expressed as T and Z score which reflect values obtained from healthy individuals

- *Z-score:* is the number of standard deviation that the patient differs from the mean value for an age, sex and race matched reference population.
- *T-score:* is the number of SD that the patient/subject differs from the peak bone mass of a young reference population matched for sex and race.

Echocardiography

This can be done to look for myocardial or valvular calcification, diastolic dysfunction and left ventricular hypertrophy.

Renal ultrasound/KUB

It would reveal Nephrocalcinosis and nephrolithiasis

After a confirmed biochemical diagnosis of PHPT is it necessary to localize the parathyroid adenoma by imaging?

If a standard 4-gland exploration is being planned then localizing studies are not mandatory. However, if minimally invasive surgery is being planned or if it is a case of re-do parathyroidectomy then localizing procedures are essential (invasive studies in re-do parathyroidectomy). The various imaging techniques utilized are :

- *USG:* though it is widely available and inexpensive, the sensitivity rates for detecting solitary parathyroid adenomas varies greatly from 20-80% as it is operator dependent. It is nonetheless the first imaging that is performed and is useful in identifying any co-existing thyroid pathology.
- ***Technetium 99m Sestamibi (MIBI):*** this is now the most commonly utilized localization procedure. The sensitivity

of MIBI for detecting a solitary parathyroid adenoma is 60-80%. A positive MIBI scan is a solitary focus of intense uptake which is seen even in late films. Causes of false-negative MIBI include small size of the adenoma, water clear cell or oxyphill adenoma and co-existing thyroid nodules. The sensitivity of MIBI can be enhanced if it is combined with SPECT study. MIBI has poor sensitivity in diagnosing multiglandular disease.
- ***MRI/CT:*** are not used routinely but are sensitive in identifying parathyroid adenomas in ectopic location particularly in the mediastinum.

How will you treat a case of PHPT?

Parathyroidectomy is the only curative treatment for symptomatic hyperparathyroidism. For asymptomatic/ minimally symptomatic patients indications for surgical treatment include:
- patients < 50 years old
- medical surveillance is difficult
- patients with serum calcium >1.0 mg/dl above normal reference range
- patients with urinary calcium level > 400 mg/24 hours
- patients with ≥ 30% reduction in creatinine clearance
- patients with osteoporosis with T-score < 2.5 SD at any site

Surgical treatment has cure rate of > 95% and can be accomplished with very low morbidity (major complications < 1 %) and virtually no mortality in experienced hands.

What are the operative considerations in PHPT?

The two important considerations are:
- surgical approach
- extent of surgery

Surgical approach

The two main approaches are :

- ***Standard 4-gland exploration:*** Utilizing standard collar incision, all 4 glands are identified after mobilization of the thyroid lobes on both side and the single offending adenoma is removed with or without biopsy of one normal gland. In advanced hyperparathyroidism, the large adenomas can be identified easily; however, the remaining 3 normal glands are very small and dissection to identify them could be tedious and may result in ischemic injury. When the adenoma is not found in the normal expected locations, one has to systematically explore the ectopic sites based on the knowledge of embryonal migration and anatomy of parathyroid gland-tracheo-oesophageal groove, para-oesophageal area, entire carotid sheath and thymus. If a thorough search does not reveal the adenoma, cervical thymectomy should be performed and operation should be terminated and further invasive localizing imaging studies should be performed.
- ***Minimally invasive parathyroidectomy (MIP):*** It involves parathyroidectomy through a small unilateral incision that allows direct visualization of the adenoma. MIP also allows focused parathyroidectomy and also parathyroidectomy under local anaesthesia on an outpatient basis (23 hour admission).
  - *Focussed parathyroidectomy:* involves small incision, usually 2.5-3 cm placed directly over the pre localized adenoma, excision of adenoma and no attempt at idenitification of any of the three normal glands. This can be performed with or without the help of intra-operative PTH (IOPTH). Advantages of focused para-

thyroidectomy is reduced risk of postoperative hypocalcemia, particularly in minimally symptomatic cases, reduced operation time, less postoperative pain and less analgesic requirement, and early return to work
– *Endoscopic parathyroidectomy*

Extent of surgery

The other consideration is the extent of surgery
- ***Adenoma:*** Excision of adenoma with or without biopsy of one normal gland
- ***Double adenoma:*** Excision of both double adenomas after confirming that the other two glands are grossly normal and hyperplasia is ruled out on frozen biopsy of one normal gland
- ***Multiglandular hyperplasia:*** In sporadic PHPT where all glands are involved, subtotal parathyroidectomy (leaving behind remnant of the most normal appearing gland) is the treatment of choice
- ***Multiglandular hyperplasia due to MEN 1:*** Total parathyroidectomy with autotransplantation is the treatment of choice.

What are the postoperative considerations in PHPT?

- Postoperative hypocalcemia may develop after parathyroidectomy, particularly if the patient had severe bone disease (low BMD, large adenomas, very high alkaline phosphatase, etc.) and is managed by calcium infusion along with high doses of oral calcium and active form of vitamin D.

- In short- and long-term follow-up most of the manifestations resolve:
  - *BMD:* There is rapid and sustained recovery, particularly in cancellous bone
  - *ALP:* Serum ALP normalization may take as much as 6-8 months and till then oral calcium replacement has to continue
  - *Renal functions:* Improve but nephrocalcinosis persists
  - *Brown tumors and fractures:* Fractures heal; brown tumors are remineralized.
  - *Hypertension:* Does not resolve.
  - *Pancreatitis:* Further attacks of acute pancreatitis do not occur.

Chapter 39

Primary Hyperparathyroidism with Pancreatitis

CASE STUDY

A 17-year-old boy presented with abdominal pain and vomiting of sudden onset and was diagnosed as a case of acute pancreatitis. He had no history of renal stones. During evaluation was found to have Hypercalcemia with values of 12, 11.6, 13.2 mg%. Subsequently PTH was done and was found to be elevated (250 pmol/L). He was referred to us for further management. Neck ultrasound, CT scan and MIBI were consistent with a right superior parathyroid adenoma. He underwent standard bilateral cervical exploration and a 700 mg right superior parathyroid adenoma was removed. Other 3 parathyroid glands were found to be normal. He was discharged on calcium and vitamin D supplementation. He did not develop any further attacks of pancreatitis.

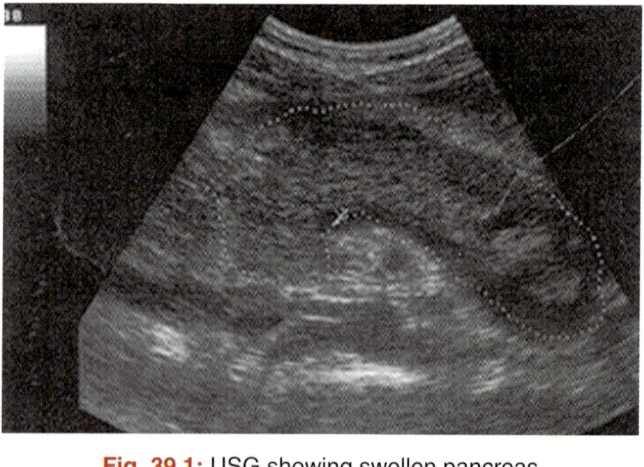

Fig. 39.1: USG showing swollen pancreas and peripancreatic fluid collection

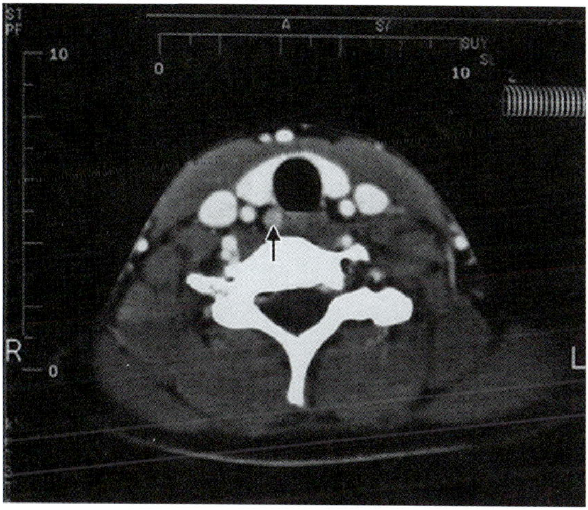

Fig. 39.2: CT neck showing right inferior parathyroid adenoma (arrow)

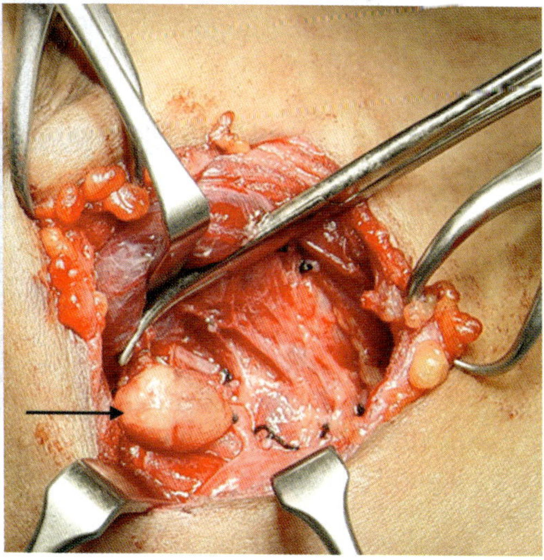

Fig. 39.3: Intraoperative photograph showing the adenoma (arrow)

QUESTIONS

What is the frequency of pancreatitis in PHPT?

In literature the frequency of this association ranges from 3.2 to 7%, which is more than the incidence of 1.5% of pancreatitis in a random hospital population.

Is there a cause-effect relationship?

The cause and effect nature of this relationship has been debated. It is now believed that pancreatitis is a consequence of PHPT as acute pancreatic inflammation appears to subside and does not recur after parathyroidectomy, and that the primary pathology is a solitary adenoma rather than parathyroid hyperplasia. However, pancreatitis is a consequence of hypercalcemia and not of high PTH levels. It has been shown that persistent hypercalcemia increases the calcium content of pancreatic juice and can lead to accelerated intrapancreatic conversion of trypsinogen to tryspsin.

When should you suspect PHPT in a patient of pancreatitis?

Whenever the serum calcium levels are found to be normal or high in a patient of acute pancreatitis, primary hyperparathyroidism should be suspected. Various subsets of pancreatitis have been reported:

1. Acute or acute recurrent pancreatitis that leads to diagnosis of PHPT and is cured by parathyroidectomy,
2. Acute pancreatitits after parathyroidectomy,
3. Acute pancreatitis occurring after non parathyroid surgery in patients with PHPT,

4. Acute pancreatitis complicating parathyroid crisis,
5. Chronic relapsing calcifying pancreatitis and finally,
6. Tertiary HPT complicating chronic pancreatitis with prolonged steatorrhea and hypocalcemia.

How should you manage such a case. Is parathyroidectomy beneficial in such cases?

Parathyroidectomy is definitely beneficial in ameliorating the acute pancreatitis and also preventing further attacks of acute pancreatitis. In a proven case of PHPT with acute pancreatitis the neck should be explored even when the acute attack is continuing.

Chapter 40

Familial Isolated Hyperparathyroidism (FIHPT)

CASE STUDY

A patient was diagnosed to be having primary hyperparathyroidism on evaluation which was initiated after his younger brother was operated for primary hyperparathyroidism. Since his younger brother demonstrated parathyroid hyperplasia on histology, evaluation of his first degree relatives was started. Though asymptomatic he was found to be having history of recurrent renal stones for which he underwent pyelolithotomy and ESWL on two occasions. He also gave history of progressive muscle weakness and fatiguability after prolonged walking. Their mother had died of chronic renal failure. On examination there were no

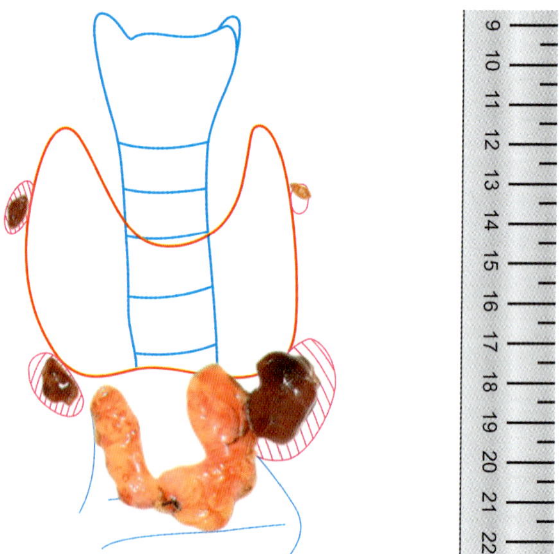

Fig. 40.1: Surgical specimen of sub-total parathyroidectomy with thymectomy in sibling of index case

neurocutaneous markers and he was normotensive. There was no thyromegaly and no jaw tumors. His abdominal examination was unremarkable. Biochemical evaluation revealed high calcium (11.6 and 11.8 mg%), low phosphorous (2.4 mg%), normal ALP (111 IU/L), elevated i PTH (410 pg/ml), low normal vitamin D (9.62 ng/ml). USG neck revealed two inferior parathyroid adenomas (1.5 × 0.78 cm and 1.2 cm) while MIBI showed scan evidence of left lower parathyroid adenoma and suspicious right lower parathyroid adenoma. USG abdomen showed bilateral Nephrocalcinosis but there were no adrenal, renal or pancreatic lesions. His 24 hour urinary metanepherine was within normal limits. The T score on BMD at hip, spine and radius were -2.1, -3.5, and-3.9 repectively. His serum

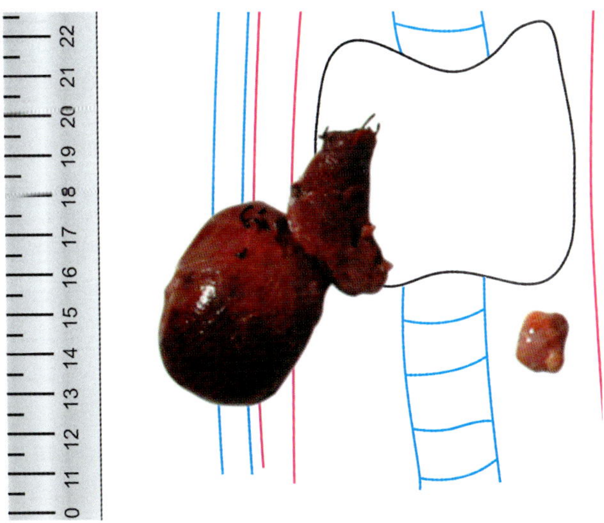

Fig. 40.2: Surgical specimen showing excision of two adenomas along with hemithyroidectomy in index case

prolactin was within normal limits and X-ray of the jaw did not reveal any jaw tumor. He underwent parathyroidectomy and standard bilateral 4-gland exploration was performed. He underwent three and half gland parathyroidectomy and transcervical thymectomy—both the inferior parathyroid adenomas were excised, right superior gland also look bigger and was excised while the left superior gland looked grossly normal; half of the this normal looking parathyroid gland was excised and sent for FS which confirmed that it was indeed parathyroid tissue. Postoperatively he was put on prophylactic calcium and active metabolite of vitamin D. The dosage of these had to be increased when he developed symptoms of hypocalcemia. The histopathology was reported as parathyroid hyperplasia involving all 4 glands but there was no supernumerary gland in the thymic tissue.

QUESTIONS

What are the settings of familial PHPT?

PHPT is usually sporadic but in < 10% cases it can be a part of hereditary syndromes, viz.,

1. MEN-1
2. MEN-2A
3. HPT-JT
4. FHH
5. FIHPT

What is familial isolated hyperparathyroidism (FIHPT)?

It is defined as hereditary PHPT without the association of other diseases or tumors. It is still not clear whethter FIHPT represents a variant/partial expression of MEN-1 or it is a distinct entity in itself.

How do you make a diagnosis of FIHPT?

The diagnosis of FIHPT is made in kindreds with PHPT in the absence of clinical, biochemical and imaging evidence of MEN-1, HPT-JT Syndrome or (FIHH). Kindreds of FIHPT do not show any cutaneous lesions and on imaging there are no pancreatic or adrenal lesions. They have a normal chest X-ray and a normal Thoracic CT. Their blood sugar is normal and on hormonal evaluation there is no evidence of excessive production of other hormones like TSH, ACTH, IGF-1, GH, VIP, Glucagon, Cortisol, FSH, LH, insulin, gastrin, and catecholamine. The ratio of renal clearance of calcium to creatinine clearance is > 0.01 and orthopentography of the jaw is normal.

Why and what genetic analysis should be done in families suspected of FIHPT?

Germline mutations of MEN-1 gene and CASR gene have been found in families of FIHPT. MEN-1 genotyping should be done in FIHPT families as the finding of mutation may predict multiglandular disease preoperatively and therefore has practical surgical implications. It also helps to identify new cases in the family and helps to start a periodic surveillance program.

What are clinical features of FIHPT?

It presents at a earlier age, usually in the third decade as compared to sporadic PHPT. Almost a third of these patients present with hypercalcemic crisis. Most of these patients have severe bone disease in the form of osteitis fibrosa cystica as well as renal disease (nephrolithiasis). Historically thought to be more aggressive than sporadic form or MEN-1.

What should the extent of parathyroidectomy in FIHPT?

The parathyroid pathology in FIHPT is heterogeneous and can range from a multiglandular hyperplasia to solitary adenoma. Supernumerary glands are common.

i. There is no role of minimally invasive surgery in FIHPT.
ii. Full bilateral exploration should be performed and all 4 parathyroid glands should be exposed along with search of supernumerary glands.
iii. Transcervical thymectomy should be performed routinely.
iv. If all 4 glands are found to be enlarged, either a subtotal or a total parathyroidectomy with autotransplantation, should be performed.
v. If a solitary adenoma or double adenoma is found with normal remaining glands then the adenoma (s) should be excised along with normal appearing ipsilateral gland. This helps to ensure that hyperplasia is not present in other glands and also ensures that parathyroid tissue is present only on one side, thus facilitating future explorations.

Are these families more prone to development of parathyroid carcinoma?

Approximately 20% of patients of families of FIHPT have parathyroid carcinoma. Such patients usually present with hypercalcemic crisis and have a palpable parathyroid tumor. However, the incidence of parathyroid carcinoma is higher in HPT-Jaw Tumor syndrome. Kindreds of HPT-JT syndrome present with jaw tumors consisting of fibro-osseous lesions of mandible and maxilla. These are different from brown tumors of PHPT in that they lack multinucleated osteoclasts and progress despite correction of the hyperparathyroid state. They are also at risk of developing polycystic kidney or renal hamartomas. There is a strong association between HRPT-2 mutations and parathyroid carcinoma in HPT-JT syndrome.

Chapter 41

Parathyroid Crisis

CASE STUDY

A 37-year-old lady presented with history of increased frequency of micturition, irritable behavior and headache for last 2 months. She was detected to be having a neck swelling by her treating physician one month back for which she got an USG done which was suggestive of a parathyroid mass. The mass was confirmed on the CT scan also. Serum calcium done at that time was significantly elevated; hence a diagnosis of hypercalcemic crisis was made and the patient was referred to us. She also gave history of severe constipation for last many years. However, there was no history of proximal muscle weakness, bone pain, easy fatiguability, fractures, renal or ureteric colic. On examination, she was found to be hypertensive and neck

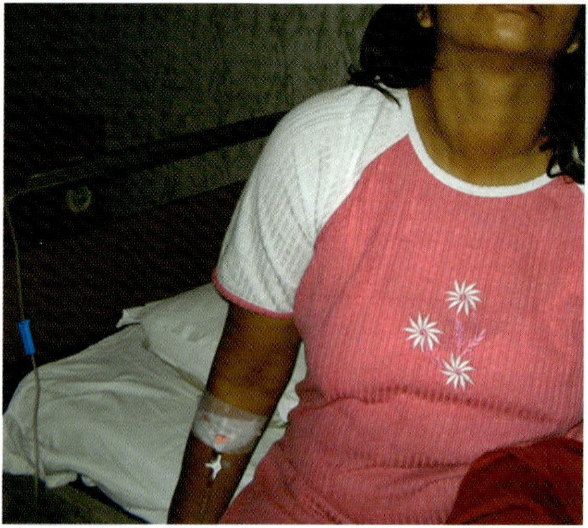

Fig. 41.1: Patient of hypercalcemic crisis on forced saline diuresis

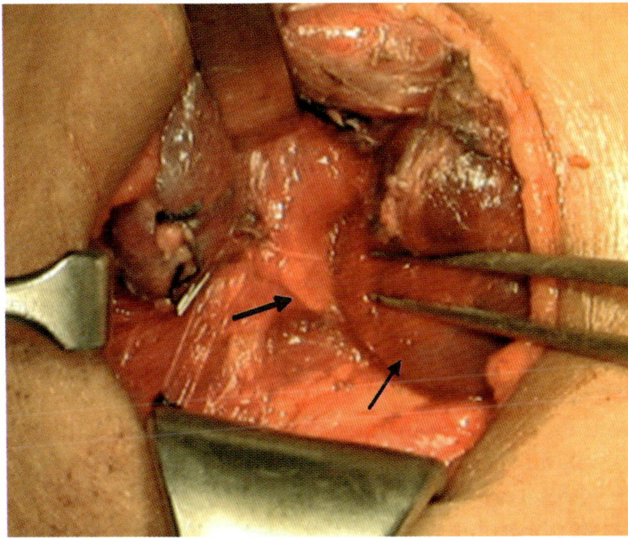

Fig. 41.2: Intraoperative photograph of the same patient showing a large adenoma (arrow) and normal parathyroid gland (thick arrow)

examination revealed a 4 × 3 cm swelling which appeared to be arising from the right lobe of thyroid and there were no neck nodes. An urgent serum calcium was done which was found to be elevated (17 mg%). The diagnosis of hypercalcemic crisis was made and she was put on forced saline diuresis and further confirmatory diagnostic work-up was started which revealed inorganic phosphorous (3.9 mg%), SALP (201 IU/L), iPTH (645 pg/ml) and vitD (30 ng/ml). She was also given bisphosphonate therapy in the form of Injection Palmidronate, 60 mg infusion over 2 hours. MIBI confirmed the presence of a right inferior parathyroid adenoma. The patient was taken up for semi-emergent parathyroid exploration. A unilateral exploration was performed and a large parathyroid adenoma, measuring 5 × 2.5 cm was removed along with the right lobe of thyroid as there were dense adhesions between the two. The right superior parathyroid gland was found to be normal. The parathyroid adenoma weighed 12 gm. Postoperatively the patient developed symptomatic hypocalcemia which was managed with calcium infusion along with oral calcium and vitamin D3.

QUESTIONS

What is the definition of parathyroid crisis?

Parathyroid crisis is an unusual state of progressive, marked hyperparathyroidism associated with rapid deteroriation of CNS (deteroriation of mental status, confusion, coma), cardiac, gastrointestinal (constipation, anorexia, vomiting, dehydration), and renal functions (decrease in renal functions) along with progressive hpercalcemia. Associated symptoms include fatigue, muscle weakness, polyuria and polydipsia. Polydipsia is due to abnormalities in urine concentrating ability on account of hypercalcemia. Usually no obvious reason could be found for this sudden progression of hyperparathyroidism but possible precipitating factors could be bacterial or viral infection, trauma or recent surgery.

Though the parathyroid crisis is usually associated with high serum calcium values of more than 15 mg/dl (3.75 mmol/L), serum calcium alone should not be the only defining criteria for a parathyroid crisis. Asymptomatic patients with serum calcium of 20 mg/dl and symptomatic patients with serum calcium less than 14 mg/dl have been reported.

What is the underlying pathology?

Almost always it is due to a solitary, large parathyroid adenoma but severe hyperparathyroidism may also be due a parathyroid carcinoma.

How will you evaluate such a case?

Management and evaluation should proceed together. Evaluation involves: estimation of PTH, high-resolution ultrasound of the neck and MIBI scan if available.

What is the emergency management?

Parathyroid crisis is potentially life-threatening condition and two-staged management is required vigorous medical management followed by emergent parathyroid surgery.

Medical management

Attention is paid towards hydration, reduction of serum calcium and stabilization of general condition. Rehydration is ensured with use of large amounts of intravenous saline with or without loop diuretics. Rehydration should proceed simultaneously with calcium-lowering treatments (bisphosphonates are the drug of choice). At the same time the diagnosis of hyperparathyroidism should be established.

Surgical management

In most cases once the clinical condition has been stabilized with rehydration, one can proceed with expeditious or emergency Parathyroidectomy. However, it should be kept in mind that even when patients are dehydrated in severe stages of this disease, operative intervention will achieve excellent results. Hence, valuable time should not be wasted in preparing the patient for surgery. Thus, operative intervention is the therapy of choice regardless of preoperative serum calcium level or associated surgical risk factors. Under no circumstance should the patient be discharged without the definitive management, which is always surgical, of the underlying cause.

Chapter 42

Persistent Hungry Bone Syndrome Following Parathyroidectomy

CASE STUDY

A 32-year-old male was referred with complaints of renal calculi since last 12 years along with multiple fractures of shaft of both femur from a trivial trauma one year back. He had history of severe bone pain and was confined to bed for last 6 months. On examination he was found to be having a palpable neck nodule 3 × 3 cm appearing to be arising from the right lobe of thyroid. Biochemical investigations revealed high serum calcium (14.1, 14.6 mg%), low phsophorous (2.5, 2.6 mg%), high Alkaline Phosphatase (1423 IU/L), high urinary calcium (1506 mg/24 hrs), elevated PTH (879 pg/ml). A biochemical diagnosis of primary hyperparathyroidism was made. On further investigations his BMD showed significant osteopenia (T-score: –3.0, –2.0). In view of impending hypercalcemic crisis, he was put on forced saline diuresis followed by diuretic therapy and palmidronate

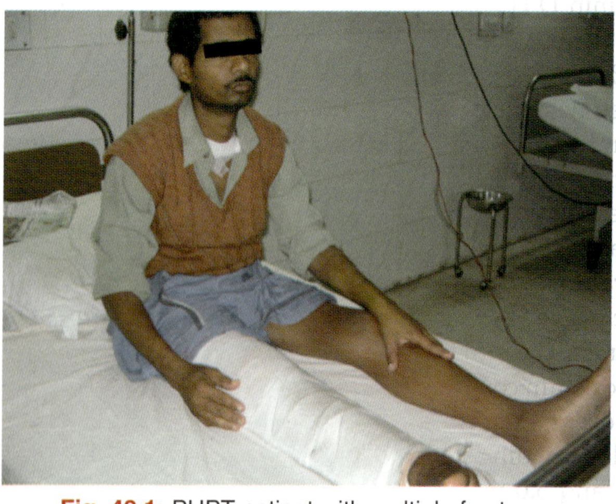

Fig. 42.1: PHPT patient with multiple fractures

infusion. His serum calcium came down to 11.2 mg%. Simultaneous evaluation revealed bilateral inferior parathyroid masses on USG while MIBI was suggestive of a large right inferior parathyroid adenoma. Since the findings on USG and MIBI were discordant, the patient was taken up for standard 4 gland exploration and operative findings included two inferior parathyroid masses while the two superior glands were grossly normal. The two adenomas were excised along with right hemithyroidectomy since the parathyroid adenoma was found to be adherent to the thyroid gland. The right inferior adenoma weighed 45 grams while the left one weighed 1.0 gram. His postoperative course was very stormy. He developed severe symptomatic and biochemical hypocalcemia (serum Ca: 7.2 mg%, phosphorous: 2.3 mg%) and hence he was put on intravenous calcium infusion in doses of 2 mg/kg/day for 4 days along with oral calcium (3 gm) and active form of vitamin D (1,25 dihydroxy vitamin D) in doses of 1mcg/day. He was discharged when his calcium stabilized to 8.6 mg%. However, he had to be readmitted after several days when he developed severe tetany. His serum calcium was found to be 5.0mg% and he was again put on intravenous calcium infusion, initially on 2 mg/kg/day which was then tapered to 1 mg/kg/day. He was also given 3 lakh units of vitamin D orally and 6 lakh units of vitamin D intramuscularly. Serum magnesium levels and urinary calcium levels were also measured and were found to be normal. The infusion had to be continued for 17 days before his calcium could be stabilized. He was discharged but had to be readmitted 2 days later with tetany, respiratory distress and impending stridor. Serum calcium levels were very low (4.1 and 5.0 mg%) and he was again put on intravenous calcium which, however, could not be tapered over next few days as he would develop symptomatic hypocalcemia once the calcium infusion was stopped. The postoperative PTH done at this time was found to be within normal range (27 pg/ml) and serum phosphorous was 4.2 mg%. He was then put on subcutaneous injection of Teraperatide in doses of 20 mcg/twice daily for 2 weeks and then tapered to once daily injection. His serum calcium then steadily rose and he was then discharged when his serum calcium was 8.7 mg%.

QUESTIONS

What is most common cause of postoperative hypocalcemia following successful parathyroid surgery?

The commonest cause of postoperative hypocalcemia in advanced cases is "hungry bone syndrome" which is characterized by hypocalcemia, hypophosphatemia and hypomagnesemia and is due to excessive and unregulated rapid bone remineralization following parathyroidectomy. In minimally symptomatic cases, postoperative hypocalcemia is due to ischemic injury to the rest of the three normal glands following 4-gland exploration.

What are the predictive factors for hypocalcemia following parathyroidectomy?

Patients who have one or more of the following features are more likely to develop severe and prolonged hypocalcemia

- High PTH values
- Severe bone disease
- High alkaline phosphatase

- Large adenomas
- Associated Vitamin D deficiency
- Impaired renal function

What is the appropriate management of such a patient?

Oral calcium: is started in high doses of 2-3 gm per day.

Oral vitamin D: especially calcitriol which is the active form of vitamin D in doses of 0.5 to 2.0 mcg/day.

Intravenous calcium: Calcium infusion of calcium gluconate (10 ml ampoule of 10% gluconate contains 93 mg of elemental calcium while 10% ampoule of calcium chloride contains 272 mg of elemental calcium; 6 amp of calcium gluconate dissolved in 540 ml of 5% dextrose would give 1 mg of calcium in 1 ml of fluid; this is infused at the rate of 1-2 mg/kg/hour over next 48-72 hours till the patient becomes asymptomatic or the serum calcium is around 8 mg%; this also gives time for the oral vitamin D (calcitriol) to achieve maximal action.

Intramuscular magnesium: Hypermagnesuria may be an important cause of resistant hypomagnesmeia after parathyroid surgery: Following successful Parathyroidectomy, hungry bone syndrome may result in unmasking of pre-existing hypomagnesemia. Hypomagnesemia evolves from a disordered flux between plasma and any one of several pools. Redistribution of magnesium from plasma into bones and soft tissues can occur afer parathyroidectomy. Also, patients treated with vitamin D and calcium are often hypercalciuric and hypercalciuria results in renal magnesium wasting. This may explain occurrence of magnesium depletion in such patients. Hypomagnesemic hypocalcemia is refractory to standard therapy but responds to magnesium replacement in the form of deep I/M injections of 50% Magnesium sulphate (2 ml amp). These injections are, however, painful. Oral magnesium 300-600 mg elemental magnesium per day in divided doses can be added.

Oral thiazide: In patients with persistent hypocalcemia addition of a thiazide diuretic in the doses of 50-100 mg per day will reduce renal excretion of calcium and may permit the use of lower doses of vitamin D.

Section 3

ADRENAL DISORDERS

Chapter 43

Conn's Syndrome

CASE STUDY

A 30-year-old female, resident of Jaipur, was referred with complaints of hypertention of 3 year duration and episodic weakness of proximal muscles of both upper and lower limb since 2½ year. She was apparently asymptomatic 3 years back when she was incidentally detected to have high blood pressure 150/100 mm of Hg on her routine check-up during 4th month of pregnancy and was prescribed anti hypertensive drugs. The highest recorded BP was 220/110 mm of Hg during the 7th month of pregnancy, which resulted in loss of precious baby. After 7 days, labor induction was done for dead fetus. After 5 days of fetus expulsion, she developed sudden onset weakness with pain in both thighs and got bed ridden. At this time she consulted an endocrinologist and was found to be hypothyroid with a

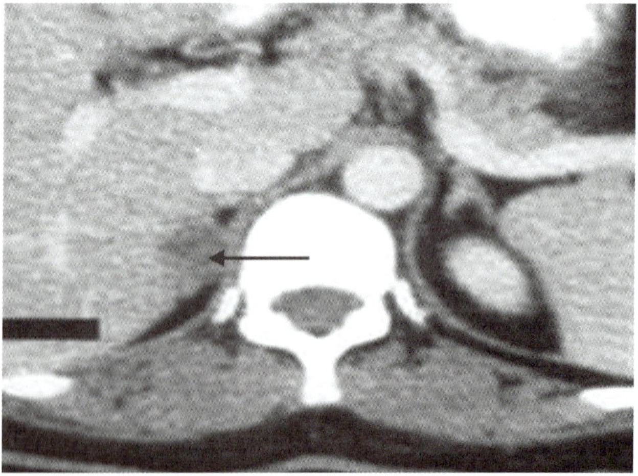

Fig. 43.1: Solitary hypodense lesion measuring 2.5 cm arising from right adrenal gland (arrow)

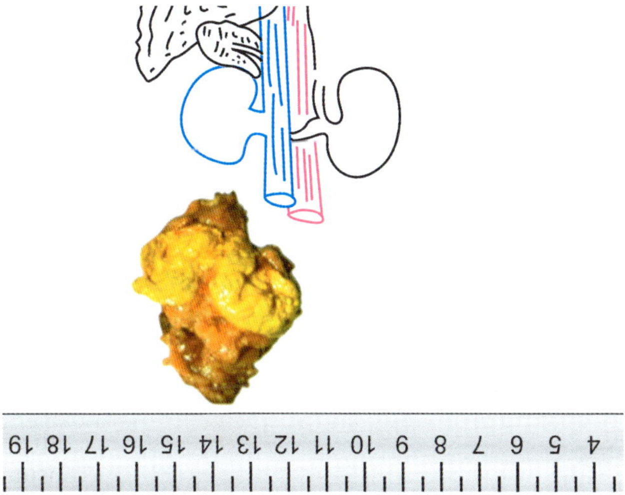

Fig. 43.2: Bisected adrenalectomy specimen showing bright yellow adenoma

TSH of 112 mmol/l and was prescribed Tab Thyroxine 100 mcg per day. She was symptom-free for 2½ years, but, again developed sponta-neous weakness of both upper and lower limbs, mainly involving the proximal muscle group, associated with myalgia. Then she went to a neuro-physician and was found to have very low potassium level (2.2 mg/dl). MRI abdomen revealed enlargement of right adrenal gland. Subsequently, she was referred to us. We reviewed the MRI plates and decided to do an abdominal CECT as the left adrenal gland looked bulky. CT scan revealed normal left adrenal gland but showed a solitary hypodense lesion measuring 2.5 cm arising from right adrenal gland. Subsequent biochemical work-up revealed high plasma aldosterone (PAC) levels-2395 p mol/l and suppressed plasma renin activity (PRA)-0.53 ng/ml/hr. There was no history s/o Cushing's disease or pheochromocytoma or adrenocortical carcinoma. Treatment history revealed treatment taken for primary infertility. At presentation she was on one antihypertensive medication with good control and 100 mcg of thyroxine. Family history suggested that both her parents were diabetic and hypertensive since last 40 years.

General and abdominal examination did not reveal any significant finding. She was put on the potassium sparing diuretic spironolactone 400 mg per day in divided doses for 4 weeks following which a lap adrenalectomy was performed uneventfully and she achieved normokalemic state on 5th postoperative day. In the postoperative period she did not require antihypertensive drugs to control her blood pressure.

QUESTIONS

What is the incidence of primary hyperaldosteronism (PHA)?

The prevalence of PHA in hypertensive patients is very low, < 2% though it is the commonest cause of surgically correctable hypertension.

What are clinical characteristics of PHA patients and are they different in Asian (Indian) patients?

- It is more common in women
- Patients are usually hypertensive: blood pressure is moderate to marked and is usually resistant to therapy
- Symptoms related to hypokalemia may be present: polyuria, nocturia and muscle cramps

- Severe muscle weakness, tetany or even spontaneous periodic flaccid paralysis can occur: this is more commonly reported from Asian countries like China and India (personal experience). Tetany is more commonly seen in women. The pathophysiologic basis lies in hypokalemic alkalosis leading to decreased ionized calcium (total calcium would be normal) which in turn results in tetany. It is a potentially life-threatening situation but if treated and recognized early patients recover completely without sequale. The diagnosis of hypokalemic periodic paralysis should be considered in any patient presenting with biochemical evidence of hypokalemia and a sudden onset areflexic pure motor weakness involving one or more limbs; there is no alteration in level of consciousness and in bladder or bowel functions. Typical abnormalities on ECG are flattening or inversion of T waves, appearance of U wave and flattening of ST segment. Treatment is replacement of potassium (either as potassium infusion or as oral syrup).

How would you screen hypertensive patients to diagnose PHA?

Following hypertensive patients need to be screened for presence of PHA

- Patients with spontaneous hypokalemia (< 3 mmol/L)
- Patients with inappropriate kaliuresis (K^+ excretion > 40 mmol/day.
- Patients with incidental imaging of adrenal abnormality
- Patients with resistant hypertension (requiring 2 or more drugs)

- Children or young adults especially with a family history of hypertension
- *Screening method:* Since 20-40% of patients of PHA would have a low normal serum potassium level, serum potassium alone is not a good screening test. Similarly serum PRA alone is also not a good and reliable method of screening. The best screening method is to estimate the plasma aldosterone (PAC): plasma renin activity (PRA) ratio. All untreated hypertensive subjects with PAC:PRA >30 merit further evaluation. However, routine screening of all hypertensive subjects for presence of PHA is not cost-effective and is not recommended.

How is the measurement of PAC:PRA useful?

If aldosterone is elevated and PRA is suppressed: suspect PHA.

If aldosterone is suppressed and PRA is also suppressed: Suspect pseudohyperaldosteronism, e.g. Cushing's syndrome, DOC producing tumor, congenital adrenal hyperplasia or Liddle syndrome.

If both aldosterone and PRA are suppressed: Suspect secondary hyperaldosteronism, e.g. diuretic therapy or rennin-secreting tumor.

What are various forms of PHA?

The various forms of PHA are:

a. Aldosterone producing adrenocortical adenoma (AHA or Conn's syndrome)	65%
b. Bilateral adrenocortical hyperplasia (IHA)	30%
c. Adrenal producing carcinoma	< 1%
d. Glucocorticoid remediable hyperaldosteronism	< 2%

e. Unilateral adrenal hyperplasia < 2%
f. Ectopic aldosterone producing tumors < 1%

How would you make a definitive diagnosis of PHA after finding PAC:PRA ratio of > 30?

If PAC is elevated and PRA is suppressed one can be almost certain of the presence of PHA and thus one can proceed directly to localizing methods like CT scan. However, definitive biochemical diagnosis can be made by dynamic testing utilizing the Salt loading test.

Salt loading test

This test is carried out either by increasing dietary sodium intake or infusing normal saline. The rationale behind this test is that when volume expansion is done with sodium, in normal subjects it will suppress both PRA and PAC. However, in patients with primary hyperaldosteronism volume expansion does not suppress the autonomous production of aldosterone. While performing this test antihypertensive medications which interfere with measurement of renin and aldosterone (like spironolactone, ACE inhibitors, diuretics, beta-blockers and calcium channel blockers) should be stopped for at least 2 weeks prior. (Spironolactone needs to be stopped for atleast 6 weeks).

Oral salt loading

Patient is kept on high sodium diet (2 to 3 grams with each meal or > 200 mEq/day) for 3 days and then the plasma aldosterone is measured. A normal person will show suppression (12 mcg/day) while patients with PHA will not show suppression.

What is the next step after confirming the diagnosis of PHA?

The next step is to differentiate APA from IHA because the former benefits from adrenalectomy while the latter benefits from medical treatment. This differentiation can be done by using the salt loading test as well as the postural test.

Postural test

With upright posture, a rise in plasma aldosterone occurs in cases of IHA but not in APA. Postural test is carried out by taking a recumbent basal sample at 8AM for plasma aldosterone and plasma cortisol and then taking a blood sample again after standing for 2-4 hours.

What localization studies need to be done after a definitive biochemical diagnosis of PHA?

Imaging with modern CT scanner (angio CT, multislice) is highly accurate in detecting adrenal masses, even those that are less than 1 cm. A typical aldosteronoma appears as a hypodense lesion, usually in one of the limbs of the adrenal gland. Infact presence of a typical hypodense lesion along with an atrophied contralateral adrenal gland in a patient with biochemically proved hyperaldosteronism is an indication to proceed surgery directly without performing any other localizing tests.

However, CT is not very specific and has to be interpreted carefully in following situations:

- In IHA, though both glands are typically enlarged, one gland may also have a nodule
- Presence of adrenal incidentaloma associated with IHA
- Unilateral aldosteronoma with a contralateral incidentaloma.

What are the indications of invasive testing like adrenal venous sampling?

These are:

- If CT is suggestive of adenoma plus hyperplasia of contralateral gland.
- Asymmetrical bilateral adrenal hyperplasia
- Bilateral multiple adrenal nodule (bilateral nodular hyperplasia).

What is the treatment of AHA?

The treatment of choice is unilateral adrenalectomy.

Preoperative preparation

The patients are prepared by keeping them on spironolactone in doses of 75-300 mg/day for atleast 4 weeks prior to surgery. This helps to minimize postoperative hypoaldosteronism and to restore potassium levels thus minimizing the risk of arrhythmias during surgery. Unilateral adrenalectomy can be performed with almost zero mortality and acceptable morbidity. The various operative approaches used are:

- Flank approach
- Posterior approach
- Transperitoneal approach
- ***Laparoscopic approach:*** This is now the gold standard in the surgical management of Conn's syndrome because it reduces hospital stay and analgesic requirement.

How do you perform laparoscopic adrenalectomy?

Position

Though semi-lateral position has been described we prefer to operate in the full lateral position as gravity assists surgery considerably in this position, particularly on the left side where the fourth port for spleen retraction is not required.

Punemoperitoneum: can be safely established by the open method:

Port placement: Ports are placed 2 finger breadth below the subcostal margin, and usually 5 cm apart. Through the open port, 10 mm port is inserted, then and then trocars are inserted on the upper mid line, one trocar in the anterior axillary line and one trocar in the midclavicular line.

Left adrenalectomy

The dissection is begun by incising the paracolic peritoneum followed by division of the splenocolic ligament. This enables to reflect the spleen along with pancreatic tail medially and then the Gerota's fascia is opened. The renal pedicle is dissected to identify the draining adrenal vein, making sure to visualize the entry of adrenal vein into the renal vein so as to avoid mistaking the renal vein for adrenal vein. The adrenal vein is clipped with 2 titanium clips on the renal vein side and another clip on the gland side and then divided. The whole of the left gland along with the adenoma is removed by ultrasonic shears-medial dissection along the aorta, superior dissection and then the inferomedial dissection between the adrenal and the kidney.

Right adrenalectomy

After incising the hepatocolic ligament using a hockey-shaped incision, Gerota's fascia is opened to identify the adrenal gland superomedial to the upper pole of the right kidney. Dissection of the medial margin of the adrenal gland, keeping just lateral to the inferior vena cava helps to identify the main adrenal vein, which is clipped and divided. The right adrenal vein is short, oblique and lies in a deeper plane.The superior and inferior pole of the gland are dissected and this usually requires clipping of one well defined vein on either pole. Finally the lateral and posterior surfaces of the gland are dissected which are usually avascular.

What are the short-term and long-term results of adrenalectomy for AHA: Do all patients become normotensive after adrenalectomy?

Hypokalemia is cured in virtually 100% patients but hypertension is cured only in 60% cases, though it improves in almost all patients. However, it should be kept in mind that hypertension improves with time as well.

Certain factors which are predictive of persistent hypertension after unilateral adrenalectomy are:

- Older age of patient at surgery
- Poor response to spironolactone
- Longer duration of hypertension before surgery
- Unilateral adrenal hyperplasia
- Male sex

What is the management of glucocorticoid remediable PHA?

This is an autosomal dominant disorder and is a diagnosis of exclusion. It should be considered in any hypertensive patient who has a biochemically confirmed diagnosis of PHA but who have normal adrenal glands on CT scan. This variety of PHA is usually seen in young adults and often in childhood. Except for hypertension, the patients are usually asymptomatic. Infact many of these patients are normokalemic. The syndrome results from a chimeric gene because of which a novel ACTH control system results. Thus, unlike other forms of PHA, in this syndrome aldosterone secretion is under the ACTH control and can be suppressed by glucocorticoid therapy. The biochemical diagnosis is established by finding normokalemia, aldosterone excess, suppressed PRA and elevated 18-hydroxycortisol and 18-oxycortisol. The definitive biochemical diagnosis is established by dexamethasone suppression test—both short-term and long-term (2 mg/day × 3 weeks). However, now-a-days the diagnosis can easily be made by genetic testing without the need for suppressive tests. The treatment includes long-term glucocorticoid suppressive therapy along with anti-hypertensives. Family screening is advised in a patient with this diagnosis.

What is the management of unilateral hyperplasia?

Rarely PHA may be caused by unilateral adrenal hyperplasia (UAH). It is important to diagnose this entity because the patients benefit from unilateral adrenalectomy unlike those of IHA which have to be treated medically only. UAH may also include micronodular, macronodular and diffuse hyperplasia if it is confined to one adrenal gland. Adrenal venous sampling or NP-59 scintigraphy is essential to show unilateral function before proceeding to surgery.

What is the medical therapy and when is it indicated?

Medical treatment for IHA involves keeping the patient on low sodium diet and use of spironalactone in doses of 25-400 mg/day. Though hypokalemia is corrected quickly, blood pressure control may take several weeks and may require the use of spironolactone in high doses. However, at higher doses of 400 mg/d, spironolactone is associated with considerable side effects like GI symptoms, impotence, gynecomastia and menstrual irregularities. To avoid this other drugs may need to be used like calcium channel blockers, ACE inhibitors or drugs that block synthesis of aldosterone like Trilostone.

Why should we treat hyperaldosteronism?

Autonomous excess production of aldosterone causes cardiovascular and renal damage both from indirect effects of hypertension and left ventricular hypertrophy and also direct effects of vascular smooth-muscle hypertrophy, endothelial dysfunction and cardiac fibrosis, proteinuria and renal vascular injury. Thus, patients with hyperaldosteronism are at higher risk for damage to both heart and kidney. Left ventricular hypertrophy regresses after adrenalectomy.

Chapter 44

Occult Ectopic ACTH Syndrome

CASE STUDY

A 26-year-old female presented with complaints of progressive weight gain, more on the trunk for 3 years, progressive darkening of knuckles, hair growth over face, back and thigh, all for last 3 years. She also noticed striae over abdomen and arms for last one year and difficulty in squatting and climbing stairs for last 1 year. She also sustained fracture in the left thigh following trivial trauma which was preceded by severe pain. On examination she was found to be having moon facies with dorsal pad of fat, supraclavicular pad of fat, acanthosis, dark knuckles and dark palmar creases; vellus hair on back and thighs. She had severe proximal muscle weakness and was found to be

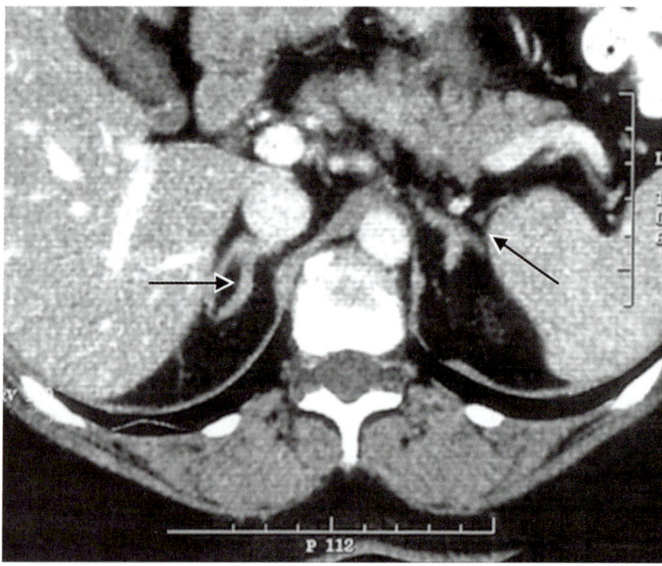

Fig. 44.1: CECT showing bilateral hyperplastic glands (arrows)

diabetic and hypertensive. She also appeared to be depressed.

A provisional diagnosis of Cushing's syndrome was made and she was evaluated as follows:

- ***Basal cortisol:*** 297 nmol/L
- ***LDDST:*** 214 nmol/L
- ***HDDST:*** 32 nmol/L
- ***ACTH:*** 48 pg/ml
- ***MRI head:*** No pituitary lesion
- ***CT thorax:*** No lesion could be identified in the lung parenchyma or in the mediastinum
- ***CT abdomen:*** Bilateral hyperplastic adrenals; no nodules

In view of elevated ACTH and a suppressible HDDST and normal MRI, the differential diagnosis between ectopic ACTH syndrome or a Cushing's disease was kept and IPSS was planned. IPSS was done through the femoral route and both the inferior petrosal sinuses were cannulated. Two samples were taken at the base line and at 4 min followed by 3 samples after stimulation with 10 microgram of Vasopressin, at 3, 5, 10 and 15 min interval. No procedure related acute complications occurred. The report of ACTH estimation was not suggestive of a pituitary lesion, hence a diagnosis of Ectopic ACTH Syndrome (EAS) was made. However, since the lesion was not localized on CECT thorax and abdomen and in view of severe osteoporosis, and her crippling state, patient was advised to undergo bilateral adrenalectomy. Meanwhile the patient was put on ketaconazole in doses of 200 mg twice daily till the time she was prepared to undergo surgery. Patient opted to undergo surgery after 6 months. She underwent bilateral adrenalectomy through the transabdominal route via the bilateral subcostal incision after adequate steroid cover.

Hyperplastic adrenal glands were removed and the procedure as well as the postoperative course was uneventful. Histopathology revealed bilateral adrenal hyperplasia without nodularity: right adrenal gland measured 4.5 × 2.5 × 2.0 cm and weighed 4 gm while left adrenal gland measured 6.0 × 4.0 × 1.0 cm and weighed 6 gm. In subsequent follow-up patient symptomatically improved with decrease in plethora, resolution of hypertension and improvement in her proximal muscle weakness and stabilization of her femur fracture so that she was now able to walk without support. She was adequately replaced with 5 mg/d of prednisolone and mineralocorticoid.

QUESTIONS

What is the Ectopic ACTH Syndrome?

Ectopic ACTH syndrome (EAS) is defined as symptom complex caused by a hormone produced by a neoplasm which is derived from tissue not normally engaged in the production of the hormone in question. In ectopic ACTH syndrome, the hormone ACTH which is normally produced by pituitary is elaborated by a neoplasm resulting in excessive stimulation of adrenal glands which in turn causes symptoms and signs of Cushing's syndrome.

Causes of EAS

Intrathoracic neoplasm: 60-80%

- Carcinoid of the bronchus
- Carcinoid of the thymus
- Carcinoma of the lung (small cell or oat cell)

Pancreatic tumors: 5-10%
- Islet cell tumor
- Carcinoid tumor

Pheochromocytoma: 5-10%
Medullary thyroid cancer: 0-5%

When should you suspect EAS?

EAS occurs in two clinical settings: Overt and occult

Overt EAS: An abrupt onset of severe Cushing's syndrome should prompt an evaluation for EAS. This form of EAS classically presents as a paraneoplastic syndrome in the context of a known malignancy with features like hypokalemia, weight loss, weakness and diabetes.

Occult EAS: Patients with this syndrome are a diagnostic dilemma. The biochemical tests like HDDST or urinary UFC are suggestive of pituitary disease but they have high ACTH levels. Also they do not show hypokalemia, hyperpigmentation or other features typical of severe ectopic ACTH secretion.

What should be done if the source of ectopic ACTH production is not localized?

Patients who have ACTH-dependent CS and no identifiable source of ACTH are a particularly challenging group. Those patients in whom an optimal and modern cross-sectional imaging techniques have failed to localize the ectopic source require control of hypercortisolism, either by bilateral adrenalectomy or drugs and also require frequent imaging studies until the potentially malignant tumor is discovered, often after a gap of 15-20 years.

What is role of bilateral adrenalectomy in ectopic Cushing's syndrome?

If curative surgery is not possible as in patients with EAS who have an unresectable or occult source of ACTH production, palliation by reducing the cortisol levels is important and this can be achieved either by medical or surgical treatment.

Medical treatment

Medical treatment involves blockade with adrenolytic drugs or chemotherapy. The drugs commonly used are metyrapone and ketaconazole. However, medical treatment has certain disadvantages. Over time ACTH levels increase and override, requiring additional increases in the dosage of enzyme inhibitor. Also, the incidence of patient intolerance and adverse effects (nephrotoxicity and hepatotoxicity) of these medications is high. Thus, few patients are able to tolerate long-term therapy with these drugs and infact over time to prevent an Addisonian crisis in patients receiving adrenal enzyme inhibitors, glucocorticoid and mineralocorticoid replacement may be necessary.

Surgical treatment

Bilateral adrenalectomy is a life-saving treatment option especially because of the minimal morbidity associated with the laparoscopic approach. Further, this procedure can treat the symptoms of hypercortisolism in patients who have disseminated malignant ectopic tumors, and thus it offers improved quality of life and effective palliation for a reasonable period of time. The indications for and timing of surgery are difficult to establish. Bilateral adrenalectomy can be recommended if the manifestations of cortisol excess progress rapidly (these patients are generally severely ill with deranged electrolyte and glucose levels) or when patients do not want to continue on adrenolytic drugs which caused unwanted side effects. Surgical intervention should be considered when blockade of adrenal steroid synthesis is successful as evident by optimal normalization of metabolic derangements. It should be realized that if medical treatment is continued beyond a certain time period a controlled situation may become worse.

Technique of bilateral adrenalectomy

The various approaches used are bilateral retroperitoneal approach, Transabdominal approach (either via a single bilateral subcostal incision or two separate subcostal incisions). However, laparoscopic approach is now the gold standard because of the minimal tissue injury associated with this procedure especially when you consider that these patients are severely ill and immunocompromised or are predisposed to delayed wound healing. In addition, in such a severely ill patient with excessively high levels of cortisol, anything less than a complete adrenalectomy would be disastrous. Because of the magnification in laparoscopic approach there is better visibility of the surgical field, thus decreasing the risk for retained remnants and adrenal rests.

Bilateral adrenalectomy (both open or laparoscopic) is technically demanding due to the increase in periadrenal fat which is unusually fragile leading to numerous small areas of bleeding even when the fat is gently manipulated. This is overcome by utilizing the technique of finger fracture to dissect the peri-adrenal fat. Another concern is that sometimes there can be real difficulty in identifying the adrenal gland because of the increased amount of intra-abdominal and peri adrenal fat and on the right side due to a fatty enlarged liver with or without metastases. Thus, laparoscopic approach has an advantage over the open approach because it permits the the use of laparoscopic ultrasound to locate the adrenal gland. A handport-assisted laparoscopic approach may avoid some of the technical difficulties in the classical laparoscopic operation. Handport technique is particulary useful if there is a large liver with secondaries from an ectopic tumor. It also allows the tactile sensation of the adrenal glands.

What is the incidence of Nelson's syndrome after bilateral adrenalectomy for Cushing's disease?

Incidence of Nelson's syndrome after bilateral adrenalectomy varies from 8 to 45%. This variation is because different authors take different criteria to define Nelson's syndrome. Some authors define NS as high levels of ACTH associated with skin pigmentation after bilateral adrenalectomy; there are others who consider the presence of pituitary tumor or expanding pituitary adenoma causing visual field disturbance as a criteria for labeling as Nelson's syndrome.

Predictive factors

High basal levels of ACTH after adrenalectomy, young age, presence of a pituitary tumor before adrenalectomy, subnormal steroid replacement and female gender.

Prevention

Prophylactic pituitary irradiation irrespective of the presence or absence of a pituitary adenoma is a protective factor against Nelson's syndrome.

Treatment

Management is difficult. The options are: pituitary surgery, radiation and medications like valproic acid or dopamine agonists.

Chapter 45

Overt Ectopic ACTH Syndrome

CASE STUDY

A 40-year-old female, from Bihar, presented with generalized body swelling along with weight gain of approximately 16 kg for the past 1 year. Weight gain was predominantly in the upper part of the body. She also had amenorrhea and darkening of skin for the past 1 year. She complained of fatiguability, difficulty in climbing stairs and getting up from squatting position for the past 6 months. She was also detected to be having diabetes mellitus and hypertension in the past 4 months. There was no history of psychotic symptoms, headache, visual disturbance or any loss of consciousness. Her obstetric profile revealed that she had 6 alive and healthy children. She underwent tubal ligation 3 years prior to her presentation. Family history was not contributory.

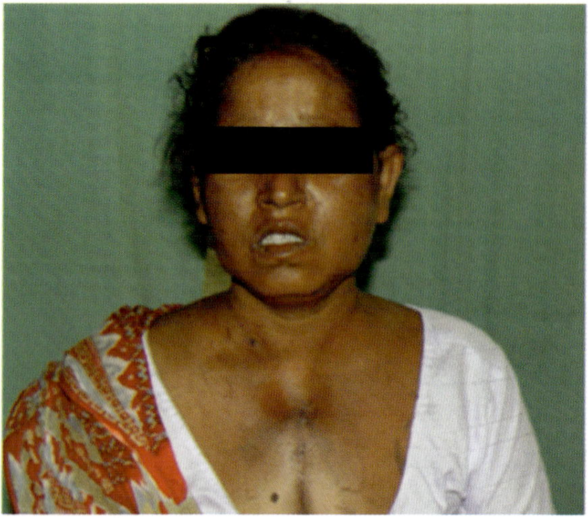

Fig. 45.1: Patient with mild features of Cushing's syndrome

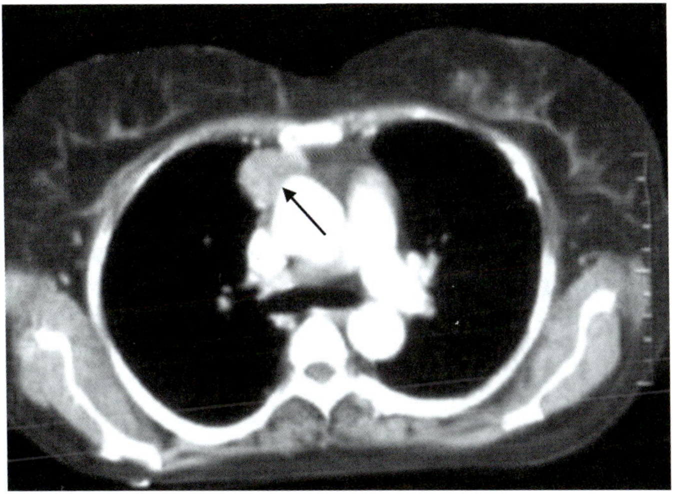

Fig. 45.2: CT scan showing anterior mediastinal mass (arrow)

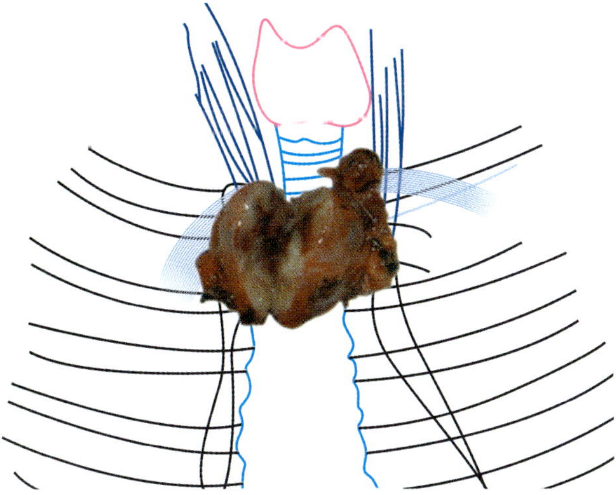

Fig. 45.3: Excised ACTH producing tumor

The patient was under the treatment of a physician at her native place. Investigative profile revealed increased levels of serum cortisol with loss of diurnal variation. An overnight dexamethasone suppression test (ONDST) done outside showed non-suppression of serum cortisol after 1 mg Dexamethasone. Following these reports, the patient was referred to us.

On examination, the patient was obese, had a round face with dark pigmentation. Skin was hyperemic and petechiae were present over the legs. Her BP was 146/94 mm Hg. Rest of the systemic examination was normal. On per abdominal examination, there were striae over the lower part of the abdomen. She had motor weakness in the lower limbs (grade 4), but the reflexes were preserved. There was no buffalo hump, pink striae over the abdomen or any behavior changes.

Investigations revealed anemia but all other hematological and biochemical parameters were normal. Liver function tests were also in the normal range. Basal Serum cortisol was 916 nmol/L (normal 110-520). ACTH levels done on the same date were 143 pgm/ml (normal 4-80). An overnight dexamethasone suppression test, (ONDST) done with 1 mg revealed cortisol levels of 793 nmol/L (normal 110-520). A day later high dose dexamethasone suppression test (HDDST) was done, which was nonsuppressible (869 nmol/L) as well.

Ultrasonography of the abdomen did not reveal any hepatomegaly or adrenal tumors. Computerized tomography of the thorax revealed an anterior mediastinal mass. An MRI of the pituitary was also normal. Inferior petrosal sinus sampling (IPPS) done to localize the source of high ACTH was not suggestive of a pituitary source of ACTH.The right and left sided ACTH levels were 216 and 234 pgm/ml respectively (normal 4-80).

In view of the reports, a diagnosis of a thymic carcinoid as an ectopic source of ACTH secretion was made. Perioperatively the patient was put on ketaconazole, which was stopped for 2 weeks prior to the LNDST and the IPSS.

The patient was taken up for surgery and was explored by a transternal route. Operative findings revealed a 3 × 3 × 2 cm fleshy tumor in the right limb and body of thymus, with pleural and pericardial infiltration. The junction of the brachiocephalic vein and the SVC was infiltrated by the tumor. The tumor was excised along with a portion of the brachiocephalic vein with primary repair. In the postoperative period she required ventilatory support for 7 days, after which she was weaned off and then discharge at 16th postoperative day on steroid replacement.

QUESTIONS

How would you confirm a diagnosis of EAS; what is the role of IPSS?

There are two main problems facing the endocrine surgeon or the endocrinologist with a patient of CS due to occult ectopic ACTH production. It is really difficult clinically and biochemically to distinguish Cushing's syndrome due to occult ectopic ACTH production from pituitary-dependent Cushing's disease.

Simple clinical findings have a good predictive value. A patient with mild to moderate hypercortisolism, a normal or slightly elevated ACTH levels and normokalemia has a

95% chance of having Cushing's disease. On the other hand, a patient with profound hypercortisolism, hypokalemia, and marked elevation of ACTH levels is more likely to have an occult ectopic ACTH-secreting tumor.

A strategy for differential diagnosis of CS starts with measurement of plasma ACTH levels. It is important to remember that ACTH is susceptible to degradation and hence the sample must be kept in an ice water bath and quickly processed (centrifuged, aliquoted, and frozen within a few hours to) to avoid getting spuriously low levels. Plasma levels > 20 pg/ml indicate ACTH-dependent CS. However, ACTH values alone cannot differentiate reliably the two forms of ACTH-dependent CS as there is a complete overlap between occult ectopic ACTH secretion and Cushing's disease. Only few patients with overt EAS tumors have extremely elevated values of plasma ACTH (>100pg/ml).

Since within the ACTH-dependent etiologies the incidence of Cushing's disease is so high (more than 4-5 times of EAS) any differential diagnostic test must be very accurate.

Pituitary imaging with MRI is the initial study required. However, only 40-50% of pituitary microadenomas causing CS in adults are visible on MRI. The use of dynamic MRI (with intravenous gadolinium) with gradient sequences may increase the sensitivity. Unfortunately, there is a 10% incidence of pituitary Incidentaloma.

Bilateral inferior petrosal sinus sampling (BIPSS)

BIPSS with CRH stimulation is the only study having the potential to yield a diagnostic sensitivity and specificity for Cushing's disease higher than its pretest probability.

Method

The test utilizes the normal venous drainage of each half of the pituitary gland into the corresponding petrosal sinus. Each petrosal sinus is catheterized separately via a femoral approach, and blood for measurement of ACTH is obtained simultaneously from each sinus and a peripheral vein at two time points before and 3, 5, and 10 min after the administration of ovine CRH (1/mcg/kg IV).

Interpretation

In case of pituitary adenoma, predictably the ACTH concentrations are greater in the central samples and also increase after CRH stimulation. In contrast, in EAS tumors, ACTH values in central and peripheral specimens are similar. Also, if we take ratios, the presence of unequivocal pituitary ACTH gradient (IPSS: peripheral ACTH) > 2.0 in the basal state and/or 3.0 after CRH yields a diagnostic sensitivity of nearly 100%.

Problems

Neurologic complications, like CVA (transient or permanent) have been reported. Diagnostic sensitivity decreases considerably if the radiologist has been able to cannulate only one petrosal sinus. Anamolous venous drainage may give rise to false-negative results. Optimal results are obtained only when CRH is used. The test is not reliable in mild or intermittent hypercortisolism. Thus it is mandatory to document hypercortisolism by determining midnight plasma cortisol or UFC excretion immediately prior to IPSS. Also, any patient without a significant pituitary ACTH gradient during IPSS should have samples retrospectively evaluated for a prolactin gradient to ensure that adequate pituitary venous effluent was obtained.

Variations

Cavernous sinus sampling and jugular venous sampling instead of petrosal sinus sampling has been tried though it is easier to perform, its sensitivity (88%)less than IPSS.

How would you localize the ectopic source of ACTH production?

Another problem in such a patient is to locate the source of ectopic production of ACTH. The radiological investigation of such patients presents a major challenge. A radiological search for occult ectopic ACTH secreting tumor should be instituted only after the diagnosis of Cushing's disease has been reasonable excluded by IPSS to avoid any false-positive studies (particularly in the chest) and subsequent surgical misadventures. The chest is the most common site of EAS tumors (80%), followed by abdomen (15%) and neck (MTC). Thus, imaging of the thorax and abdomen with CT will yield the highest detection rate in search for an occult EAS tumor. In the chest, the commonest tumor is the bronchial carcinoid (55%), followed by thymic carcinoid while in the abdomen the common occult EAS tumors are the islet cell tumors and adrenal pheochromocytoma

However, the bronchial carcinoids are usually very small (0.2 to 2.0 cm) and their detection requires careful analysis of subtle abnormalities to allow the differentiation of tumor from incidental pulmonary opacities and normal vascular structures. Co-existent calcified lesions (especially with rampant tuberculosis in India) may be mistakenly diagnosed, as tumors. Chest radiograph is usually normal. Thin-section, high resolution contrast-enhanced CT imaging is, therefore, required. MRI of the chest may also be of additional value as some bronchial carcinoids have a central location and may be mistaken on CT scanning for a blood vessel.

CT is also able to identify small thymic carcinoids which do not distort the mediastinal contour and also allows delineation of normal vascular structures.

Abdominal ultrasonography and CT

This is performed with particular attention to adrenal and pancreas as possible sites for primary EAS tumor or liver for metastatic disease.

Pancreatic islet tumors are usually small and it should be kept in mind that this EAS tumor may not distort the pancreatic margins and may only be identified as tumor blush on CT angiogram.

Pheochromocytoma as an ectopic source of ACTH is rare but if present can be picked up on CT or MRI. Adrenal tumors in EAS usually appear as a nodular hyperplasia compared to the mild smooth enlargement of the gland seen in Cushing's disease. The nodules are usually small but sometimes can reach upto 4 cm to give an appearance of a adenoma but the rest of the gland appears hyperplastic.

Other imaging tests

If above studies fail to yield a positive finding, following further studies may be done but are usually not helpful: Somatostatin receptor scintigraphy, PET scan and Systemic venous sampling for ACTH levels.Tumor markers such as plasma calcitonin, gastrin, glucagon or somatostatin may often be elevated but they rarely help in locating the neoplasm.

It is often necessary to repeat the radiological tests at regular intervals if the findings are normal or non-specific.

What is the surgical management?

After the localization of the lesion responsible for ectopic secretion of ACTH, the optimal management is complete surgical excision, a goal that cannot be always be achieved, because by the time these tumors manifest they are already locally infiltrating.

What is the outcome of surgical management?

Patients not treated surgically have much shorter survival. Prognosis of patients is correlated with the tumor histology. Patients with small cell carcinoma (SCC) have the worst prognosis while patients with other tumors, especially bronchial carcinoid tumors show prolonged survival.

Chapter 46

Benign, Functioning Adrenal Adenoma

CASE STUDY

A 48-year-old female patient presented with complaints of low backache which was mild and intermittent since 3 years but had become severe and almost continuous for last one and half months. The backache was aggravated on forward bending and was relieved by taking analgesics. She also gave history of having non-radiating pain in left hip joint which had started only recently. She also had difficulty in getting up from sitting position and in climbing stairs. She also had history of easy bruisability of skin. She did not give any significant history of recurrent pyrexia or joint pains. However, she did complain of burning during micturition as well as increased frequency of mic-turition for last 2 months. On detailed history taking it was revealed that in the past she had been continuously on steroids for last 10 years which were prescribed by a skin specialist for her skin disease (pemphigus), though she had stopped taking steroids for last 3 months. She had been a known hypertensive since 7 years but was on treatment for only last 3 years. On examination she was found to be hypertensive (180/100 mmHg) having cushingoid facies, facial plethora but no buffalo hump. Thyroid was normally palpable. There was

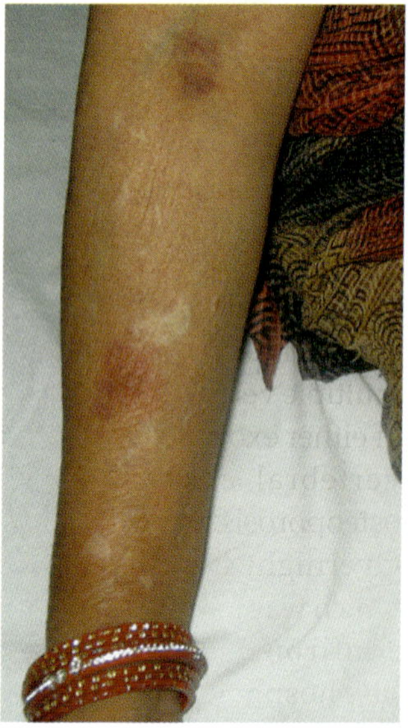

Fig. 46.1: Cushing's patient with fungal infection

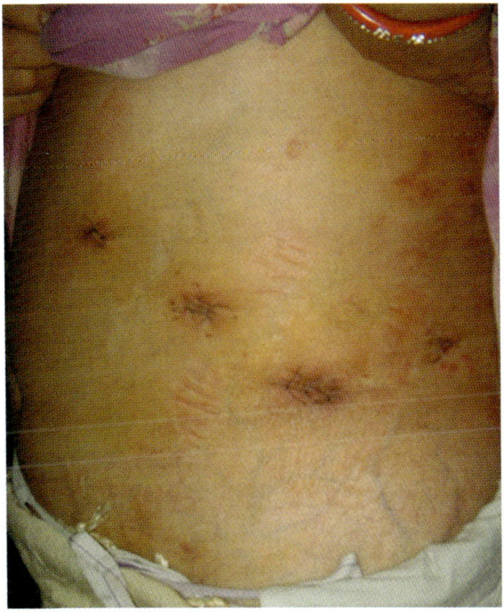

Fig. 46.2: Postoperative photograph following laparoscopic adrenalectomy showing the port sites

thinning of skin and ecchymotic patches all over her body and nonviolaceous striae over lower abdomen. There was spine tenderness at L 2, 3, 4 levels and X-ray spine revealed multiple vertebral collapse fractures. A differential diagnosis of either exogenous or endogenous Cushing's with multiple vertebral collapse resulting from steroid induced osteoporosis was made. She was evaluated by performing Overnight Dexamethasone Suppression Test (ONDST) which was found to be non-suppressible (268 nmol/L). BMD confirmed severe osteoporosis and she was given bisphosphonate therapy (4 mg of Zoledronic infusion). Subsequent investigations revealed normal serum ACTH levels (16 pg/ml) and non-suppressible LDDST (496 nmol/L), non-suppressible HDDST (432 nmol/L). The diagnosis of ACTH-Independent Cushing's syndrome was made and a CECT was ordered which revealed a moderately enhancing and partially calcified mass, 3.2 × 2.4 × 1.0 cm, in relation to the left adrenal gland while the contralateral gland was suppressed. She was optimized for surgery by vigorous chest physiotherapy, broad spectrum antibiotics, antifungal therapy (ketaconazole), antihypertensives and DVT prophylaxis. She underwent a successful laparoscopic left unilateral adrenalectomy utilizing 4 ports through the right lateral transperitoneal approach. The specimen weighed 14 gm and cut section revealed two nodules 3 × 2.2 and 1.2 × 1.0 cm with a calcified area in one nodule. The histopathology was consistent with adrenocortical adenoma and the patient made an uneventful recovery.

QUESTIONS

What is the CT anatomy of normal adrenal gland?

Right adrenal gland is in the shape of inverted V. The junction of medial and lateral limbs usually lie posterior to IVC. Medial limbs of a normal right adrenal gland measure 3-4 mm. Conventionally it has been compared with adjacent right crus of diaphragm. A rule of thumb is that the limbs of adrenal gland should be no thicker than the nearby crura of the diapghram. The left adrenal gland has the shape of an arrowhead and is somewhat difficult to identify as compared to the right gland.

How can you differentiate between an adenoma and carcinoma on CT scan?

With modern machines, CT can image adrenals in almost 100% cases and can be performed in a single breathhold using a multislice machine. The abnormal/normal adrenal gland can be optimally evaluated with thin sections of the order of 3-5 mm. Sections should begin and end few cms above and below the visualized adrenal gland so that exophytic masses are not missed.

An adrenal mass is evaluated by CT densitometry and CT density washout. On a plain CT scan (i.e. contrast minus, -C1) adenomas typically have a low HU, usually 10 HU (this is because of presence of fat in adenoma; a typical soft tissue mass has density of 40-50HU while fat has a lower CT value, generally of the order of-4 to-100HU). Another important index is CT density washout measurement though both adenomas and carcinomas enhance, there is rapid washout of contrast in benign adenomas as compared to malignant ones.

What are the causes of calcified adrenal masses?

Adrenal cyst is the commonest calcified adrenal mass seen in adults while neuroblastoma is the commonest calcified adrenal mass in children. Calcification may also be seen in hydatid cyst, carcinoma and adrenal hemorrhage. However, calcification within an adrenal mass is nonspecific. One-third of adrenal adenomas may show calcification on CT, especially if they are large and show degenerative cystic changes. Adrenal oncocytoma, a rare lesion, may show characteristic peripheral curvilinear or onion-peel calcification.

What is the treatment of choice for benign adenomas?

Unilateral adrenalectomy, either by open transperitoneal, retroperitoneal or laparoscopic approach is the treatment of choice.

How do you evaluate these patients in postoperative period and in follow-up?

Postoperative hypocortisolism (morning plasma cortisol < 3.6 mcg/L) indicates cure of Cushing's disease. Patients are usually discharged on either prednisolone or hydrocortisone, in doses of 12-15 mg/m^2 usually given in two divided-doses. Generally split dose strategy is followed in which one-third of total daily dose is given between 3-6 PM. The time to recovery of adrenal axis in patients undergoing unilateral adrenalectomy is between 6-12 years. Hence, all such patients should carry a medical information bracelet or tag stating the need for taking steroids. The patients should be forewarned about the need for taking steroid daily, the need for doubling the dose in cases of fever, nausea and dirrhoea. They should also be forewarned about the need to consult a physician for parenteral administration of steroids during vomiting, trauma and other medical stresses like operation.

How do you monitor the recovery of adrenal axis?

Clinical assessment is done be assessing the patient's well-being and taking weight and blood-pressure. Estimating cortisol response to synthetic ACTH (cosynotropin 250 mcg) is done 6 months after surgery and then at regular intervals. If the cortisol response in > 9 mcg/dL, weaning from steroid can be started.

Chapter 47

Adrenocortical Carcinoma Presenting as Adrenal Incidentaloma

CASE STUDY

A 41-year-old lady presented with history of pain in abdomen and gaseous distention since 2 months predominently on left side. She was evaluated by a physician who ordered an ultrasound of the abdomen which detected a left adrenal mass. He then ordered a CE CT scan abdomen and guided biopsy which was inconclusive. She was non hypertensive/non-diabetic with no significant family history. On examination she was found to be anemic and on local examination of abdomen a vague lump in left hypochon-drium was found which was mobile, moving with respiration, firm in consistency, ballotable and only lower border could be felt. Subsequent investigations revealed anemia with normal clinical chemistry 24 hour urinary Metanephrine was less than twice normal (1.44; upper value 0.84). Basal cortisol was not elevated and serum electrolytes were normal. CECT revealed a large, nodular and inhomogenous mass with irregular borders as well as irregular enhancement. There was no local invasion or lymphadenopathy. A presumptive diagnosis of adreno-cortical carcinoma (ACC) was made and open left adrenalectomy was performed. There was no invasion of kidney and the weight of the specimen was 490 gram. Her postoperative period was uneventful. She received external beam radiotherapy but died 18 months later due to widespread metastases.

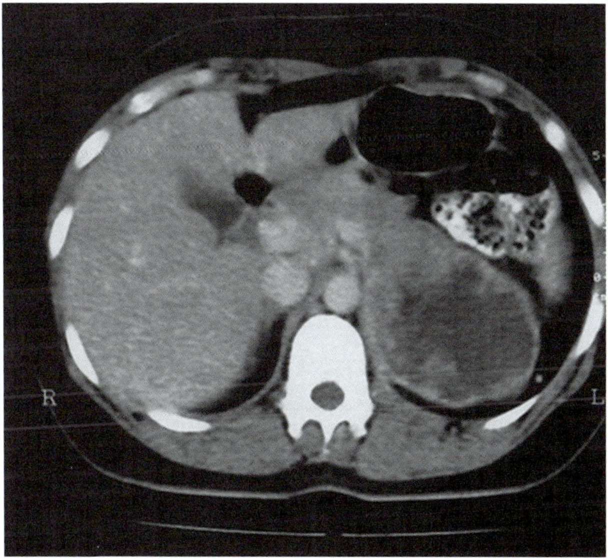

Fig. 47.1: CT scan showing a large mass with heterogeneous density, peripheral enhancement and nodular borders

QUESTIONS

What is the clinical presentation of adrenocortical carcinoma (ACC)?

ACC is more common in two age groups with different clinical presentation: in children less than 10 years of age and in the fifth decade.

Adult		Children	
Functioning (60%)	*Non-functioning (40%)*	*Functioning (90%)*	*Non-functioning (10%)*
Mixed Cushing's syndrome and virilization (35%)		Virilizing ACC (55%)	
Cushing's syndrome (30%)		Mixed Cushing's and virilization (30%)	
Virilization (20%)		Cushing's syndrome (<5%)	
Malignant aldosteronoma (<1%)			
Feminizing or oestrogen secreting ACC (1%)			

40% of adult ACC are non-functioning and are detected incidentally as large masses on imaging during evaluation of nonspecific complaints like abdominal pain, nausea, vomiting, flank pain or abdominal fullness, etc. However, non-specific tumor symptoms like anorexia, weight loss or fever are less common.

When would you suspect adrenocortical carcinoma?

Functioning ACC:

Rapid development of Cushing's syndrome (CS)
CS with virilization

Non-functioning ACC:

Large tumor (> 6 cm)

CT characteristics suggestive of malignancy are: inhomogenous density, irregular margins, irregular contrast enhancement, and delayed attenuation. Of course, local invasion, tumor extension into IVC, lymph nodes and distant metastases (lung and liver) are strong pointers of advanced malignancy.

How can you evaluate the benign or malignant character by imaging?

- The gold standard is contrast enhanced thin collimation CT
- The following factors together are taken into account: Size, attenuation co-efficient, washout values, tumor tissue heterogeneity and contrast enhancement.
- ***Size:*** The size of the adrenal mass remains the single best indicator of malignancy. The likelihood of ACC increases to 35-98% in patients with an adrenal mass > 6 cm.
- ***Attenuation co-efficient:*** Benign adrenal adenomas are lipid rich and thus have low attenuation values (i.e., low HU). On an enhanced CT, adenomas have values less than +10 HU whereas carcinomas have values greater than +20. This criteria has a sensitivity of 73% and specificity of 96%.
- ***Delayed contrast-enhanced CT:*** This can be used to further characterize lesions with higher HU in unenhanced scans. CT images obtained 1 hour after the injection of contrast show enhancement of 11+-13 HU (< 30HU) for adenoma and a value of 49+-8.3HU (> 30HU) for carcinoma with a sensitivity of 95% for distinguishing adenomas from carcinomas and specificity of 99%. Adenomas also exhibit

greater than 50% washout within 15 min of contrast injection, whereas carcinomas exhibit greater retention of contrast.

- *Other features:* ACC are typically inhomogeneous (because of necrosis), with irregular margins and irregular enhancement of solid components after contrast. Calcification is sometimes visible. Local invasion into surrounding structures like kidney or tumor extension into inferior vena cava as well as lymph node metastases may be found in ACC.
- *MRI:* With the advent of dynamic gadolinium enhanced- and chemical shift technique MR, characterization of adrenal masses has improved significantly. Lipid-rich adenomas show a 34% change in relative signal intensity between in-phase and out-of-phase imaging, whereas carcinomas do not change. MR is superior to CT in detecting tumor extension into the inferior vena cava.
- Adrenal Scintigraphy with NP-59 is not widely available and has no superiority over CT or MRI.
- *FDG-PET:* Can differentiate between benign and malignant lesions and can also be used to detect metastatic disease.

What is the role of FNAC?

It is not recommended due to the risk of complications, in particular needle tract metastases and its controversial diagnostic value.

How would you stage the ACC?

According to Mc Farlane classification (modified by Sullivan)

Stage	Size	Lymphadenopathy	Local invasion	Metastases
I	< 5 cm	-	-	-
II	> 5 cm	-	-	-
III	Any size	+	+	-
IV	Any size	+	+	+

In a non-functioning ACC is there a need for peri-operative steroid supplementation?

In a biochemically proved non-functioning ACC, the opposite adrenal gland will not be suppressed, hence there is no need for peri-operative steroid cover when a patient of non-functioning ACC is to be operated.

What is the adjuvant or medical treatment of ACC?

Radiation therapy

ACC was thought to be radio-resistant but with modern equipment better responses may be possible. Thus RT may have a role as adjuvant postoperative radiation therapy in patients at high risk for local recurrence such as: stage III ACC or stage II patients with tumor diameter >12 cm, high mitotic index, violation of tumor capsule or frank evidence of tumor spillage during surgery. Also, palliative radiotherapy could be effective in metastatic disease and is the treatment of choice for bone metastases.

Mitotane therapy

Mitotane has been consistently used in the treatment of metastatic ACC but the clinical efficacy of mitotane remains disputed.

- It can be used either as adjuvant therapy after complete surgical removal (because of high risk of loco-regional recurrence) or in metastatic ACC.
- However, as an adjuvant therapy mitotane has failed to show a beneficial effect in extending life expectancy but since the adjuvant treatment options are limited, mitotane continues to be used in this setting.

Inhibitor of steroidogenesis

A variety of inhibitors of adrenal function have been used to suppress steroid hormone production in functioning ACC and improve the clinical manifestations of the disease, thus improving the quality of life. These include ketaconazole, etomidate, metyrapone and aminoglutethimide.

- ***Ketaconazole:*** It is the most frequently used drug. It is an important inhibitor of adrenal and gonadal steroidogenesis and may even possess antiproliferative activity. It has been used to treat patients with Cushing's syndrome and virilization caused by adrenal tumors. The doses used are 400-1200 mg/day. Adrenal insufficiency requiring hormone replacement and hepatotoxicity are the most frequent side effects. Adrenal insufficiency can be avoided by decreasing the dose sufficiently to maintain normal cortisol levels. Other frequent side effects are nausea and vomiting, abdominal pain and pruritus.
- ***Etomidate:*** It is the most potent adrenostatic drug and is the treatment of choice for severe life-threatening hypercortisolism.
- ***Aminoglutethimide:*** The drug has been used in both adults and children in doses of 500 mg to 2 g per day. Besides neurologic and GI side effects, it can cause hypothyroidism and a skin rash.

How would you follow-up such patients?

Follow-up is life-long. Because recurrent or metastatic disease is common, close biochemical and radiology follow-up is mandatory. The risk factors are: stage III tumors, a tumor diameter more than 12 cm, a high mitotic index and intratumoral hemorrhage. In order to detect loco-regional recurrence even after a presumed complete excision, CT should be performed after every 3-4 months during the first 2 years after complete tumor removal after which intervals may be increased. In functioning tumors DHEAS may be used as a tumor marker because in cases of recurrence or metastases it may rise again after surgery long before tumor tissue becomes detectable by CT.

What is the prognosis of ACC?

The prognosis of ACC is still very poor. Patients with untreated ACC have a median survival of 3 months only whereas in treated ACC the overall 5-year survival ranges between 23 to 60% in different series. Survival is higher in patients who receive surgical treatment. Therefore, the two most important prognostic factors are: early stage at presentation and complete tumor removal. Endocrine activity has no general influence on prognosis as compared to nonfunctioning ACC. However, there is some evidence that tumors secreting androgens or steroid precursors only have a better prognosis than cortisol-secreting ACC or tumors secreting both cortisol and androgens.

Chapter 48

Metastatic Adrenocortical Carcinoma

CASE STUDY

A 41-year-old female complained of on and off fever for last one year and anorexia for one month. During the evaluation of her complaints ultrasound abdomen was done which revealed an incidental left suprarenal mass and hence the patient was referred to SGPGI for further evaluation and management. A clinical diagnosis of adrenal incidentaloma was made. She was found to be normotensive and did not have any features of Cushing's disease. Hormonal evaluation revealed suppressible ONDST and normal 24 hour urinary metanephrine (0.77 mg/day). CECT was done which revealed multiple space occupying lesions in right

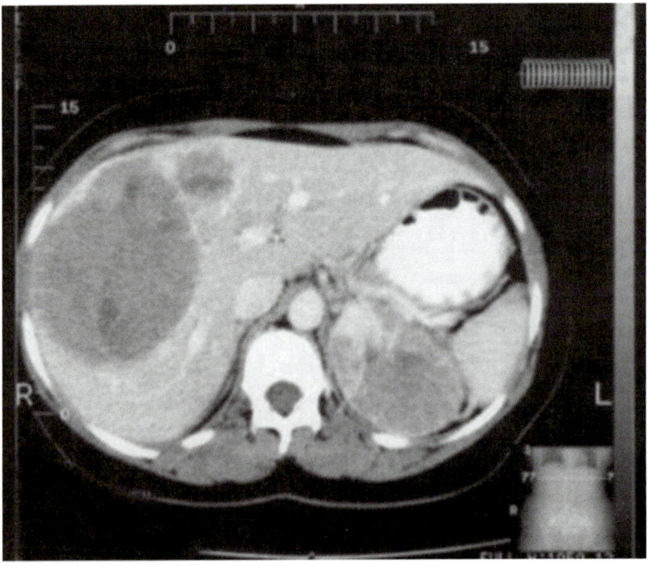

Fig. 48.1: CT scan showing a large adrenal mass with multiple metastases to the liver

lobe along with a large adrenal mass which showed heterogeneous enhancement suggestive of necrotic areas. A clinical suspicion of non-functioning adrenocortical carcinoma was made and an FNAC was ordered from the adrenal mass as well as from the liver lesion. The smears from adrenal and liver aspirate showed tumor cells in large clusters, groups and lying singly. The tumor cells display abundant finely vacuolated cytoplasm with round to mildly pleomorphic nuclei, coarse chromatin with prominent nucleoli in a few of them. Some binucleate forms as well as few stripped nuclei were discernible in the background. The cytology was thus suggestive of adrenocortical carcinoma with metastases to liver. The patient and her relatives were counseled regarding the inoperability and its futility as well as poor survival. Patient and relatives were advised mitotane therapy as well as cytotoxic chemotherapy. They, however, decided against any form of treatment.

QUESTIONS

What are the common sites of metastases of ACC?

The most frequent sites of metastases are the lung, liver, lymph nodes, and bones. 50% of patients in stages I,II, and III are alive at 40 months after diagnosis while only 10% of patients in stage IV are alive at that time.

What is the role of surgery in such a case?

In cases of synchronous metastases one option is to perform an adrenalectomy along with excision of isolated hepatic or pulmonary metastases. However, survival is very dismal and hence non-surgical treatment such as thermoablation for metastatic disease is preferred.

What is the medical management of metastatic ACC?

Mitotane therapy

Mitotane has been consistently used in the treatment of metastatic ACC but the clinical efficacy of mitotane remains disputed.

- Mitotane is an adrenolytic drug with selective action on the adrenal cortex. It acts after metabolic transformation into active metabolites within the adrenal gland.
- Mitotane has been associated with partial or complete response in only33% of patients with ACC.
- It can be used either as adjuvant therapy after complete surgical removal (because of high risk of loco-regional recurrence) or in metastatic ACC.
- However, as an adjuvant therapy mitotane has failed to show a beneficial effect in extending life expectancy but since the adjuvant treatment options are limited, mitotane continues to be used in this setting.
- ***Dosage:*** Treatment is started with doses of 1g twice daily and gradually increased to tolerance. Drug monitoring is important. It has been found that drug levels>14 mg/l are required to induce tumor regression. It is either given as tablets or as capsules of micronized mitotane mixed with cellulose acetyl phthalate, with a lower absorption rate, but possibly a better gastrointestinal tolerance. The drug is best administered with fat containing foods. Due to long half-life, the highest trough levels are achieved only after several months of therapy.
- ***Toxicity:*** Mitotane causes significant toxicity in therapeutic effective doses. The adverse effects are dose

dependent and are often dose-limiting. These effects are GIT (diarrhea, nausea, anorexia), CNS (lethargy, somnolence, ataxia, dizziness, and confusion), hepatotoxicity, skin rash, bleeding, gynecomastia and leukopenia. For management of nausea, 5-HT blockers may be useful. The adverse effects are frequent when the doses exceed 6 g/day and unfortunately this is the dose required to achieve therapeutic blood levels of 14mg/l. Long-term treatment with mitotane induces adrenal insufficiency, thus high-dose glucocorticoid replacement becomes necessary. Hydrocortisone in doses of 50 mg per day is the treatment of choice. With larger doses of mitotane, replacement with fludrocortisone may also be necessary, guided by the blood pressure, serum potassium levels and plasma renin activity.

Cytotoxic chemotherapy

In patients with extensive local disease not amenable to surgical resection or in metastatic disease, cytotoxic chemotherapy may be tried. However, the results are not very encouraging because in ACC there is strong expression of the multidrug-resistance gene mdr-1 which results in high levels of p-glycoprotein; the latter acts as a drug efflux pump and may cause chemotherapy failure.

- The highest response rate so far has been observed using the combination of etoposide, doxorubicin and cisplatin given together with continuous mitotane
- Oral mitotane together with intravenous streptozocin can also increase survival

Other agents: used are SURAMIN and GOSSYPOL alone or in combination with mitotane.

What are the newer modalities of treatment of ACC?

Because of low prevalence, the progress in management of ACC is still limited. In stage IV ACC it is important to resolve whether mitotane alone is better as compared to mitotane plus chemotherapy. The innovative treatment includes:

- Overcoming drug resistance in ACC
- Vascular targeted therapies in ACC using antiangiogenic drugs
- Inhibition of IGF-II signaling
- Use of Tyrosine kinase inhibitors
- Gene therapy
- Immunotherapy.

Chapter 49

Functioning Adrenocortical Carcinoma in Children

CASE STUDY

A 14-year-old girl presented with complaints of weight gain over one year and increased hair growth for one year. The child had gained 10-15 kg over 1 year, though it was not quantified. She also gave history of rapid hair growth over face, chin, abdomen, thighs and arms. There was positive history of irritability, anxiety and labile behavior. She also gave history of repeated syncopal attacks with spontaneous recovery after 5-10 min. There was history of headache, especially after crying. She also gave history of repeated itching of skin lesions in perineal area. There was negative history of diplopia, galactorrhea, abdominal pain. There was history of primary amenorrhea. However, she did not remember the age of pubarche or thelarche. On examination her height was 147 cm and weight 61 kg. She was conscious and, cooperative. Her pulse rate was 122/min, regular, BP: 150/100 mm Hg. She had acanthosis, buffalo hump, truncal obesity, facial plethora, facial puffiness, cushingoid facies, 4 cm ecchymotic patch present over left loin, no skin tag, no galactorrhea, no field cuts and skin was of normal thickness 0.5 cm square and 1 cm long erythematous striae was present over lower back. The Tanner staging of her pubic hair was stage 4; clitoris: 20 mm long and 12 mm wide while FG Score for distribution of hairs was: 21

Upper lip : 2
Chin : 3
Chest : 2
Upper abd : 2
Lower abd : 2
Upper back : 2
Lower back : 2

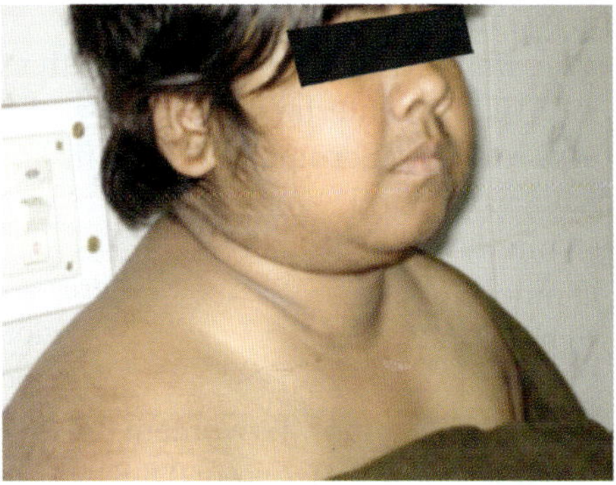

Fig. 49.1: Cushing's patient with typical features-hirsutism, buffalo hump and facial plethora

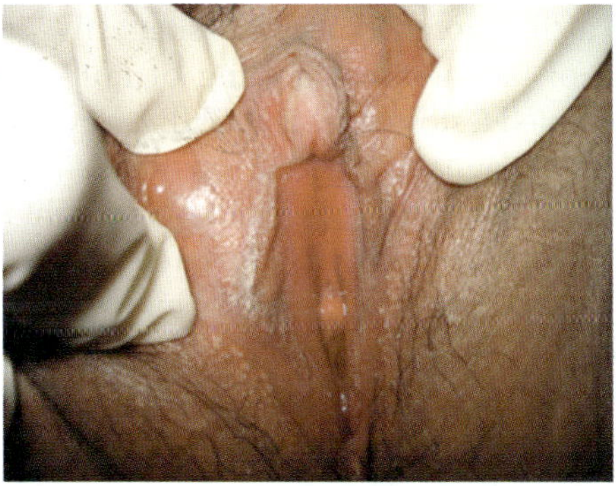

Fig. 49.2: Clitoromegaly

Thighs : 2
Arms : 2

Thyroid: Normal in size and consistency, no hyperpigmentation, nails were normal

CVS: S1, S2 normally heard, no murmur

Resp: Trachea central, movements equal B/L, no creps/rhonchi

Oral cavity: Normal
Clinical impression: Cushing's syndrome with virilization. Possibility of ACC was entertained.
Investigations revealed: Serum ACTH: WNL
Basal cortisol: 540 nmol/L
ONDST: 568 nmol/L
LDDST: 605 nmol/L
HDDST: 596 nmol/L
TSH: 2.5
Serum testosterone: 7.1 nmol/L (women: 0.7-2.8)
DHEAS: 29.30 micromol/L (women: 0.8-8.99)
USG abdomen: revealed 8cm right adrenal mass
CT abdomen: 8.9 cm right adrenal mass with heterogeneous intensity, calcification and necrosis; suggestive of ACC

In view of biochemical finding of non-suppressible HDDST, elevated testosterone and DHEAS levels and a large adrenal mass, diagnosis of ACC was made and the child was taken up for surgery. She underwent right adrenalectomy via a transabdominal approach utilizing a right subcostal incision. The tumor was not infiltrating the kidney or the liver. A 12 × 9 × 8 cm mass weighing 410 gm was resected. Outer surface was nodular and cut surface revealed a grayish white growth with areas of hemorrhage and cystic degeneration. A thin adrenal gland could be identified at the periphery. On microscopic examination, there were features of malignancy such as areas of necrosis, high nuclear grade, high mitotic rate and presence of abnormal mitoses. However, there was no evidence of capsular or vascular invasion.

Postoperative course: The postoperative period was uneventful and the paitent was discharged on 14th postoperative day after suture removal. Postoperative endogenous cortisol was collected on 14th day of surgery and was found to be subnormal (< 27.59 nmol/L).

QUESTIONS

How would you clinically evaluate such a case?

Signs of virilization in a child, especially if associated with signs of Cushing's syndrome should alert the physician about the possibility of adrenal carcinoma. Signs of androgen hypersecretion should be sought for such as tall stature, muscular hypertrophy and development of axillary and pubic hair. In girls usually there would be enlargement of labia majora and clitoral hypertrophy along with secondary amenorrhea. In boys there would be deepening of voice and precocious growth of phallus.

Signs of hypercortisolism: The four cardinal symptoms of CS in children are:

- *Growth failure:* Is the commonsest symptom and sometimes is the only presenting feature.
- *Obesity:* Progressive obesity giving a lemon on stick appearance is very common.
- *Hypertension:* More commonly seen in children than in adults. Headaches are not observed.
- *Hirsutism:* Premature appearance of pubic and axillary hair.

What is the hormonal work-up required in a suspected case of ACC; is there a tumor marker for ACC?

- Overnight or Low dose dexamethasone suppression test; 24 h urinary free cortisol (UFC).

- ***Baseline serum DHEAS:*** In the presence of adrenal lesion, elevated serum dehydroepiandrosterone sulphate levels suggest an ACC.
- ***Baseline serum 17 alpha oestradiol (in men only):*** it is a typical marker of estrogen-secreting ACC in men.
- ***Basline serum testosterone and androstenedione:*** in women with virilizing tumors
- Urinary excretion of 17 ketosteroids, 17 alpha-OHprogesterone, 11-deoxycortisol, deoxycorticosterone (DOC): these additional steroids should be measured as they may also serve as tumor markers during follow-up.
- In advanced ACC serum LDH may serve as a marker of disease progression.
- 24-h urinary metanephrine excretion or plasma metanephrine: for exclusion of pheochromocytoma in all cases.
- ***PRA and serum aldosterone:*** only in patients with hypokalemia and hypertension.

How would you prepare the patient for surgery?

i. *Vigorous chest physiotherapy:* because of intercostal muscle weakness these patients have poor respiratory efforts.
ii. Prophylactic therapy for venous thromobembolism
iii. Correction of electrolyte imbalance
iv. Control of blood pressure and blood glucose
v. Prophylactic antibiotics and antifungal therapy
vi. Starting inhibitors of adrenal function like ketaconazole in doses of 200-600 mg/day.

What is the perioperative and postoperative steroid schedule of this patient?

Time after operation (days)	*IV steroids*	*Oral steroids*	*Oral fludrocortisone(mg/d)*
On the day of operation	30 mg/hr for 6 hrs, then 10 mg/hr for 18 hrs	—	—
+1	200 mg/24 hrs	—	Nil
+2	100 mg/24 hrs	20 mg 6 hrly	Nil
+3	Nil	25 mg 6 hrly	0.1
4 to 7	Nil	20 mg 6 hr	0.1
8 to 10	Nil	20 mg 8 hr	0.1
11 to 14	Nil	10 mg 6 hr	0.1
15th day onwards	Nil	10 mg 8 hr	0.1

Is the histopathological diagnosis of ACC difficult?

The diagnosis on histopathology may remain difficult. Tumor weight is important: most ACC weigh more than 100 gram For histopathological diagnosis, different diagnostic scores (Weiss, Hough, Saeger, etc.) have been used. Histological features suggestive of malignancy are:

i. ***Nuclear atypia:*** moderate to strong.
ii. ***Mitosis:*** High mitotic rate > 5/50 HPF
iii. Atypical mitosis
iv. Clear cells < 25% of the tumor
v. Diffuse architectural pattern
vi. Venous invasion
vii. Sinusoidal invasion
viii. Capsular invasion
ix. Foci of confluent necrosis
x. Fibrous bands

In Weiss Scoring system, each of these characteristics is given a score of 1. If the sum is between 1-3 then it is likely to be benign, whereas if the sum of the score is ≥ 4 then it is likely to be malignant.

What is the importance of postoperative endogenous cortisol levels?

Endogenous cortisol should be measured 10-14 days after surgery. After presumed complete tumor excision, post-operative endogenous cortisol should be subnormal, otherwise patient is labeled as stage IV even if no metastates are detected on MRI and/or CT.

Chapter 50

Adrenocortical Carcinoma Presenting as Cushing's Syndrome in Adults

CASE STUDY

A 30-year-old male presented with following complaints: weight gain, moon facies, abdominal obesity and red skin marks for last 15 days. He also had increased fatiguability for 3 months and adominal pain for one month. Patient was apparently asymptomatic 3 months back when he noticed progressive mooning of the face, swelling of the face and increased abdominal fat along with increasing fatigue. He also noticed red marks on the abdomen for last 15 days. He was also recently found to be hypertensive. There was no history of bone pains, loss of apetite, difficutly in climbing stairs, skin or nail infections, hyperpigmentation, paralytic attacks or polyuria. He was never diabetic and there was no history of any drug or alcohol intake. Family history was not contributory.

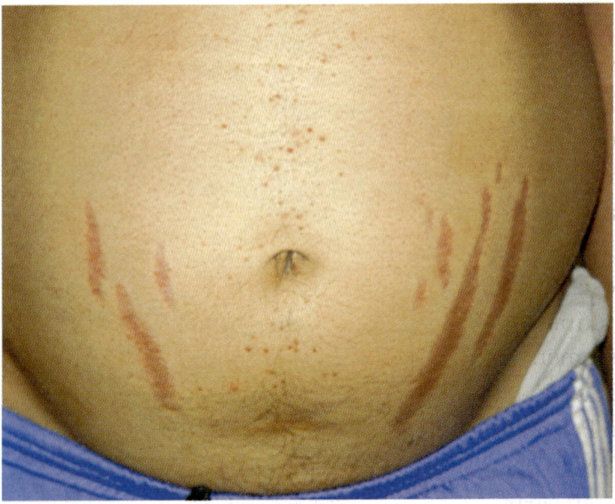

Fig. 50.1: Cushing's patient with truncal obesity and abdominal striae

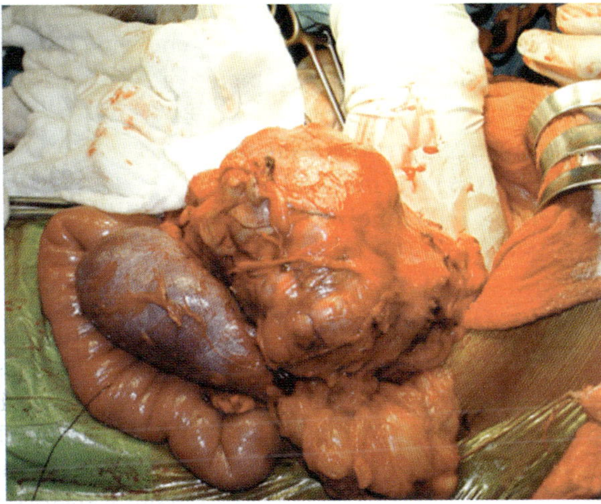

Fig. 50.2: Intraoperative photograph showing large nodular adrenal mass with infiltration into kidney

O/E: BP: 130/80 mm Hg (on drugs)

P/R: 86/min

Plethoric face, moon facies

Mild buffalo hump

Black comedones over trunk

Acanthosis nigricans absent

Ptosis of right eye

Multiple striae: deep, broad(>1cm), violaceous over lower abdomen and axilla

Abdominal obesity present

No Proximal muscle weakness (PMW)

P/A: No organomegaly, no FF

Chest: clear

Skin: dry and thin, no pigmentation, no fungal infection

A clinical impression of Cushing's syndrome was made and in view of short history a suspicion of ACC was kept in mind.

Following investigations were ordered

Serum ACTH: 0.83 pg/ml (4-80 pg/ml)

Basal cortisol: 1600 nmol/L

LDDST: 1583.0 nmol/L

HDDST: 1615 nmol/L

DHEAS: 24.70 micromol/L (3.6-11.9)

PRA/ALDO: 38.73/68

The diagnosis of Cushing's syndrome was confirmed and the etiology was likely to be of adrenal origin in view of unsuppressible HDDST. An ultrasound of the abdomen revealed a large 10 × 10 × 9.8 cm left adrenal mass.

CECT: confirmed a large nodular mass with heterogeneous intensity, calcification and necrosis; also suggestive of infiltration to superior pole of left kidney.

In view of elevated DHEAS, and CT findings a preoperative diagnosis of ACC was strengthened. Renal study with GFR was done to establish the function of the opposite kidney. Patient was explored through the open, transabdominal approach utilizing a left subcostal incision. On initial exploration there were no liver or peritoneal metastases. However, the large adrenal mass was found to be adherent to superior pole of left kidney but could be freed from the spleen, tail of the pancreas or left lobe of liver. A nephroadrenalectomy was performed and a 15 × 15 × 10 cm adrenal mass weighing 1000 grams was removed.

The outer surface of the tumor was nodular and the cut surface revealed a nodular, grayish white mass with myxoid and necrotic areas. The tumor was well demarcated with no tumor infiltration into the kidney. On microscopy the features suggestive of ACC were: presence of thick fibrous bands, atypical mitoses, large areas of necrosis, hemorrhage and calcification, and presence of 6-7 mitotic figures/50 HPF.

Postoperative period was uneventful and the patient was discharged on 10th postoperative day and subsequently sutures were removed with a good scar. Patient continued to be on steroid and mineralocorticoid supplementation. The postoperative endogenous cortisol was < 27.59, i.e. subnormal at 6 months and then at 2 years.

QUESTIONS

What is the role of extensive surgery in ACC?

- Radical resection often provides the only chance for cure or atleast for long survival. A margin free resection (R0) is a strong predictor of long-term survival.
- Surgical strategy must be planned in advance based on a recent CT scan
- *Exposure:* Wide exposure of the mass is important to limit the possibility of rupture of tumor capsule. For tumors less than 10 cm a bilateral subcostal incision is preferred while for larger tumors a thoraco-abdominal approach should be used.
- To avoid tumor spillage, the tumor capsule must remain intact. Invasion by or adherence of the carcinoma into adjacent structures often requires en bloc excision of the kidney, the spleen, partial hepatectomy or pancreatectomy in addition to lymphadenectomy.
- The invasion of the adjacent structures must be carefully evaluated intraoperatively. The kidney is the organ most often involved. If there is a suspicion of this, a nephro-adrenalectomy should be performed (although there is

no survival advantage in routine concomitant nephrectomy). Evaluation of the functional status of the contralateral kidney is mandatory. Liver and spleen are frequently involved by local extension. But often a cleavage plane can be found under the liver capsule and major resections are rarely required.

- ***Invasion/thrombus of IVC:*** This may occur in 15-20% cases, especially on right side. If the invasion is limited to vena cava, venovenous by pass is sufficient to perform either a wedge resection or segmental caval resection or flushing a limited intracaval thrombus. But, if the tumors extend into the right atrium, cardio-pulmonary bypass is necessary and the bilateral subcostal incision is combined with a sternotomy.
- ***Palliative surgery:*** The role of tumor debulking in the presence of metastatic disease is a matter of debate. However, tumor debulking does help in controlling hormone excess in functional tumors.

What is the role of laparoscopic surgery in ACC?

Laparoscopic surgery in ACC is fraught with the danger of tumor capsule violation, tumor fragmentation and the potential difficutly to perform a definite margin-free R0 resection.

Chapter 51

Sporadic Pheochromocytoma

CASE STUDY

A 15-year-old girl presented to us with complaints of headache, decreased vision and on and off palpitation for last one year. The headache was continuous, mainly on the right side in the temporoparietal region and was not associated with vomiting. She did not give any history of increased sweating. She had been seen by an internist 6 months back and was found to be hypertensive for the first time (BP: 140/100 mmHg) and was put on two anti-hypertensive drugs. She was also evaluated by an USG which revealed a hypoechoic mass in right adrenal gland measuring 11.8 × 7.2cm and hence referred to us with a working diagnosis of pheochromocytoma. Detailed history and physical examination was performed to rule out any

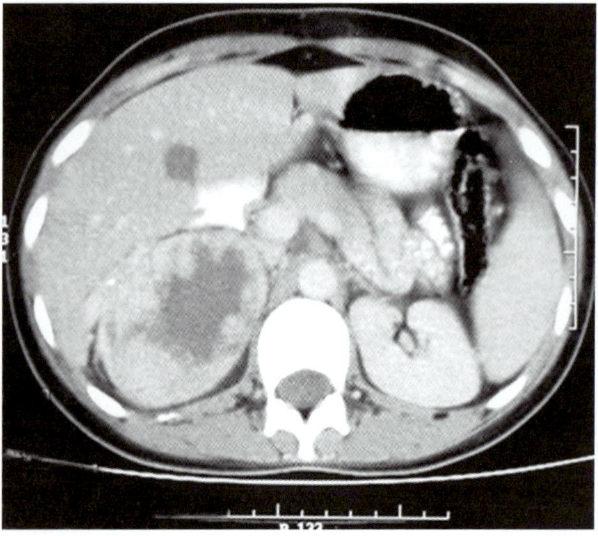

Fig. 51.1: Large adrenal mass with central cystic necrosis

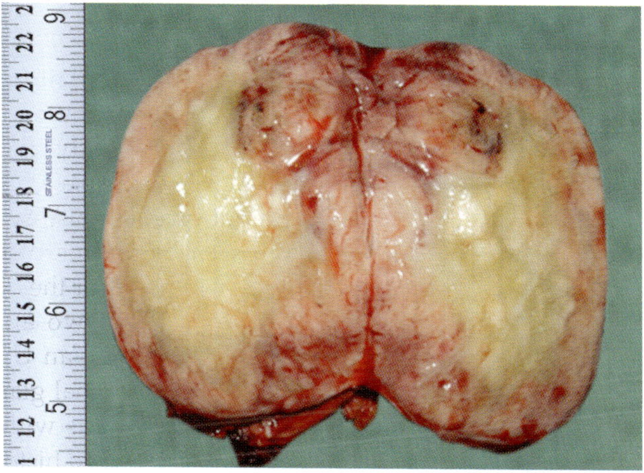

Fig. 51.2: Cut section of adrenalectomy specimen showing cystic area

feature of MEN but none could be found 24 hour urinary metanephrine estimation was done and was found to be significantly elevated (5.20 mcg/24 hours, range: upto 1.0 mcg/24 hrs). CECT was performed which confirmed the presence of an adrenal mass with central necrosis and a normal contralateral adrenal gland. She was started on alpha blockade with prazopress with starting dose of 0.5 mg at bedtime and was gradually increased to a maximum of 10 mg/day over a period of 20 days. During this period she was given blood transfusion and extra salt. She did not have any postural drop during the pre-operative period. She did not develop tachycardia though she did have occasional nasal stuffiness. Beta blockers were added 24 hours prior to surgery. She underwent laparoscopic adrenalectomy, but had to be converted to open unilateral adrenalectomy due to technical difficulty on account of difficult dissection

ALPANA CHAURASIA 2002 [illegible] 80784

SANJAY GANDHI POSTGRADUATE INSTITUTE OF MEDICAL SCIENCES, LUCKNOW.

Department of Endocrine Surgery

Pheochromocytoma- Preoperative preparation chart

Date	Dose of Alpha Blocker	Weight (Kg)	Pulse (/min.)	BP Supine	BP Standing	Postural drop	Nasal Stuffiness	Hb (gm%)	HCT	Other drugs	Dose	Remarks
31.07			96/min	110/70	—	—	–ve	8.7	30.8	×	×	? Incidentaloma
01.08	[illegible] PRAZOSIN	[illegible]	90/min	120/76	100/60	10/16	–ve	—	—	×	×	? [illegible]
02.08	PRAZOSIN [illegible]		96/min	110/80	100/70	10/10	–ve	—	—	×	×	
3.08	1mg–1mg	38.5	106/-	110/70	100/70		–ve					
4.08	2mg 2mg	38	104	110/70	100/70	10/0	—	–	–	—	–	1 U transfused
5/08	6mg		110/min	100/80	90/70	10/10	occasionally					preop.
6/08	3-2-3	39.0	90/-	110/70	100/70	10/0	(–)	9.0	30.7	×	×	-
7/08	9mg	39.0	86/-	120/80	110/70	10/10	(–)	-	-	Dex [illegible]	×	
8/08	9mg.		120/min	110/80	100/70	10/10	—					
9/8/02	9mg	40kg	110/m	120/86	110/80	10/[illegible]0	-				×	× 2 [illegible]
10/8/02	9	30.5	104/-	100/70	90/60	10/10	—	.			×	
												operated 12.08.02

Name of Patient: ALPANA CHAURASIA
CR No.: 2002180784
Date of Operation:
Date of Admission: 31-07-2002
Date of Discharge:

Tumour size:
On CT- 44 × 38 × 38 mm.
Per operative- 5×5.5×3.6 cms.

Urinary Metanephrine: 11.54 mg/day

Fig. 51.3: Preoperative chart of a patient undergoing alpha-blockade

because of the large size of the lesion. Intraoperative hemodynamic alteration in the form of accelerated hypertension (max BP was 222/140 mmHg) which was managed by sodium nitroprusside infusion. At the time of closure she developed hypotension which was managed by infusion of colloids as well as noradrenaline; the latter was tapered off within next 12 hours. She was kept for observation in the postoperative recovery room during which her CVP was maintained to 12-14 cm of H_2O by infusion of colloids. She made an uneventful recovery and was discharged on the 6th postoperative day. The histopathology was confirmatory of pheochromocytoma and her 10th postoperative day urinary metanephrine estimation was within normal limits.

QUESTIONS

What is pheochromocytoma?

Pheochromocytoma are catecholamine producing neuroendocrine tumors arising from chromaffin cells of the adrenal medulla or extra-adrenal paraganglia.

What is the basic pathophysiology of pheochromocytomas?

The receptors on which the catecholamine acts are:

Adrenergic receptors

Alpha

- α-1 : NE > E
- α-2 : E > NE

Beta

- β-1 : E > NE
- β-2 : E > NE

The anatomic concept of prejunctional α2 and postjunctional α1 receptor has been abandoned in favor of pharmacological and functional classification. There are physiologically distinct receptors for neurally released Nor Epinephrine (NE) as well as circulating epinephrine (E). The location of receptors is as follows: Alpha-1 and Beta-1 receptors populate tissues with rich SNS innervation (heart and gut) and are situated strategically to be activated during stimulation of these nerves. Alpha-2 and Beta-2 receptors are situated in post-junctional regions remote from sites of release of NE. They populate tissues with little sympathetic innervation (skeletal, uterine and tracheal muscles). There are different roles of SNS as well as circulating catecholamine. Because of enhanced SNS activity and excessive stores of NE in sympathetic nerve terminals any direct or reflexly mediated stimulus to SNS could release excessive quantities of NE into the synaptic cleft and produce a hypertensive crisis. The easier access of NE released from the post-ganglionic neuron at its receptor site on effector cells can result in marked symptoms with relatively small increments in circulating NE.

What are the hemodynamic characteristics of the circulation in pheochromocytoma?

The concept has evolved that pheochromocytoma is associated with a hyperkinetic, vasoconstrictive and hypovolemic form of hypertension (HTN). The increased peripheral resistance is primarily responsible for maintenance of HTN.

How does a patient of pheochromocytoma present?

Pheochromocytoma has diverse manifestations because of variation in hormones it releases, because of variation in patterns of release and because of individual to individual differences in catecholamine sensitivity. Therefore, pheochromocytoma is known as "The GREAT MIMIC". The various manifesta-tions are:

CVS manifestations
Endocrine/Metabolic manifestations
Associated Syndromes
Incidentaloma

The symptomatic triad of headache, sweating attacks and tachycardia in a hypertensive patient has a sensitivity of 90.9% and specificity of 93.8%.

Describe the hypertension of pheochromocytoma?

Hypertension could be

Paroxysmal (NE+E):	48%
Sustained (NE):	29%
Normotensive (E):	10-15%

The most dramatic presentation of pheochromocytoma is an explosive clinical syndrome characterized by severe hypertension, diaphoresis, headache, tachycardia or arrhythmias. In contrast to adults, HTN is more likely to be sustained in children; headache, sweating and nausea are three most common symptoms experienced by children with pheochromocytoma.

What are the major complications that can arise as a result of pheochromocytoma?

Myocardial infarction (MI)

Either due to myocarditis or coronary spasm. Both of these may cause release of cardiac enzymes and produce ECG pattern resembling those of MI.

Cardiac arrhythmias

Atrial and ventricular fibrillation due to sudden release of catecholamine which may be precipitated by anesthetic agents or during surgery for unrelated conditions.

Acute pulmonary edema

Cardiogenic: Secondary to LVF from dilated congestive cardiomyopathy or non-cardiogenic resulting from transient increases in Pulmonary Capillary Wedge Pressure (PCWP).

Hypertensive crisis

May result from: Drugs like tricyclic anti-depressants, anti-dopaminergic agents like metoclopramide, and naloxone or when beta blockade is started without prior adequate alpha-blockade.

Stroke

Hypertensive encephalopathy

Presenting as altered mental status, focal neurologic signs and symptoms, and seizures.

Shock

Patients with pure epinephrine producing tumor may be hypotensive because of epinephrine-induced peripheral vasodilatation. Acute hemorrhagic necrosis of the tumor may present as an acute surgical abdomen associated with marked HTN followed by hypotension and even shock and sudden death. The latter is a consequence of marked arterial and venous dilatation due to sudden withdrawal of catecholamine, desensitization of adrenergic receptors or hypocalcaemia. Hypovolemia or chronic treatment with alpha-blocking drugs further compounds this problem.

Intense peripheral arterial vasoconstriction might also produce apparent shock.

Orthostatic hypotension

Some patients also present with unexplained orthostatic hypotension that, on a background of HTN, provides an important diagnostic clue for the presence of a pheochromocytoma.

What are metabolic abnormalities seen in pheochromocytoma?

i. ***Lactic acidosis:*** In the absence of shock it should arouse suspicion of pheochromocytoma.
ii. ***Hypercalcemia:*** May be related to excessive production of PTH
iii. ***Diarrhea:*** due to production of VIP
iv. ***Hypokalemic alkalosis:*** Due to ectopic production of ACTH by a pheochromocytoma
v. ***Glucose intolerance:*** Catecholamine induced suppression of insulin release or an inhibiting action of epinephrine on insulin-stimulated glucose uptake by skeletal muscle coupled with direct alpha-adrenergic stimulation of hepatic glucose production results in glucose intolerance.

When should you suspect and screen for presence of pheochromocytoma?

The following patients should receive priority of evaluation:

- Episodic symptoms of headache, tachycardia and diaphoresis (with or without associated hypertension)
- Family history of pheochromocytoma
- Signs and symptoms suggesting a MEN syndrome

- Incidental suprarenal or abdominal masses
- Hypertension associated with equivocal increases in catecholamine
- Adverse cardiovascular manifestations during pregnancy, in response to anesthesia, to any surgical procedure or to certain medications known to precipitate symptoms in patients with pheochromocytoma
- Spells or attacks occurring during exertion, twisting or turning of torso, straining, coitus or micturition

How do you establish the biochemical diagnosis of pheochromocytoma?

Biochemical diagnosis

Because pheochromocytoma are a heterogeneous group of hormone-secreting tumors, no single analysis can achieve 100% sensitivity. Debate over the relative merits of various tests will continue. The most important consideration is the reliability of the test for exclusion of pheochromocytoma. A missed diagnosis due to a false-negative result can have catastrophic consequences for the patient. The high diagnostic sensitivity of plasma-free metanephrine or urinary-fractionated metanephrine mean that negative test results reliably exclude the presence of virtually all pheochromocytomas

Sensitivity and specificity of biochemical tests

Biochemical test	*Sensitivity*	*Specificity*
Plasma free metanephrine	99%	89%
Plasma catecholamine	84%	81%
Urinary catecholamine	86%	88%
Urinary-fractionated catecholamine	97%	69%
Urinary total metanephrine	77%	95%
VMA	64%	95%

How do you localize the pheochromocytoma?

Localization is mandatory because of the variable location of these tumors. Should ideally only be initiated once there is unequivocal biochemical evidence for pheochromocytoma. The distribution is:

Abdomen	: 97%
Thorax	: 2.3%
Neck	: 1%
Currently used techniques	: CT/MRI/MIBG

CT

Widely used CT scan of entire abdomen (including pelvis) with and without contrast. Patient should be protected from a hypertensive crisis or cardiac arrhythmia by combined blockade by α and β blocking drugs. It can detect tumors >1 cm.

MRI

T2 weighted MRI with gadolinium enhancement has a similar diagnostic sensitivity to CT. Preferred, as localization of extra-adrenal pheochromocytoma is better, no exposure to radiation, do not require intravenous contrast, procedure of choice for pregnant women and produces in vivo tissue characterization.

MIBG

Provides both anatomical localization and functional characterization of tumor. Additional multifocal or metastatic tumors can be easily detected. However, not warranted before surgery in all patients with biochemical proven pheochromocytoma. Some drugs can interfere with tumor uptake or retention of MIBG- labetolol, tricyclic antidepressants, guanethedine.

Phenozybenzamine, prazosin, propranolol and calcium antagonists DO NOT interfere neither with metanephrine estimation nor with MIBG scanning.

Imaging	*Sensitiviy(%)*	*Specificity(%)*
CT	98	70
MRI	100	67
MIBG	78	100

MIBG is not sensitive enough to exclude pheochromocytoma; CT and MRI have poor specificities, as low as 50% in some series. This is an important problem because of the relative high frequencies of adrenal masses that are not pheochromocytoma

- ***Echocardiogram:*** to be undertaken regardless of blood pressure levels. This evaluation is to ensure that chronic exposure to high levels of circulating catecholamine has not resulted in dilated cardiomyopathy.

How do you manage the pheochromocytoma?

Management consists of:

i. Preoperative α and β–blockade
ii. Intraoperative management
iii. Postoperative management
iv. Surgical techniques

Preoperative α-blockade

The major aim of medical pretreatment is to prevent catecholamine –induced serious complications during surgery –hypertensive crisis, cardiac arrhythmias, pulmonary edema, and cardiac ischemia. With adequate preoperative preparation, perioperative mortality has fallen to less than 3%. Even if a diagnosis is considered in a very rare life-threatening conditions (e.g. shock due to a hemorrhagic necrosis or rupture of a pheochromocytoma) stabilization with subsequent medical pretreatment and elective surgery is preferred, since emergency tumor resection without proper preparation results in poor survival. Traditional regimen include:

- ***Non-competitive blockade:*** Phenoxy benzamine
- ***Competitive blockade:*** Prazosin, doxazosin
- ***Alternative drugs:*** Calcium channel blockade or labetolol, either alone or in combination with alpha blockade.

Phenoxybenzamine (PXB)

It blocks alpha receptors noncompetitively and makes it difficult for released catecholamine to have a physiologic effect. It also permits intravascular volume expansion. Its half life is >24 hours. The effect of PXB dissipate over 36 hours, and large volumes of IV fluids are often required in the postoperative period. Patients are often somnolent in the first 24 hours after surgery, which may be due to persistent central alpha-2 adrenergic blockade. The disadvantage is that marked orthostatic hypotension and tachycardia can occur in the preoperative period. Preoperative blockade can be performed on outpatient basis but is preferable in hospital settings. The initial dose is 10 mg BD, PO, combined with noninvasive monitoring of arterial BP in supine and standing position. Dose is increased by 10 mg increments daily. There is no evidence that preoperative PXB therapy for >14 days was more effective than 7-10 days. PXB produces a nonspecific, complete and prolonged blockade.

Selective alpha-1 antagonists

These have several potential advantages:

- Do not produce reflex tachycardia
- Have a shorter duration of action and can be adjusted rapidly before surgery and the duration of postoperative hypotension is decreased.
- Preoperative α-adrenoreceptor antagonists are rendered unnecessary (unless the patient has E + producing tumor) because alpha-2 receptors which regulate NE release at cardiac adrenergic nerve ending) are not antagonized.

  The various agents in this group are Doxazosin, Prazosin and Terazosin

Prazosin

- It has a short elimination half life (2-3 hrs) and thus blood concentration may decrease to ineffective levels at the time of surgery if the last dose was given on the previous night.
- Requires frequent dosing. The initial dose is 1 mg, 3-4 times a day with an average dose of 12-16 mg.
- Doxazosin has a long duration of action, allowing once daily dosing and may have a near ideal profile for pre-operative patients
- ***Calcium Channel Blockers:*** They control BP and symptoms by relaxing arteriolar smooth muscle. In more resistant cases, calcium-channel antagonists can be combined with specific alpha-1 antagonists with successful control of BP. Their other advantages include their usefulness for normotensive pheochromocytoma and their utility in managing patients with cardiovascular complications because they prevent catecholamine-induced coronary vasospasm and myocarditis.

How will you know the patient has been adequately blocked and can be taken up for surgery?

The Roizen's criteria can be used to assess the adequacy of blockade:

i. No BP reading > 160/90 mmHg should be evident for 24 hours before surgery.

ii. Orthostatic hypotension with readings> 80/45 mmHg should be present.

iii. The ECG should be free of ST, T changes for at least one week.

iv. The patient should have no more than one premature ventricular contractions (PVCs) every 5 min.

What additional things are to be done during pre-operative blockade?

- Risk of excessive orthostatic hypotension can be kept to a minimum by the increase of salt and fluid intake.
- If control of BP is a problem, the addition of a calcium antagonist may help reduce BP to a reasonable level obviating the need to increase the dose of alpha-blockers with its attendant risk of postoperative hypotension.
- For the patient with intermittent hypertension, use of a calcium antagonist may be an alternative approach.
- Propranolol, 40 mg, three times a day or atenolol 25-50 mg once daily could be included after several days of alpha blockade.
- This addition is especially useful in patients who have tachyarrhythmia. However, the efficacy of routine use of beta-blockade in preventing intraoperative tachyarrhythmia has been questioned.

- Blockade of beta-receptors should never be initiated before blockade of alpha-receptor since the loss of beta-receptor mediated vasodilatation leaves alpha-adrenergic stimulation unopposed, which could result in hypertensive crisis.
- Beta adrenergic blockade should be avoided in patients with catecholamine-induced cardiomyopathy.

What preparation is to be done intraoperatively?

Intraoperative management requires close, collegial communication which is crucial to the success of intra-operative management of patients undergoing pheochromocytoma resection. The important considerations are:

- Anesthetic consideration
- Vasodilators
- Beta antagonists
- Fluid management

What are the anesthetic considerations?

- Administer an anxiolytic.
- Place an intra-arterial catheter before induction.
- Place an intravenous catheter for antihypertensive administration(SNP, NTG).
- Place a central venous catheter for intravascular volume monitoring.
- Treat hemodynamic fluctuations with antihypertensives and beta-adrenergic antagonists.
- Monitor for hypotension and hypoglycemia after tumor excision.
- Measurement of pulmonary capillary wedge pressure (PCWP) and cardiac output (CO) may be helpful because

these patients may exhibit a discrepancy between right sided and left sided filling pressure. PCWP and CO should particularly be monitored in the presence of heart disease.

- *General anesthesia:* Depth of anesthesia is generally more important than the specific agent.
- *Inhalation agents:* Isuflurane and Enflurane, servoflurane can be safely used. Halothane results in severe arrhythmias and should be avoided.
- There are no contraindications to the use of Nitrous oxide.
- *Intravenous agents:* Induction with propofol or thiopental is safe. Ketamine and ephedrine should be avoided. Morphine causes histamine release which is a known trigger of pheochromocytoma crisis. Droperidol should be avoided.
- *Neuromuscular blockers:* Vecuronium has little or no autonomic effects and does not release histamine and is the drug of choice.

How do you manage the hemodynamic alteration during surgery for pheochromocytoma?

The hypertensive peaks are managed by various vasodilators. The hypertension during surgery has two distinct origins: noxious stimuli such as tracheal intubation, skin incision and abdominal exploration cause catecholamine release from excessive stores in adrenergic nerve endings. Deepening the level of anesthesia may block the cardiovascular response to noxious stimuli. The hypertensive response to tumor manipulation also results from marked increase in plasma NE and E concentration. They are best treated with vasodilators.

- *Direct vasodilators:* Sodium Nitroprusside (SNP) and Nitroglycerine (NTG).
- *SNP:* Should be used in patients with pheochromocytoma and complicating acute MI or CHF to obtain a gradual reduction of arterial BP. It decreases preload and after load. Its onset is immediate and recovery occurs in 1-2 min. At higher doses, toxic metabolites, such as cyanide and thiocyanate, are a concern.
- *Beta-antagonists:* Alpha-adrenergic antagonists can help control tachycardia or tachyarrhythmia. Esmolol is a selective alpha-1 antagonist with a short duration of action. It has hemodynamic effects that may be uniquely suited for the intraoperative management of pheochromocytoma.
- Successful surgery requires co-operation of the endocrine surgeon, the anesthesiologist and the endocrinologist.
- Surgery for pheochromocytoma is technically demanding and preferably is done in centers that have experience with this disease.

What are various surgical approaches and techniques to manage pheochromocytoma?

Anterior or transabdominal approach

- Used most frequently especially for large masses
- Patient is placed in supine position
- Flank elevated 30 deg on a pillow
- Use of fixed subcostal retractors

Technical aspects of anterior approach (Right adrenalectomy)

- Mobilizing the hepatic flexure of the colon and retracting it inferiorly exposes the adrenal tumor/gland.

- Hockey stick incision is given and duodenum is mobilized medially by the Kocher maneuver to expose the IVC.
- If (R) gland is high or the tumor is large, the (R) triangular ligament is incised to mobilize and retract the (R) lobe of liver anteriorly (caution: do not injure right hepatic vein or compress IVC).
- Gerota's fascia is incised and surrounding fibro fatty tissue is dissected free.
- Right adrenal vein (SHORT, THINWALLED, OBLIQUE and enters IVC posteriorly) is identified and ligated. It is located at the superomedial aspect of the gland.

Technical aspects of anterior approach (Left adrenalectomy)

- Enter the lesser sac by dividing the gastrocolic omentum or by medial visceral rotation (by dividing the splenorenal and splenocolic ligament) and mobilize the spleen + pancreas from the retroperitoneum toward the midline.
- Left adrenal vein leaves the gland at its inferomedial aspect and enters the left renal vein. Always make certain that the adrenal vein is entering the gland before ligating.

Other approaches

- Posterior approach is not recommended
- Thoracoabdominal for large, malignant pheochromocytoma

Laparoscopic adrenalectomy

- Less postoperative pain, shortened hospital stay and fewer incisional complications.
- Procedure of choice except in the case of invasive carcinoma or masses >15 cm.
- Conversion rate in experienced hands is <5%.
- It is safe, has similar operative time and shows no difference in BP and heart rate increments when compared with open operations.

- Infact, in patients undergoing laparoscopy, intraoperative hypotension was less severe and hypotensive episodes were less frequent.

In the postoperative period what precautions should be taken?

After surgery, patients need to be under close surveillance for the first 24 hr in an intensive or intermediate care unit. The two important events one should be careful are:

- ***Hypotension:*** due to hemorrhage, sudden increases in venous capacitance, inadequate volume repletion or residual effects of preop alpha-adrenergic blockade that can last for 48-72 hrs (especially common after Phenozybenzamine)
  - ***Mx:*** fluids should be administered first especially colloids, keeping in mind that those patients require large amounts of volume after tumor resection. Pressor agents are not usually effective in the presence of hypovolemia. Pressor agents used are epinephrine or if epinephrine infusion is ineffective, vasopressin might be used.
- ***Hypoglycemia:*** Slow emergence from anesthesia or persistent lethargy or somnolence after extubation should arouse suspicion of hypoglycemia. It is due to:
  - Rebound hyperinsulinism that occurs when the inhibitory effect of NE on insulin secretion is suddenly gone.
  - Preoperative stimulation of glygenolysis and lipolysis by catecholamine.
  - Alpha-adrenergic blockers may also impair recovery from hypoglycemia (by decreasing release of gluconeogenic substances and inhibiting glycoge-

nolysis) and can mask the clinical manifestations of hypoglycemia.
- These patients should therefore be monitored for blood glucose levels for at least 48 hr postoperative.

What is the microscopic picture and can histopathology give a definitive diagnosis of malignant pheochromocytoma?

- Encapsulated tumor
- Nests, trabeculae
- Separated by delicate vascular channels.
- Anisomorphic nuclei, vesicular chromatin, conspicuous nucleoli.
- Abundant granular eosinophilic to amphophilic cytoplasm
- Hyalinization and hemorrhage

The histopathology cannot give a defintive diagnosis of malignancy but there are certain criteria for malignancy:

- Capsular invasion (CI)
- Vascular invasion (VI)
- Extension into periadrenal adipose tissue
- Expanded large and confluent nests (at least 3 times the size of zellballen in normal sympathetic paraganglia)
- Diffuse growth
- Necrosis
- Increased cellularity
- Tumor cell spindling
- Profound cell and nuclear pleomorphism
- Cellular monotomy with high N/C ratio
- Nuclear hyperchromasia
- Macronucleoli
- Increased mitotic figure (more than 3/10 or 20HPF)

- Atypical mitoses
- Absence of hyaline globules

Score 1 CI, VI, profound pleomorphism, nuclear hyperchromasia

Score 2 For all other features

Score of 4 or more suggests potential malignant biological behavior.

What are the features of malignant pheochromocytoma?

Successful surgical excision of an apparently benign tumor may be followed by a diagnosis of malignancy as long as 15 years later. It remains impossible to predict the subsequent development of malignant disease based on histological findings in a resected tumor. Only the presence of metastases of chromaffin tissue at sites where no chromaffin tissue should be expected establishes a definite diagnosis of malignant pheochromocytoma. Suggested adverse prognostic factors:

1. Large tumor size (>5 cm)
2. Local tumor extension at the time of surgery
3. Extra-adrenal location
4. Ploidy pattern of DNA: tetraploid or aneuploid tumors have a more malignant course
5. Paraganglionoma in patients with SDHB mutations
6. Increased plasma/urinary concentration of dopamine and dopa.

The common sites of metastases are bones, lungs, liver, lymph nodes. The 5-year survival is < 50% but they can be slow growing and patients may have minimal morbidity and survive for as long as 20 years. Wherever possible surgical excison/debulking should be done. Symptomatic treatment involves: alpha-blockers and alpha-methyl paratyrosine in selected patients. MIBG therapy is another alternative.

Combination chemotherapy

Cyclophosphamide, vincristine and doxorubicin. RF ablation of hepatic and bone metastases. Combination treatment with MIBG and myeloablative chemotherapy and stem cell rescue.

What are the causes of persistent hypertension after successful surgery for pheochromocytoma?

Persistent hypertension may represent

- Fluid excess
- Return of autonomic reflexes
- Inadvertent ligation of a renal artery
- Presence of residual tumor
- Residual nonparoxysmal hypertension is found in 27-38% after pheochromocytoma removal and may be due to: familial hypertension, and increased age.

How do you follow-up such patients?

Repeat measurements of plasma catecholamine and 24-hr urinary metanephrine should be obtained 7-10 days after surgery and annually thereafter for at least 5-10 years, even if the patient remains asymptomatic. Patients with extra-adrenal or familial pheochromocytoma should be followed up indefinitely and all family members should be screened. Recurrences occur more often in patients with extra-adrenal disease (33%) than in those with adrenal disease (14%), and more often in the familial population (33%) than in the non-familial populations (13%).

Chapter 52

Hereditary Pheochromocytoma: Von Hippel Lindau (VHL) Disease

CASE STUDY

A 20-year-old boy was seen for evaluation of his hypertension which was detected only 8 months back on account of severe headache. The headache occurred daily and was of maximum intensity in the night. It was mainly frontal, lasting for 30 min and then subsided on its own. It was not associated with chest pain, anxiety or flushing. However, increased sweating was noted during these episodes. The maximum blood pressure recorded during such episodes was 190/105 mmHg. However, no postural giddiness was present. He also had history of breathlessness on exertion (NYHA Class III) due to pleural effusion for which he was taking emperical anti-tubercular treatment for last 3 months but without much symptomatic relief.

There was no family history of hypertension. On examination he was found to be having marfanoid habitus with height of 171.5 cm and arm span of 177cm and high arched palate with positive wrist sign. Blood pressure recorded at that time was 180/110 mmHg. However, there were no mucosal neuromas or neurofibromatosis. But he had café-au-lait spots over the abdomen. There were no cerebellar signs and he had no proximal muscle weakness. Thyroid was normally palpable. During evaluation of his hypertension, CECT of the abdomen was done which revelaed a 5 cm soft tissue attenuating lesion arising from right adrenal showing moderate post contrast enhancement with central necrosis. 24-hour urinary normetanephrines were estimated and were found to be significantly high (16117.9 mcg/24 hours, normal range: 88-444) with normal metanephrine. For evaluation of his headache he had also undergone MRI of the brain which revealed hemangioblastoma of the left cerebellar hemisphere. In view of two

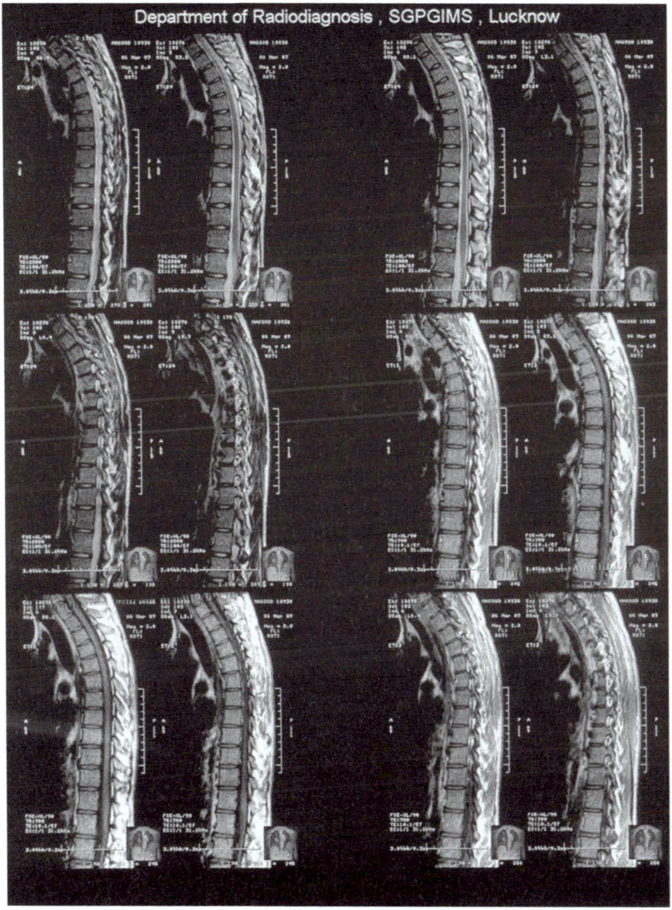

Fig. 52.1: MRI (T1 weighted image) showing spinal hemangioblastoma

associated lesions in a young patient a possibility of Von Hippel Lindau disease was kept and he was further investigated as follows: Fundus examination was done to

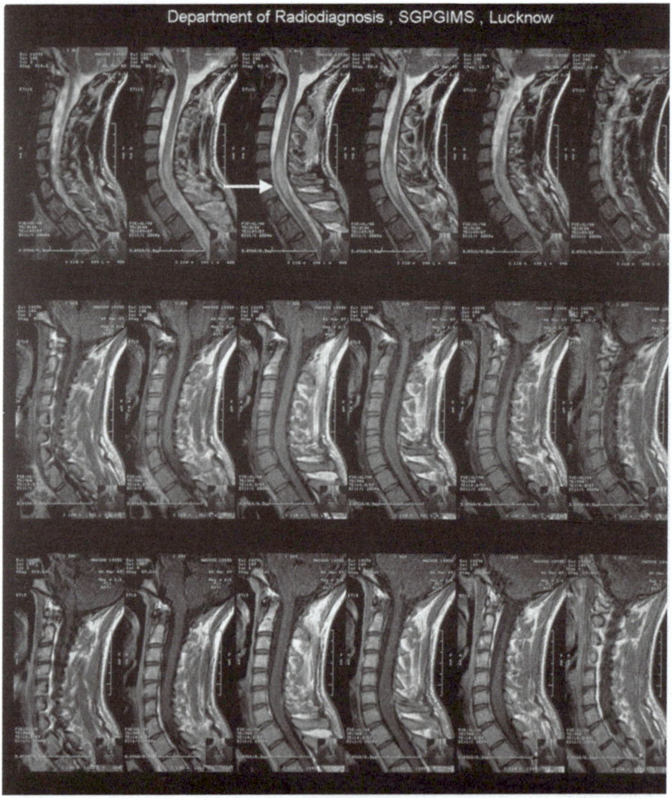

Fig. 52.2: MRI (T2 weighted image) showing spinal hemangioblastoma (arrow)

look for retinal hemangiomas which was, however, negative. MRI of the spine also revealed hemangioblastomas. CECT of the abdomen was reviewed and it showed multicystic lesion, measuring 2.5 cm involving the pancreatic tail. Family history revealed that his sister, brother and mother were

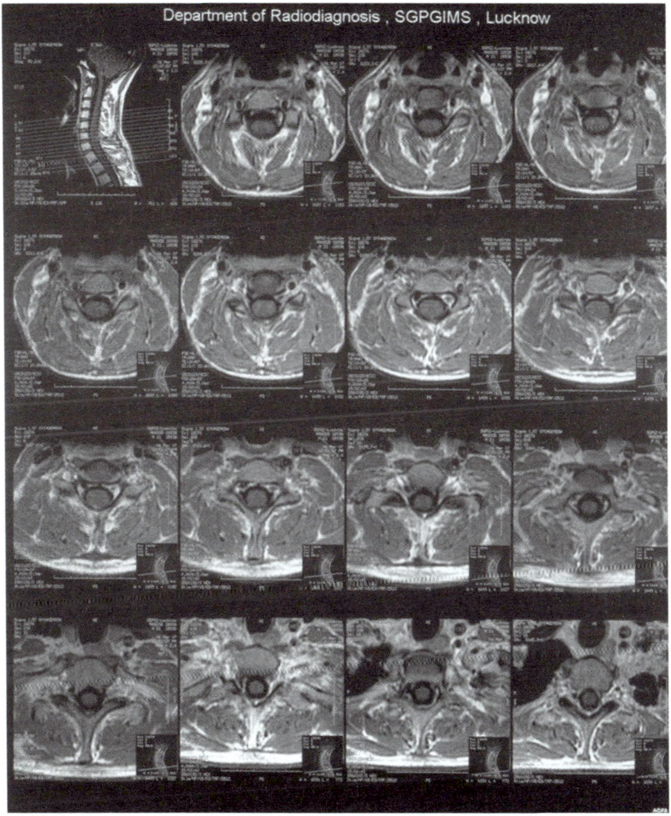

Fig. 52.3: MRI (coronal section) showing spinal hemangioblastoma

operated for brain tumors (details were not available). Thyroid Ultrasound was normal but thyroid function tests showed hypothyroidism (f T4: 9.25, T4:45.73 and TSH: 8.27). CT thorax confirmed presence of miliary tuberculosis and pleural tap was positive for AFB, though culture was negative for AFB. He is still under evaluation and treatment for pulmonary tuberculosis and is planned for adrenalectomy after alpha blockade.

QUESTIONS

What are the various syndromes forms of pheochromocytoma?

There are 5 genetic syndromes in which pheochromocytoma can occur:

VHL syndrome	VHL gene
MEN2 syndrome	MEN 2 gene
Von Recklinghausen's disease (NF Type I)	NF-I gene
Familial paraganglionoma syndromes (PG)	SDHB gene
Familial paraganglionoma syndromes (PG)	SDHD gene

All these differ in their potential for malignancy, bilaterality, multiplicity, recurrence potential and age of presentation

What is the incidence of familial pheochromocytoma?

Accumulating evidence suggests that familial pheochromocytoma is more frequent than previously thought, accounting for upto 25% of patients with pheochromocytoma but with no obvious initial evidence of a syndrome or family history.

Should all apparently sporadic pheochromocytoma undergo genetic analysis or screening?

It is recommended that all presumed sporadic pheochromocytoma should undergo analysis of mutation of RET, VHL, SDHD and SDHB gene especially in following situations:

When to consider familial pheochromocytoma
Multifocal pheochromocytoma
Extra-adrenal pheochromocytoma
Young age
Family history of pheochromocytoma
If other tumors are also present in the index case like that of brain, spinal cord, eyes, ears, thyroid, parathyroid, kidney, pancreas, epididymis, skin
Relatives with these tumors

When a patient presents with a family history in which the primary manifestation is pheochromocytoma, VHL is the likely cause; on the other hand when MTC is the primary manifestation, MEN 2 is the likely cause.

What kind of genetic testing should be done in a suspected familial PCC?

In adrenal PCC start with RET and VHL followed by SDHD and SDHB.

For extra-adrenal tumors: RET can be postponed.

For neck paraganglionoma one should analyze SDHD and SDHC.

In malignant PCC/paraganglionomas SDHB and VHL should have preference.

What is VHL disease?

It is an autosomal, dominant inherited disorder with a prevalence of 2-3/100000 patient. A germline mutation in VHL gene predisposes carriers to highly vascularized tumors in multiple organs viz:

Tumors in VHL disease
Brain and spinal cord hemangioblastoma (HB)
Retinal hemangioblastomas/angiomas
Pheochromocytoma (PCC)
Renal cell carcinoma (RCC)
Cyst and cystadenomas of epididymis, kidneys, pancreas, broad ligament
Islet cell tumors of pancreas

Describe the VHL gene?

The VHL gene is a tumor suppressor gene and is involved in blood vessel formation by regulation of activity of hypoxic inducible factor (HIF)-1 alpha.

It is a relatively small gene that covers approx.14 500 bp of genomic DNA. The protein–coding region is contained in 3 exons.

VHL germ line mutations are consistently detected in 100% of classic families with more than one affected family member or classic sporadic patients with multiple VHL related tumors. The mutation spectrum is heterogeneous. The commonest (40%) mutations are missense mutations followed by microdeletions, large deletions, insertions, splice site or nonsense mutations

What are the clinical subtypes of VHL disease?

There are 4 subtypes

Type I : without pheochromocytoma
Type II : with pheochromocytoma
IIA : PCC with HB(CNS)
IIB : PCC with RCC with HB (CNS)
IIC : only PCC

How do you suspect VHL clinically in a patient?

Patients with positive FH: If the patient has a typical VHL tumor such as retinal, spinal or cerebellar HB, or RCC, PCC, multiple pancreatic cysts or endolymphatic tumors
Patients with negative FH: VHL should be suspected when they exhibit two or more HB or a single HB with either RCC or PCC.

What are the characteristics of PCC associated with different syndromes?

Characteristics	*VHL*	*MEN2*	*NF-1*	*PGL*
Gene	VHL	RET	NF-1	SDHD, SDHB, SDHC
Chromosome	3p25-26	10q11.2	17q11	11q23
Exons	3	21	59	4-8
Typical tumor	Adrenal and extra-adrenal	Adrenal	Adrenal and extra-adrenal	Adrenal, extra-adrenal, thoracic, head and neck para-ganglionoma
Associated lesion	CNS hemangio-blastomas, RCC, etc	MTC, PHPT, ganglio-neruoma	Neurofibromas, pigmented spots, Lisch-nodes of Irish nodules	No
Malignant potential	<5%	<5%	No	High
Hormone secretion	NE	E + NE	–	–
Age	<30 years	–	–	–
Symptoms	Fewer			
Bilaterality, mutlifocality	High	High	–	–

How can you confirm the clinical diagnosis of VHL?

This can be done by mutation analysis of VHL gene

Persons eligible for VHL gene mutation analysis

- Patients with classic VHL disease and/or first degree family members
- A person from a family in which VHL gene mutation has been identified
- A VHL-suspected patient, i.e.
  - a multicentric tumor in one organ,
  - bilateral tumor,
  - two organ system affected,
  - one VHL-associated tumor at young age (<50 years for HB, PCC and <30 years for RCC)

What should be the protocol for evaluation of a suspected VHL disease?

Protocol for VHL

- Ophthalmoscopy
- MRI of brain
- MRI of spinal cord
- MRI of abdomen
- Plasma free metanephrine/24 hour catecholamine measurement
- 24 hour BP monitoring
- Audiometry
- USG of testis
- Thyroid function tests
- DOPA or dopamine-PET

Protocol for MEN 2A/MEN 2B

- Stimulated calcitonin assay
- Serum calcium
- Serum intact PTH

Protocol for PGL syndromes

- MRI of skull base and neck
- MRI thorax
- MRI abdomen
- Plasma free metanephrine
- DOPA or dopamine PET

Protocol for NF-Type I

- Ophthalmoscopy
- Skin investigations

How do you establish the biochemical diagnosis of pheochromocytoma in VHL?

Measurement of plasma free metanephrine promises to be the best screening biochemical test for familial PCC because of high sensitivity (97%) and good specificity (90%). This provides early detection before signs and symptoms occur, when tumors are small and not secreting large amounts of catecholamines.

How does the treatment of familial pheochromocytoma differ from sporadic pheochromocytoma?

Pheochromocytoma and paraganglionoma, although rare, pose a significant threat because of sudden and unsuspected release of catecholamines particularly in the perioperative and postoperative periods. Their lesions, though small can suddenly become symptomatic and life threatening at the time of any surgery for another VHL tumor. Hence, it is recommended that pheochromocytoma be tackled first before the hemangioblastoma. Previously bilateral adrenalectomy in bilateral tumors and unilateral adrenalectomy for unilateral tumors were the gold standard.

However, because of the absence of adrenomedullary hyperplasia and low malignant potential as well as reported low recurrence rate, cortical sparing adrenal surgery, open or laparoscopic, is now the preferred approach. Centralized multi-disciplinary approach, because of the accompanying risk due to spinal or brain HB, is needed whenever operating a pheochromocytoma associated with VHL.

Routine prophylactic bilateral adrenalectomy is not warranted in familial PCC.

What determines the prognosis in VHL?

The prognosis is mainly determined by RCC and HB. RCC is the main tumor that metastasizes to other organs in VHL disease. Secondly, morbidity resulting from postoperative complications is caused by spinal cord/cerebellar HB.

Chapter 53

Unusual Presentation of Pheochromocytoma: Patient Presenting with Hemiparesis

CASE STUDY

A 22-year-old boy was detected to be hypertensive 2 years back during a routine medical evaluation for purpose of going overseas. Further evaluation at that time revealed LVH on CXR, positive TMT, and hypoechoic lesion inferior to right lobe of liver on USG and hypertensive retinopathy. He took irregular treatment for hypertension. Two years later he suddenly developed hemiparesis while going to sleep and was bedridden for 10 days. CT scan done at that time revealed a massive left basal ganglia bleed. Following this, patient recovered and became ambulant but with mild diminution of power and some residual speech defect. Patient was subsequently referred to us for management of

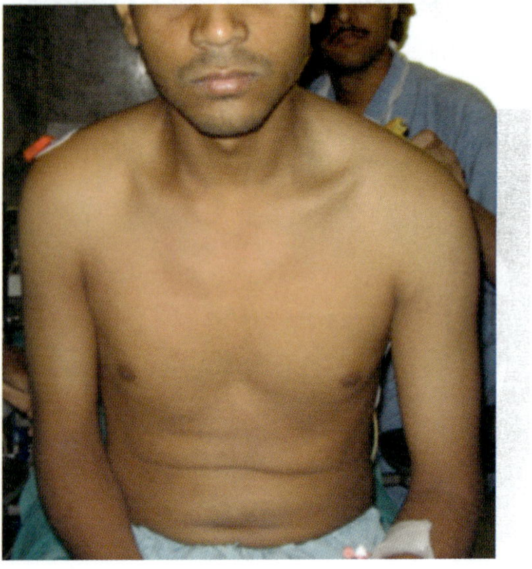

Fig. 53.1: Young hypertensive patient with right hemiparesis

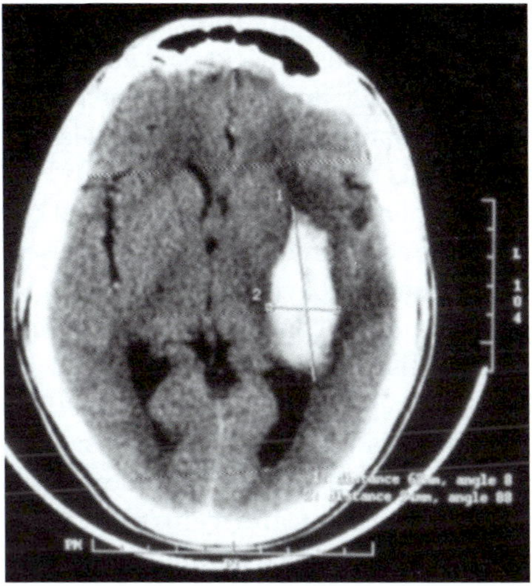

Fig. 53.2: CT head showing massive left basal ganglia bleed

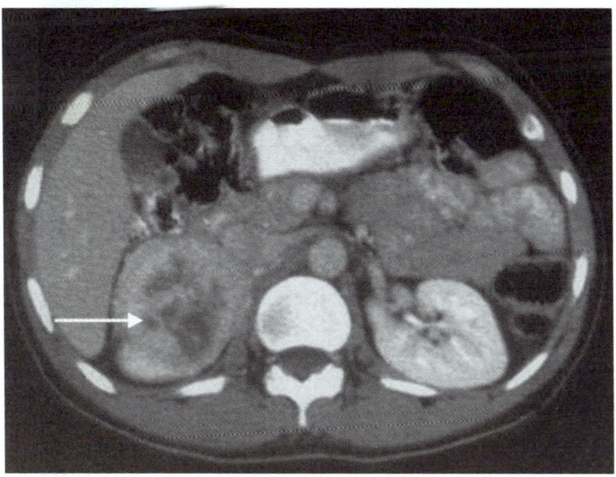

Fig. 53.3: CECT abdomen showing large right adrenal mass with central necrosis (arrow)

his hypertension and evaluation of adrenal mass. At presentation to us he was conscious, mildly aphasic with a standing BP of 160/120 and supine BP of 180/120 mmHg with normal pulses and no radio-femoral delay. There were no neurocutaneous markers. Cardiomegaly was present along with a systolic murmur. A neurological consultation was sought but no active intervention was advised. A strong suspicion of pheochromocytoma was kept. In view of his resolving stroke, urgent control of his blood pressure was given priority. His medication was altered in order to prepare him for metanephrine testing. Beta blocker was stopped and he was put on vasodilators. A CECT was ordered which revealed a large right adrenal mass with peripheral enhancement and central hypodense area suggestive of pheochromocytoma. Echocardiography revealed concentric LVH, normal LV size and systolic function but with diastolic dysfunction. Serum chemistry revealed normal blood sugar and potassium levels. After stabilization of his blood pressure he was discharged and advised to come for metanephrine testing after two weeks. Patient was readmitted after two weeks for 24 hour urine collection for metanephrine estimation which was found to be elevated, 4774 microgram/24 hours. His thyroid was not enlarged and serum calcium and calcitonin were estimated to rule out MEN association and were found to be normal. Patient was put on alpha-blockade with prazopress for18 days with a maximum dose of 20 mg. Beta blockers were added a day prior to surgery. He underwent unilateral adrenalectomy via the transperitoneal route using a right subcostal incision. Intra-operatively maximum blood pressure elevation was seen on tumor manipulation (180/120 mmHg) and following adrenal vein ligation his BP dropped to 90/70 mmHg). Hypertensive peaks were managed by Sodium Nitroprusside infusion. Post-operative hypotension was managed by infusing colloid like blood and plasma. Grossly the tumor was globular, encapsulated, measuring 9 × 6 × 4.5 cm, weighing 150 gm and cut surface revealed hemorrhagic areas with myxoid tumor and compressed peripheral adrenal tissue. The microscopic picture showed intermediate to large polygonal cells arranged in well-defined nests (Zellballen) bounded by a fibrovascular stroma. Tumor cells varied in size and shape and had finely granular basophilic or amphophilic cytoplasm. The nuclei were round to oval with coarsely clumped chromatin and a single prominent nucleolus. Nuclear pseudoinclusions and intracytoplasmic hyaline globules were also seen. Some of the tumor cells showed nuclear pleomorphism and hyperchromasia. The areas of hemorrhage, necrosis and foci of lymphocytic infiltrate were also seen in the stroma.

QUESTIONS

Which are the drugs that interfere with the biochemical estimation of metanephrine/catecholamine?

- Tricyclic antidepressants block norepinephrine reuptake, causing rise in plasma and urinary norepinephrine, normetanephrine, and VMA
- Phenoxybenzamine blocks presynaptic alpha-2 adrenoreceptors, causing increases in plasma and urinary norepinephrine, normetanephrine, and VMA

- Monoamine oxidase inhibitors blocks deamination, causing up to five-fold increases in plasma and urinary metanephrines
- Levodopa is metabolised by enzymes that also convert catecholamines
- Alpha-methyldopa is metabolised by enzymes that also convert catecholamines
- ***Stimulants (e.g. Caffeine, nicotine):*** Increase plasma and urinary catecholamines.
- ***Sympathomimetics:*** Increase plasma and urinary catecholamines (e.g. Amphetamines, ephidrine)
- ***Calcium-channel blockers:*** Increase plasma catecholamines due to sympathetic activation (dehydropyridines)

What is the etiology of a stroke in a patient of pheochromocytoma?

The nature of the cerebrovascular disease that results in stroke includes possibilities like:

i. emboli from a cardiac source (if the patient is having dilated cardiomyopathy with mural thrombus),
ii. thrombosis in situ,
iii. intracranial hemorrhage due to severe or malignant hypertension,
iv. cerebral infarction as a result of enhanced coagulation, vasopspasm or both due to catecholamine effects, and
v. rarely due to cerebrovascular diseases such as fibromuscular hyperplasia and complex migraine.

What is the pathophysiology of stroke in pheochromocytoma?

Cerebral vasospasm can be either due to excess catecholamine or secondary to the other secretory products of the adrenal tumor such as neuropeptide –Y. Vascular spasm in peripheral, coronary and cerebral arteries has been induced with sympathomimetic agents, either intentionally as in the treatment of epistaxis or as an unintended complication of use of these agents. In fact, cerebral infarct and gangrene of the extremities secondary to vasospasm has been reported in some patients with pheochromocytoma. Spasm is known to cause either transient impairment of circulation or infarcts with reversible dementia. Patient may have multiple infarcts corresponding to paroxysm of hypertension.

What is the recovery pattern of these patients?

Usually there is complete recovery even after documented infarct in the brain. However, such patients should undergo evaluation and treatment for pheochromocytoma as early as possible to avoid a rebleed.

Chapter 54

Unusual Presentation of Pheochromocytoma: Fainting during Micturition

CASE STUDY

A 40-year-old male presented with history of headache for last one year. Headache was holocranial, throbbing type and intermittent. The frequency of headache was once in a week but lasted for hours. During one of these episodes of headache, he was found to be having high blood pressure (240/140 mm of Hg) and was started on antihypertensives. Blood pressure was not controlled on even maximum doses of three antihypertensives. He also complained of spasmodic pain for the last four months, mainly in hypogastric region with no localizing symptoms. He also complained of fainting during micturition, especially whenever he strained. There was no family history of hypertension. He underwent

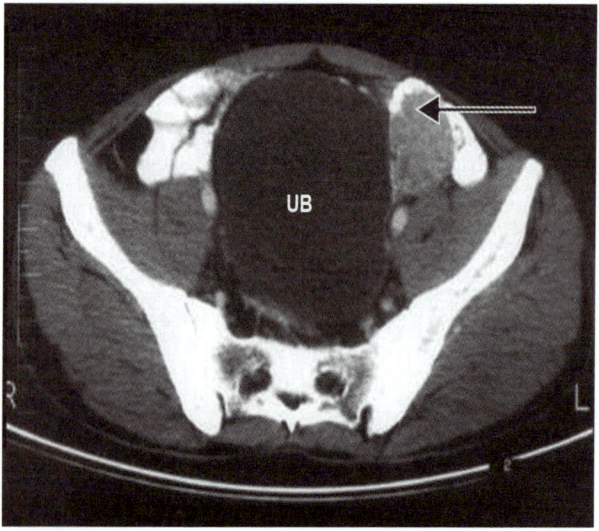

Fig. 54.1: CT showing mass (arrow) arising from left wall of Urinary bladder (UB)

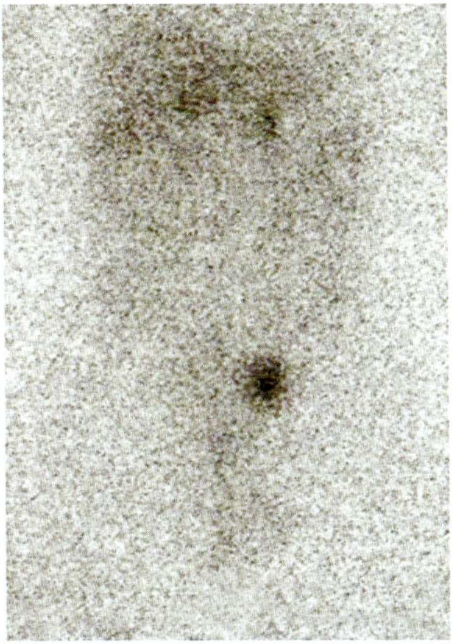

Fig. 54.2: MIBG scan showing increased focus of uptake in the area of lcft wall of urinary bladder

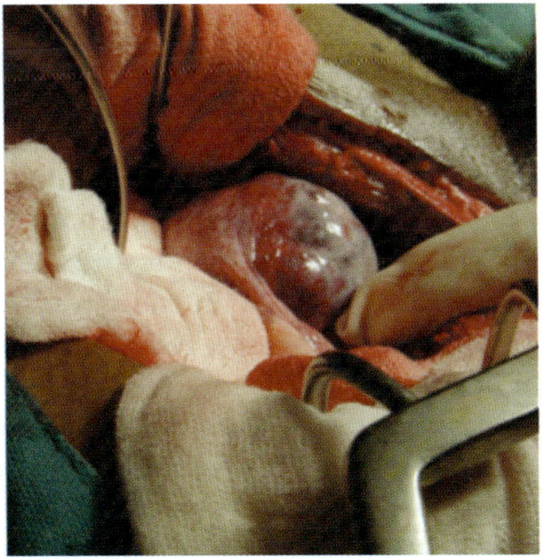

Fig. 54.3: Intraoperative photograph showing mass from UB

ultrasound examination of the abdomen that showed 46.3 x 38.8 mm, well circumscribed hypoechoic lesion in left half of urinary bladder showing moderate vascularity. CT scan showed mass arising from the left pelvic region possibly arising from urinary bladder wall. Both adrenals were normal. 24 hr urinary VMA was 19.32 mg/g of creatinine (normal 1.6-4.2). Total urinary norepinephrine (1088.91 µg/24 hr (12.1-85.5)) and dopamine (663.98 µg/L (65-400)) were also elevated. MIBG whole body scan was done after 600 µCi of I 131 MIBG which showed increasesd tracer uptake in the left suprapubic region. There was normal whole body tracer uptake including the adrenal glands. Bladder mucosa was free from the tumor on cystoscopic examination but increased vascularity was noted on left wall of bladder. He was preoperatively blocked with alpha blocker prazopress for 12 days and he required maximum doses of 15 mg of prazopress for adequate alpha blockade. Bladder was approached through extraperitoneal approach after midline incision. A well encapsulated tumor (5.5 × 4 × 3 cm, weight 46 gm), brownish red colour tumor at the dome and left wall of bladder was seen. Peritoneum was invaded at the dome of diaphragm, hence a partial cystectomy (full thickness excision) of the dome of urinary bladder was done with primary repair. Intraoperative hemodynamic changes were noticed with maximum blood pressure of 200/120 mm of Hg which was managed with sodium nitroprusside infusion. Minimum blood pressure recorded was 90/50 mm Hg after surgical excision.

Histopathology examination showed encapsulated tumor with cells arranged in variably sized nests separated by thin fibrovascular septae. Tumor cells displayed round to oval nuclei with finely granular chromatin, inconspicuous nucleoli and moderate amount of granular eosionophilic cytoplasm. Occasional mitotic figures were evident. There was no evidence of capsular or vascular invasion. Postoperatively he required single antihypertensive for adequate control of blood pressure.

QUESTIONS

What is the origin of pheochromocytoma of the bladder?

It is a rare tumor that accounts for less than 1% of all cases of total pheochromocytoma. It can arise from the chromaffin tissue of the sympathetic nervous system within any of the layers of the bladder wall.

When should it be suspected?

Hematuria and intermittent hypertension during micturition are the usual symptoms. Still they can have diagnostic dilemma for localization when they present with classical symptoms of pheochromocytoma due to raised catecholamines such as hypertension, headache and flushing.

They frequently produce a characteristic syndrome in that a typical paroxysmal attack usually occurs during or shortly after micturition or with distension of bladder due to liberation of catecholamines by compression of tumor.

In addition to classical symptoms of pheochromocytoma, postmicturition syncope and hematuria are also present. Approximately half of the patients do not have classical symptoms and are suspected when patient has inadvertent change in blood pressure during surgical procedures.

How do you establish the biochemical diagnosis?

The diagnosis of pheochromocytoma is based on elevated 24 hr urine catecholamines (epinephrine and norepinephrine) or their metabolites (metanephrine, normetanephrine and vanillyl mandelic acid). Plasma metanephrine is considered to be more sensitive than plasma catecholamine measurement.

Is it necessary to perform localization studies?

Anatomical localization of tumor is required after biochemical confirmation of pheochromocytoma. It is necessary because of variable location of tumor and in preparation for surgical excision of tumor. USG and CT can localize the tumor only if size of tumor is greater than 1 cm. MRI is now replacing CT because of its diagnostic accuracy, non-invasive nature and because it avoids the possible risk of hypertensive crisis that may be precipitated by intravenous contrast medium. I^{131} MIBG is considered superior to CT and MRI in diagnosis and localizing of tumor. Some have recommended I^{123} for better image quality and short exposure. I^{131} and I^{123} MIBG have a molecular structure resembling that of norepinephrine and specifically localizes in adrenergic tissue. Although highly specific (95 to 100%) for pheochromocytoma, MIBG scintigraphy, which requires imaging for 24 to 48 hour period, has demonstrated only moderate sensitivity (77 to 90%).

What is the surgical management?

The treatment of paraganglioma of the urinary bladder is essentially surgical. The preferred approach is tumor excision with partial cystectomy. Total cystectomy is performed only in cases of infiltrative or multiple tumors. Paragangliomas are generally considered to be radio and chemoresistant. Chemotherapy has been tried with variable success including combination of etopside, 5-FU and cisplatin.

What is the prognosis?

Most paraganglioma follow a benign clinical course, only 10% being malignant. Local recurrence or metastases have been reported to occur as late as 30 years after surgery, with regional lymph nodes, lungs and bones being the commonest sites.

Chapter 55

Pheochromocytoma Presenting with Glycosuria

CASE STUDY

A 32-year-old lady presented with complaints of polyuria and nocturia. Her subsequent investigations revealed significant glycosuria, though her fasting and post-prandial glucose values were normal. An ultrasound abdomen was asked for which revealed a cystic adrenal mass of the right adrenal gland, measuring 7.6 × 5.4 cm. She was then referred to us for further management. On history taking she complained of retrosternal chest pain for last 3 months with no other significant history. Subsequent hormonal evaluation revealed elevated 24-hour urinary metanephrine and a diagnosis of pheochromocytoma was made and she was put on alpha blockade in preparation for surgery.

QUESTIONS

What abnormalities of blood sugar metabolism can be associated with pheochromocytoma?

These are:

- fasting hyperglycemia
- impaired glucose tolerance, and
- glycosuria

However, these abnormalities are usually mild to moderate in severity.

What is the pathogenesis of glucose intolerance associated with pheochromocytoma?

The underlying mechanisms could be:

- Inhibitory effect of epinephrine on insulin stimulated glucose uptake by skeletal muscles.

- Catecholamine- induced suppression of insulin secretion
- Direct stimulation of hepatic glucose synthesis by alpha stimulation
- Decreased peripheral sensitivity to insulin due to elevated plasma Free Fatty Acids (FFA).

Is development of ketoacidosis common in pheochromocytoma?

Ketoacidosis rarely develops in patients with pheochromocytoma because adequate endogeneous insulin is present.

Does the blood glucose abnormalities revert after removal of pheochromocytoma?

Patients become normoglycemic after removal of pheochromocytoma.

Chapter 56

Pheochromocytoma Presenting as Orthostatic Hypotension

CASE STUDY

A 23-year-old male presented with history of postural giddiness and blurred vision for last 2 months. Each episode lasted for 10-20 min and he had 3-5 episodes per day. He gave the history of severe giddiness the moment he tried to sit up or stand. He was found to be hypertensive but he was not on any medication. There was discrepancy in blood pressure measurements in both upper limbs-BP in right upper limb was 110/90 mmHg while in left limb was 130/110. Also while recumbent his BP was 220/160 while on sitting position it was 110/90. He was carrying an ultrasound which revealed a retroperitoneal mass in the aortocaval region; however, no comment was made on the adrenal glands. He had also undergone a urinary VMA measurement which was reported as normal with a value of 5.8mg/day (normal range was upto 7.1 mg/day). On examination he was found be severely emaciated and a vague mass could be felt in the epigastric and umbilical region. The impression was a young hypertensive with orthostatic hypotension and possibility of pheochromocytoma was kept. 24 hour urinary metanephrine was done which was found to be significantly elevated, 12.39 mg/24 hrs. CECT taking 5 and 8 mm sections was done which revealed bilateral normal adrenals along with a large, 4.7 × 3 × 5 cm hypodense mass in the retroperitoneum between IVC and aorta at the level of left renal hilum with enhancing vessels around the mass. MIBG scanning was done which revelaed increased radiotracer concentration in the retroperitoneum. Workup for hereditary pheochromo-cytoma was found to be normal. A diagnosis of sporadic extra-adrenal pheochromocytoma was made and the patient was explored via the transperitoneal route using

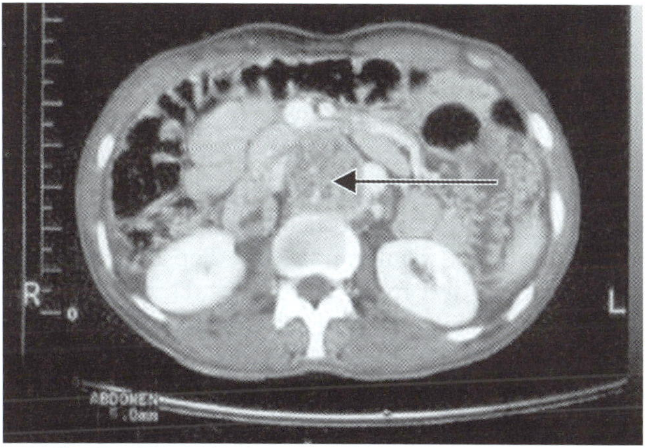

Fig. 56.1: Large, 4.7 x 3 x 5 cm hypodense mass in the retroperitoneum between IVC and aorta at the level of left renal hilum (arrow)

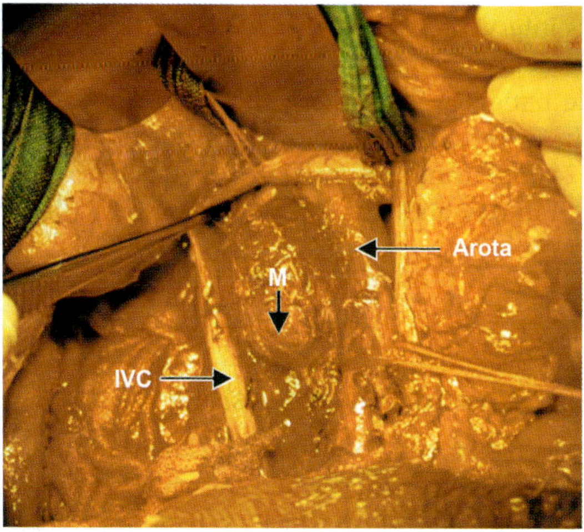

Fig. 56.2: Intraoperative photograph showing the inter aorto-caval mass (M)

a roof-top incision with a superior midline extension (Mercedes Benz incisions). Left colon, spleen, pancreas were rotated medially. Left kidney mobilized and left renal vein identified arching over the tumor. The root of mesentry was opened and right colon also mobilized to visualize the IVC. Superior mesenteric artery identified and preserved. Tumor dissected off the IVC and aorta after repairing two rents in the IVC with 5-0 prolene suture. The hemodynamic alteration included hypertensive peaks during tumor manipulation to the extent of 230 mmHg systolic and 140 mmHg diastolic. After tumor removal patient developed hypotension (90/50 mmHg) which was managed by giving colloids in the form of blood transfusion and plasma. In the postoperative period for the first 24 hours his CVP was kept around 12-14 cm by giving him large quantities of crystalloids and colloids. His blood sugar was monitored at 2 hours interval for the first 10 hours and then at 4 hourly interval. Subsequent postoperative period was uneventful and the patient was discharged on the10th postoperative day. The histopatho-logy was suggestive of a paraganglio-noma. 24 hour urinary estimation of metanephrine was done on the 10th day and was found to be normal, 0.58 mg/24 hrs.

QUESTIONS

What is orthostatic hypotension?

The blood pressure in both the sitting and standing position may be much lower than when the patient is recumbent. Such patients usually give a history of giddiness or fainting attacks on sitting or standing up. Orthostatic hypotension in a patient who is not on any hypertensive medication is suggestive of pheochromocytoma.

What is the pathophysiology of patients of pheochromocytoma presenting with orthostatic hypotension?

The two major factors responsible for this pathophysiology are : diminished blood volume and suppressed sympathetic reflexes. Excessive circulating catecholamines depress the sympathetic reflex that maintains the blood pressure in the upright position. The drop in blood pressure is usually to normotensive levels or sometimes below it.

Chapter 57

Pheochromocytoma Presenting as Unexplained Shock

CASE STUDY

A 44-year-old man was admitted in the intensive cardiac unit with shock syndrome. Investigations revealed severe lactic acidosis, hyperglycemia and myocardial damage. He was managed by volume therapy and high doses of dobutamine and noradrenaline. However, despite aggressive vasopressor and volume therapy overt left ventricular failure persisted. Abdominal imaging to exclude aortic dissection revealed a 5 cm right adrenal mass. The endocrinologist was consulted and intravenous alpha blockade therapy was started which resulted in hemodynamic stabilization and gradual recovery. Subsequent 24 hour urinary metanephrine estimation was done and was found to be elevated. A diagnosis of pheochromocytoma was made and patient was planned for surgery.

QUESTIONS

What is the pathophysiology of this unexplained shock or circulatory collapse?

Rarely pheochromocytoma can present as profound circulatory shock; hence clinicians should remember that unexplained circulatory collapse may signal an unrecognized pheochromocytoma. The underlying pathophysiology could be:

i. Hemorrhage or necrosis within a large pheochromocytoma
ii. Retroperitoneal hemorrhage secondary to a ruptured adrenal gland

iii. Following severe and prolonged hypertensive crisis. It is possible that a marked decrease in circulating catecholamines at the termination of a paroxysm of hypertension may result in a state of inadequate vasoconstriction, the so called "epinephrine shock". Various other factors contribute to this circulatory collapse, viz.
- Reduced cardiac output
- Arrhythmias
- Myocardial damage
- Low plasma volume
- Desensitization of cardiovascular receptors to excessive catecholamine
- Profound release of vasodilator substances.

How does such a patient present?

A patient who presents with unexplained shock would have significant abdominal pain, signs of pulmonary edema, intense mydriasis, profound weakness, diaphoresis, cyanosis, hyperglycemia and leucocytosis. The symptoms are so profound so as to suggest a diagnosis of adrenal insufficiency.

What is the management of such a situation?

It is a challenging situation. The following should be instituted:

1. Volume replacement
2. Early institution of alpha-1 adrenergic receptors
3. Correction of metabolic acidosis
4. Careful monitoring of intra-arterial BP, CVP monitoring, arterial pH, blood gases and ECG.

5. If digitalis is indicated it should be kept in mind that myocardium of such patients is already sensitized by excessive circulating catecholamines
6. CT scan as early as possible to localize the pheochromocytoma
7. 24 hour urinary metanephrine/plasma metanephrine as soon as the patient stabilizes and the stress is abolished
8. Early surgery

Chapter 58

Extra-adrenal Pheochromocytoma

CASE STUDY

A 45-year-old lady was being operated for a retroperitoneal mass by a general surgeon when she developed hypertensive crisis and pulmonary edema during surgery which had to be then aborted. She was then referred to us for further management. On history taking it was revealed that she had history of episodes of headache, sweating and palpitations for one year. However, she was never found to be hypertensive. She had then also noticed an abdominal lump for which an USG was done which showed a retroperitoneal mass. IVP done at that time showed deviation of the left ureter consistent with a left retroperitoneal mass. There was no other positive history and her family history was also not contributory. On examination, she was found to be normotensive, there were no neurocutaneous lesions and

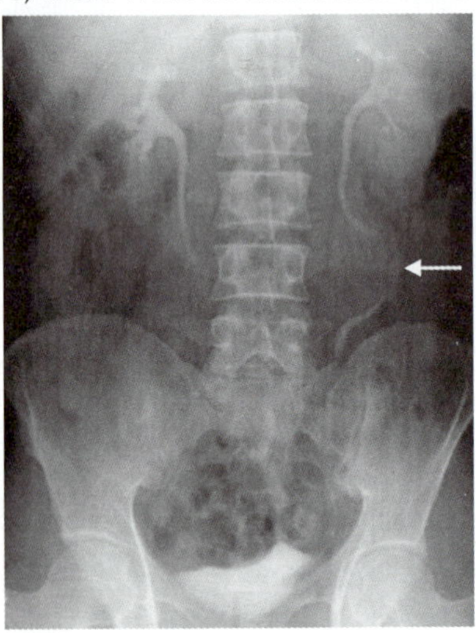

Fig. 58.1: IVP showing deviation of the left ureter consistent with a left retroperitoneal mass (arrow)

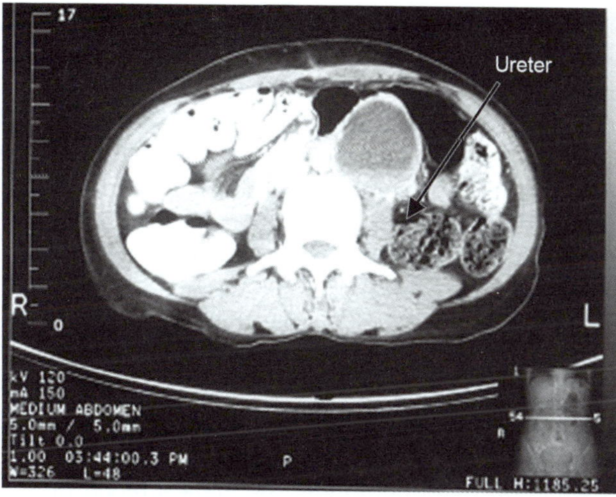

Fig. 58.2: Non enhancing hypodense lesion 5.1 x 4.7 cm with mild enhancing periphery in the left para-aortic region anterior to left ureter

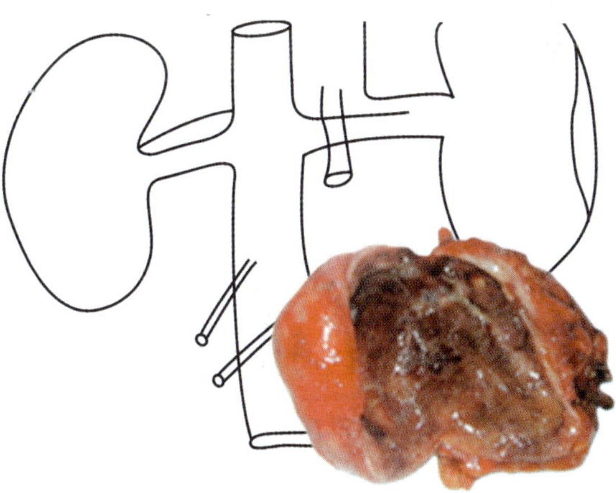

Fig. 58.3: Operative specimen

no thyroid swelling. Examination of the abdomen revealed a well-healed midline scar and a firm, well-defined 4 × 4 cm lump in the left hypochondrium. A CECT was asked for which showed a non-enhancing hypodense lesion, 5.1 × 4.7 cm with mild enhancing periphery in the left para-aortic region anterior to left ureter. Both adrenal glands appeared normal. Both 24 hour urinary metanephrine (227 mcg) and normetanephrine (328 mcg) were elevated. A diagnosis of extra-adrenal pheochromocytoma was made and she was put on alpha blockade for 12 days with maximum dose of prazosin of 11 mg. She was explored by a separate left oblique muscle cutting incision. At surgery the extra-adrenal pheochromocytoma was found to be arising from the organ of Zuckerkandl. It was highly vascular and the left ureter was stretched over the tumor. The highest blood pressure recording was 180/100 mmHg while after the excision of the tumor the BP fell to 82/42 mmHg. The postoperative period was uneventful and the histopathology confirmed the diagnosis of pheochromocytoma.

QUESTIONS

What are the sites of extra-adrenal pheochromocytoma?

Twenty percent of pheochromocytoma are extra-adrenal. Extra-adrenal pheochromocytoma can be divided into:

- Functioning : 95%
- Non-functioning: 5% (also known as paraganglinomas)

Functioning extra-adrenal pheochromocytoma

The distribution is as follows:

- Abdomen : 85%

- Thoracic : 10%
- Head and neck : 1%
- Bladder : < 5%

The abdominal extra-adrenal pheochromocytoma can be either suprarenal or infrarenal in location. The common sites are the perihilar, Para-aortic, interaorto-caval and the organ of Zuckerkandl.

What are characteristics of extra-adrenal pheochromocytoma?

- Multicentricity is high, 20-25%
- More common in children 20%
- Malignancy is higher, 20%
- Secrete exclusively NE
- Usually smaller in size
- MIBG is the best imaging modality to localize the tumor

What precautions should be taken while operating upon extra-adrenal pheochromocytoma?

- Because of anatomic location and surrounding vital structures, laparoscopic removal may be difficult.
- Infra-renal pheochromocytoma is intimately related to the ureter and one should be careful while dissecting. Usually there is a plane of cleavage and ureter can be separated out. If on CT there is no plane between the extra-adrenal pheochromocytoma and the ureter, one can put a ureteric stent just prior to exploratory laparotomy.
- While dissecting and removing the extra-adrenal pheochromocytoma, care should be taken to do a reasonably wide excision of tumor and its surrounding tissue to avoid fragmentation and subsequent implantation and recurrence.

What is organ of Zuckerkandl?

It is a collection of chromaffin cells located anterior to abdominal aorta just above its bifurcation and extending to origin of inferior mesentric artery. Extra-adrenal pheochromocytoma arising from the organ of Zuckerkandl unlike those of other extra-adrenal sites does secrete epinephrine because it contains the enzyme PNMT. It is one of the commonest location of extra-adrenal pheochromocytoma.

Chapter 59

Paraganglioma

CASE STUDY

A 70-year-old man presented with history of gradually increasing swelling in the left submandibular region for last 8 months. On examination, he was found to be normotensive and local examination revealed a 8 × 8 cm lump in the submandibular triangle which was bidigitally palpable, had limited mobility, was firm in consistency and was non-tender. There were no neck nodes. Clinical impression of submandibular carcinoma was made and FNAC was ordered which was suggestive of low-grade adenocarcinoma. CECT was done which revealed a infiltrating mass in the submandibular region showing central necrosis along with mild destruction of a part of hyoid bone. He was taken up for surgery. Intraoperative findings included a normal, though bulky submandibular gland and a large mass deep to the submandibular gland extending upto the digastric muscle and the hypoglossal nerve was stretched over the tumor. Excision of the mass along with removal of the submandibular gland was done. The histopathology was suggestive of paraganglionoma and the detailed report was as follows: Sections from the swelling outside the submandibular gland show the structure of an encapsulated tumor composed of polygonal cells disposed in nests separated by highly vascularized fibrous septae. The tumor cells display abundant eosinophilic granular cytoplasm and mildly pleomorphic nuclei with stippled to peripherally marginated chromatin and small nucleoli. Occasional mitotic figures and areas of hemorrhage are present. There is no evidence of vascular invasion. Sections from the submandibular gland show lobules of seromucinous acini displaying focal parenchymal atrophy and lymphoid

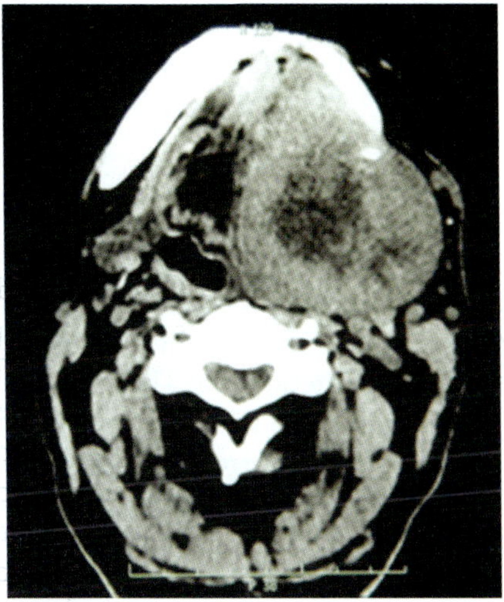

Fig. 59.1: Infiltrating mass in the submandibular region showing central necrosis along with destruction of a part of hyoid bone

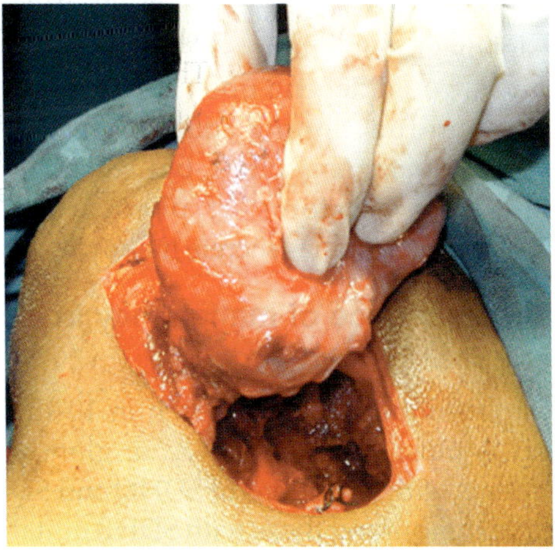

Fig. 59.2: Intraoperative photograph

aggregates. There is presence of periductal fibrosis accompanied by focal ductal dilatation and inspissated secretions.

QUESTIONS

What are paragangliomas?

These are vascular neuroendocrine tumors developing in the extra-adrenal paraganglion tissue along the sympathetic and/or the parasympathetic chain.The commonest of these are the carotid body tumors followed by those developing in jugular bulb (gloumus juglare), tympanic plexus (globus tympanicum) and the vagal nerve (gloumus vagale), paranasal sinuses, sympathetic ganglia and larynx as well as host of other sites.

What is the clinical presentation of Paragangliomas?

These are slowly growing tumors but are locally aggressive and symptoms would depend upon the site of origin. Most of these are non-functioning tumors, particularly the parasympathetic paragangliomas, but some may present with signs and symptoms of pheochromocytoma. Functioning paragangliomas secrete mainly noradrenaline.

What is the incidence of malignancy in paragangliomas?

Malignant transformation can be seen in 10-15% of these tumors and is most commonly seen in glomus jugulare tumors. Patients with mutations of SDHD and SDHB genes have multiple tumors and those with SDHB mutations have a high incidence of malignant tumors.

What is the management of paragangliomas?

Localization is done with CT and MRI of thorax and the neck. If anatomical imaging is negative, functional imaging should be done. PET with fluoro DOPA is superior in imaging neck paragangliomas.Though surgery is the main stay of the treatment, it is associated with considerable morbidity in the form of cranial nerve palsies. The other forms of treatment which are effective are radiotherapy and treatment with radiopharmaceuticals like MIBG.

Chapter 60

Normotensive Pheochromocytoma

CASE STUDY

A 20-year-old girl was referred with an ultrasound finding of a right adrenal mass. She gave history of headache off and on for last one year, associated with giddiness and vomiting. She also had epigastric pain associated with nausea and vomiting with history of significant weight loss. There was no other significant personal or family history. On examination she was found to be normotensive with no postural drop. There were no other significant findings. A clinical diagnosis of adrenal incidnentaloma was made. Her hormonal profile revealed suppressible ONDST, normal serum potassium values, but her 24 urinary metanephrine was very high, 11.54 mcg/24 hrs (normal: upto 1.0 mcg/24 hr). CECT was aksed for which revealed a 4.2 × 4.4 right

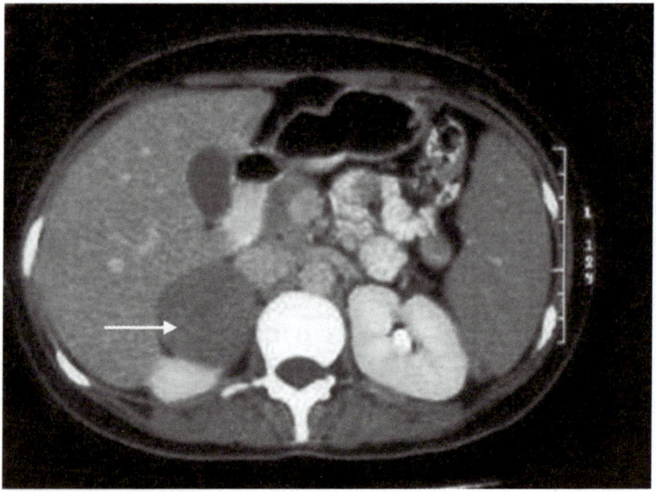

Fig. 60.1: CECT showing right adrenal mass in a normotensive patient (arrow)

adrenal mass. She was then put on alpha blockade for 12 days with maximum doses of prazosin of 16 mg/day. She was taken up for surgery via a transperitoneal approach and right adrenalectomy was performed. During surgery, hemodynamic alteration did occur in the form of hypertension with maximum BP recording of 210/160 mmHg. She developed hypotension following tumor excision with BP of 62/40 mmHg which was managed by volume expansion and vasopressors.

QUESTIONS

What is normotensive pheochromocytoma and what is the prevalence?

The term normotensive pheochromocytoma, also known as subclinical pheochromocytoma refers to the situation in which a biochemical and histopathological proven pheochromocytoma is totally asymptomatic in a normotensive patient. Historically, 10% of all pheochromo-cytoma are thought to be normotensive but recent series suggest the figure may be around 20-24%.

What is the pathophysiology of normotensive pheochromocytoma?

The resulting hypertension in a pheochromocytoma is a consequence of different combination and concentration of hormones released by pheochromocytoma. Normotension in a patient may be due to a combination of factors, viz.

i. Such patients have low blood volume due to persistent vasoconstriction.

ii. Due to down regulation or desensitization of cardiovascular receptors (decrease in number as well as sensitivity) so that the catecholamine response is blunted.
iii. Increased rate of catecholamine inactivation.
iv. The predominant secretion by the tumor may be vasodilator compounds like dopamine, calcitonin gene-related peptide, VIP, adrenomedullin, metenkephalin, atrial natriuretic peptide and neuropeptide Y.
v. If the predominant catecholamine secreted by the tumor in epinephrine patient is likely to be normotensive.

Do these patients need to be prepared with alpha blockade prior to surgery?

It is important to realize that even normotensive pheochromocytoma may produce profound intraoperative hemodynamic alterations, sometimes as explosive as the hypertensive ones; hence it is essential that all such patients should receive alpha blockade prior to surgery as is applicable to hypertensive pheochromocytoma. Certain points, however, need to be kept in mind. Normotensive patients can be better prepared with calcium channel blockers as these do not cause profound hypotension after surgery. Also, the endpoint of alpha blockade is difficult to determine in such patients but one should always try to avoid excessive blockade.

Chapter 61

Adrenal Incidentaloma

CASE STUDY

A 40-year-old lady presented with history of an episode of severe abdominal pain for which she had undergone an USG examination of abdomen which revealed a right suprarenal mass, 7.5 × 6.0 cm. She was never detected to be hypertensive and also gave no history of episodes of palpitation, headache or increased sweating. She did not have any features of Cushing's syndrome and she did not have any proximal muscle weakness. On examination she did not have any neurocutaneous markers and was normotensive. She was further evaluated by hormonal work-up and CECT. Her overnight dexamethasone suppression test was negative,

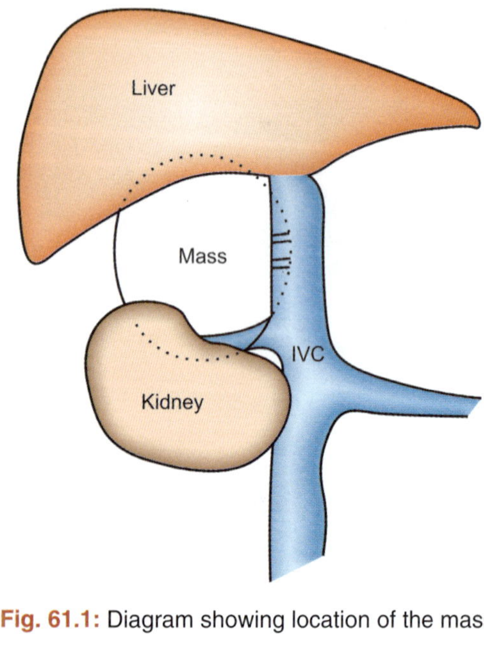

Fig. 61.1: Diagram showing location of the mass

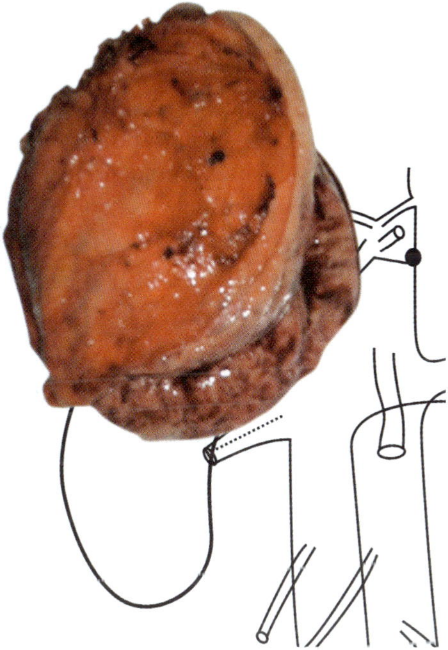

Fig. 61.2: Operative specimen of incidentally detected pheochromocytoma

serum potassium was within normal limits but 24 hour urinary metanephrines were very high (477 microg/24 hrs). CECT revealed evidence of large hypodense mass, 7.5 × 6.5 × 7.0 cm (30-35 HU) containing eccentric calcification. Mild contrast enhancement was seen in the tumor (30 HU) with few non-enhancing areas. Mass was seen displacing liver, kidney, duodenum and IVC but no obvious infiltration was seen. Left adrenal was normal in size and shape. A diagnosis of normotensive pheochromocytoma was made and she was explored via the transperitoneal route using a right subcostal incision. Right unilateral adrenalectomy was done an a 8 × 8 × 6 cm mass was removed which weighed 200 gm. During surgery, maximum BP was 210/130 mmHg which was managed by NTG. At closure, hypotension was observed (BP: 90/50 mmHg) which was managed by nor adrenaline. The postoperative period was uneventful and the histopathology was confirmatory of pheochromocytoma. Postoperative metanephrine estimated at the 10th day became normal.

QUESTIONS

How do you define adrenal incidentaloma?

An adrenal incidentaloma is an adrenal mass that is inadvertently discovered during a radiological examination performed for indications other than for an evaluation of adrenal disease. The definition excludes patients undergoing imaging procedures as a part of staging and workup for cancer.

The probability of finding an adrenal incidentaloma increases with age.

Why should adrenal incidentaloma be further evaluated?

1. To determine whether the lesion is hormonally active or nonfunctioning.
2. To determine whether it is benign or malignant.
3. To determine subclinical disease: 20% will have some form of subclinical hormonal dysfunction, particularly Sub Clinical Cushing's syndrome (SCS).

What pathologies may present as adrenal incidentaloma?

The following lesions can present as adrenal incidentaloma

a. Adrenal adenoma
b. Pheochromocytoma
c. Myelolipoma
d. Ganglioneuroma
e. Adrenal cyst
f. Hematoma
g. Adreno-cortical carcinoma
h. Adrenal metastases from other cancers

In cancer patients 75% of adrenal incidentaloma would turn out to be metastatic lesions. In contrast, without history of cancer, 65% of adrenal incidentaloma would be benign adenomas

Prevalence of ACC is directly related to size. If an incidentaloma is between 4-6 cm, the probability of it being a primary ACC is only 2%; on the other hand, if the size of the incidentaloma is more than 6 cm, the probability increases to 25%.

- 70% masses are non-functioning
- 5-10% present with SCS
- >10% turn out to be pheochromocytoma

How will you evaluate an adrenal incidentaloma?

Detailed history and physical examination is required to elicit signs and symptoms suggestive of adrenal hypersecretion or adrenal malignancy. Thus, one should look for signs and symptoms of Cushing's syndrome, pheochromocytoma, primary hyperaldosteronism, adrenocortical carcinoma and any history of extra-adrenal cancer.

What is the natural history of adrenal incidentaloma?

- 5-25% of adrenal masses increase in size by at least 1 cm
- Upto 20% masses become hyperfunctioning and masses more than 3 cm are more likely to develop hyperfunction compared to smaller tumors

What further biochemical tests would you order for an adrenal incidentaloma?

1. ***ONDST (1 mg test):*** If serum cortisol is > 5 mcg/dl then the test is considered positive for Cushing's disease.
2. ***Fractionated urinary and/or plasma free metanephrines:*** Plasma free MN (MN and NMN) can be measured with high diagnostic sensitivity (99%) and good specificity (90%).
3. In hypertensive patients only, serum potassium and PA/PRA ratio should be determined. Since 40% of patients with APA may have normal levels of serum potassium, most reasonable screening test is the PA/PRA ratio. PA/PRA ratio >30 and a plasma aldosterone concentration >0.5 nmol/L (20 microg/dl) are highly suggestive of Conn's syndrome.

Why is it important to exclude or confirm adrenal hypersecretion?

1. To uncover the subclinical Cushing's syndrome. These patients do not have the full blown CS but they continue to be exposed to the deleterious effects of continuous endogenous hypercortisolemia such as hypertension, osteoporosis, obesity and diabetes. Hence, it is important that these patients are diagnosed early and appropriate treatment is instituted as early as possible.

2. To uncover normotensive pheochromocytoma. Approximately 10-15% of adrenal incidentaloma turn out to be pheochromocytoma. It is important that these patients are diagnosed preoperatively so that they are adequately blocked and operated successfully. Mortality and morbidity of operation on unprepared pheochromocytoma is significant.
3. To uncover primary hyperaldosteronism. Though only < 1% of adrenal incidentaloma prove to be Conn's adenoma, it is important to diagnose and treat them as hypersecretion of aldosterone is associated with increased risk of cardiovascular disease and periodic paralysis.

What further radiological tests would you order for an adrenal incidentaloma?

The CECT or MRI should be carefully read primarily to assess the malignant potential of the adrenal mass

1. ***Size of the mass:*** The size may help in distinguishing between the benign and malignant lesions. The greater the size, the more likelihood of it being a malignant lesion
2. ***Imaging phenotype:*** After size, one should look for the appearance of the mass. The two important CT features that one should look for are:
   a. ***Lipid content of adrenal mass:*** This is measured as CT attenuation value and conventionally expressed in Hounsfield units (HU). Because of the high lipid content of benign adenomas, they have a low attenuation value, usually <10 HU on an unenhanced scan. However, this may not be universally applicable as 30% adenomas may not contain enough lipid to give a low HU and thus may be undistinguishable from malignant masses.

b. *Rapidity of washout of the contrast:* More reliable than the CT attenuation value is the rapidity of washout of contrast on delayed enhanced CT films. Adenomas typically show rapid washout of contrast media. Thus, at 10 min after injection of contrast an absolute washout of > 50% is virtually diagnostic of adenoma.
c. *Miscellaneous features:* A smooth border is suggestive of adenoma while a nodular adrenal mass is likely to be malignant. Presence of necrosis and lymph nodes also suggests malignancy.
d. *Chemical Shift MRI:* A benign adenoma shows a typical signal drop on out-of-phase images. However, chemical shift MRI does not provide additional information beyond that which is exhibited by unenhanced CT.

What are imaging characteristics of common adrenal pathologies?

- *Adrenal adenoma:* usually small, < 4 cm, rounded or oval with smooth borders with a homogeneous texture with attenuation values < 10HU and 50% washout at 10 min. Calcification and necrosis are rare.
- *Adreno-cortical carcinoma:* usually large, > 4 cm with irregular or nodular borders and a heterogeneous texuture; attenuation values are typically > 10 HU and they show < 50% washout. Necrosis is fairly common.
- *Pheochromocytoma:* On T2 weighted image on MRI it is typically hyperintense in relation to liver. CT may show heterogeneous enhancement with central cystic necrosis.

Imaging like NP-59, MIBG and PET are not widely available and convincing data about their usefulness is lacking, hence they are not recommended for evaluation of adrenal incidentaloma in a patient who has no history of malignant disease.

What is the role of FNAC in evaluation of adrenal incidentaloma?

There is no role of FNAC in the evaluation of adrenal incidentaloma. Image guided FNAC may be helpful in evaluation of a patient with a history of malignant diseases (especially kidney, lung, colon, breast, oesophagus, pancreas, liver and stomach) with no other signs of metastases and a radiologically suspicious adrenal mass. The primary role of FNAC in such a situation is to distinguish between metastatic disease or infective disease. Also, FNAC in adrenal lesions has a high false negative rate and may result in complications like adrenal hemorrhage, pain, hematuria, pancreatitis, pneumothorax, abscess, needle tract implantation and hypertensive crisis in a pheochromocytoma.

What are characteristics of metastatic disease to adrenal gland?

The adrenal incidentaloma in a patient who has a known history of extra-adrenal malignancy has 50% chance of turning out to be a metastatic deposit. Adrenal metastatsis are usually bilateral, and rounded. FDG PET has a very high sensitivity in detecting metastases to adrenal gland.

What criteria would you apply for the appropriate management of adrenal incidentaloma?

1. If the detailed history and physical examination reveals that the patient is having signs and symptoms of hypersecretion which is also confirmed biochemically, then adrenalectomy is the treatment of choice.
2. Unilateral adrenalectomy is also the treatment of choice in asymptomatic patients who have biochemical evidence

of hormone hypersecretion, e.g. subclinical pheocchromocytoma or hyperaldosteronism. The exact role of adrenalectomy in cases of sub-clinical Cushing's syndrome (SCS) is not well-defined. A reasonable approach would be to consider adrenalectomy for patients < 40 years of age and in those with recent onset/worsening of diabetes mellitus, hypertension, osteoporosis or obesity.

3. In non-functioning adrenal incidentalomas, one should consider the size, imaging phenotype characteristics of the lesion to distinguish between benign and malignant lesions:
   a. Lesions more than 6 cm should be surgically removed by unilateral adrenalectomy.
   b. Lesions < 4 cm can be followed-up by serial imaging, USG or CT, and proper counseling. Follow-up protocols are not well-defined. A reasonable strategy is to repeat the imaging studies at 6, 12 and 24 months. Hormonal analysis in a non-functioning lesion should be done only annually for the first 5 years.
   c. Lesion between 4-6 cm present with a dilemma. Adrenalectomy should be considered if imaging findings are suggestive of a malignant lesion or if the size increases by 1 cm during follow-up period.

Chapter 62

Bilateral Adrenal Masses

CASE STUDY

A 39-year-old male patient was referred for surgical management of bilateral adrenal masses (thought to be carcinoma) detected on CT examination. On evaluation, he was found to be having history of anorexia, weight loss, vomiting and dizziness for last 3 months. He had been taking anti-tubercular treatment for last 3 months but had not responded to it. Review of CT films revealed bilateral large irregular masses with heterogeneous enhancement and central necrosis in right adrenal mass. An impression of infective pathology was made and US-guided FNA was ordered which revealed non-Hodgkin's lymphoma of the adrenal gland. His hormonal work-up was normal. He also tested positive for HIV. He was transferred to the immunology department and was started on anti-retroviral therapy.

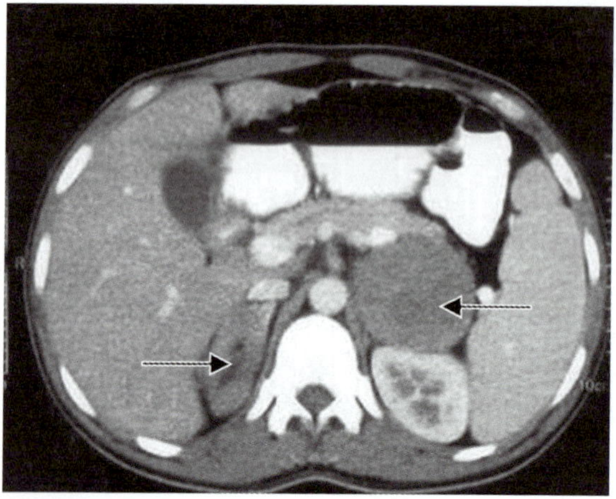

Fig. 62.1: Bilateral large irregular masses with heterogeneous enhancement and central necrosis in right adrenal mass

QUESTIONS

What are the different causes of bilateral adrenal masses/enlargement?

The different causes are:

1. **Malignant tumors**
   i. *Primary:* Lymphoma, malignant pheochromocytoma, adrenocortical carcinoma.
   ii. *Secondary:* From lung, breast, kidney, colon, melanoma.
2. **Infective**
   i. Tuberculosis, Fungal infections (histoplasmosis, cryptococcosis, blastomycosis, coccidioidomycosis).
3. **Functional**
   i. Macronodular hyperplasia, CAH, benign pheochromocytoma, Cushing's disease, ectopic ACTH syndrome.
4. **Miscellaneous:** incidentaloma, myelolipoma, hemorrhage, amyloidosis.

How will you evaluate a case of bilateral adrenal mass/enlargement?

A. *Hormonal evaluation:* To rule out functionality
   - Evaluation for Pheochromocytoma
   - Evaluation for Subclinical Cushing's syndrome
   - Evaluation for Ectopic ACTH syndrome.

B. *FNAC:* The main and the only aim of FNAC is to differentiate a primary adrenal tumor from a metastases.

C. *Imaging:* CT thorax for ectopic ACTH producing tumor or to rule out a primary lung cancer.

What are features of different causes of bilateral enlargement of adrenal glands?

Infective causes

1. ***Tuberculosis:*** In endemic areas like ours, it is the most common cause of primary adrenal insufficiency along with bilateral enlargement of adrenals. In most cases, primary pulmonary lesions are present. Calcification is commonly seen in tubercular involvement of adrenals.
2. ***Fungal involvement:*** Bilateral involvement can occur in disseminated fungal infections. All clinically important fungi except Candida can cause adrenal insufficiency and the common ones are: histoplasmosis, blastomycosis, coccidioiodomycosis and cryptococcosis. Systemic symptoms like fever, weight loss, cough, anemia, hepatosplenomegaly may be present. Diagnosis is established by FNAC which would reveal the offending fungi.

   In both of these granulomatous diseases, CT provides useful information. Bilateral enlarged glands with inhomogeneous texture indicates caseous necrosis. Glands retain their triangular shape as opposed to cases of adrenal insufficiency from bilateral metastases in which case the glands are replaced by round masses.
3. ***Haemorrhage:*** Demonstration of bilateral dense adrenal masses accompanied by acute adrenal insufficiency is virtually diagnostic of hemorrhage. Such hemorrhage results from sepsis, anticoagulant therapy, collagen vascular disease, postpartum state or as a result of idiopathic adrenal apoplexy.
4. ***Adrenal lymphoma:*** Adrenal involvement in widespread non-Hodgkin's lymphoma occurs in 4% cases as assessed

by CT and in 25% at postmortem examination. On the other hand, primary adrenal lymphoma (almost always non-Hodgkin's) is still less common. 50% of cases of primary adrenal lymphoma are accompanied by adrenal insufficiency. The clinical picture of primary adrenal lymphoma is dominated by signs and symptoms of adrenal insufficiency besides systemic symptoms like fever, weight loss, malaise, GI symptoms, hyponatremia, hypotension, hyperkalemia and rarely skin pigmentation. CT picture is of large lobulated masses with variable density. FNAC or sometimes trucut biopsy is virtually diagnostic where it reveals large cell lymphoma of B-cell lineage. Role of adrenalectomy is limited to establishing the diagnosis if FNAC/trucut biopsy is noncontributory. The prognosis is very poor and more than 90% patients die within one year of diagnosis.

How will you test for adrenal insufficiency?

This is done by the CORTROSYN TEST. This is done by administering synthetic ACTH 250 mcg, intravenously, any time of day and a blood sample is drawn after 45 min for serum cortisol. Values greater than 20 mcg/dL are normal and values less than this suggest dysfunction of the hypothalamic-pituitary-adrenal axis.

Chapter 63

Cushing's Syndrome due to Bilateral Adrenal Lesions

CASE STUDY

A 55-year-old male presented with complaints of headache, pedal edema for 4 years and history of hypertension, facial puffiness, weight gain for 2 years, and easy bruisability for 1 year. He was also detected to be diabetic 6 months back. He also gave history of proximal weakness. He had negative history of visual blurring/diplopia, recurrent vomiting, hematuria/decrease urine output or steroid intake. There was no positive family history. He also gave history of bilateral renal stones for last 6 years. He had also suffered from a cardiovascular accident for 2 years back. On examination:

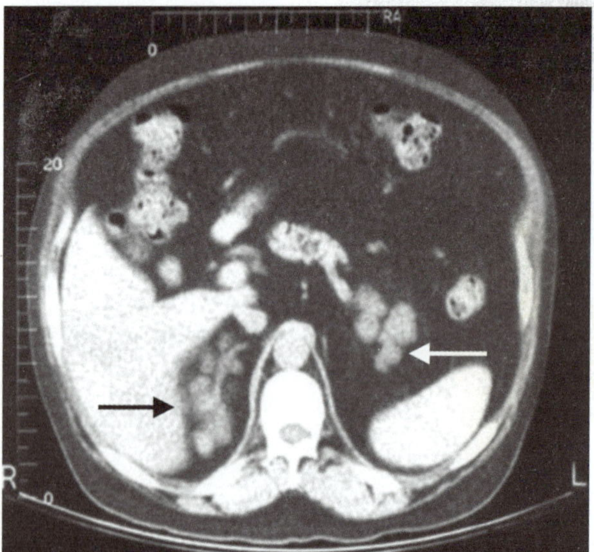

Fig. 63.1: CT scan showing, bilateral multitabulated adrenal masses "bunch of grapes" appearance (arrows)

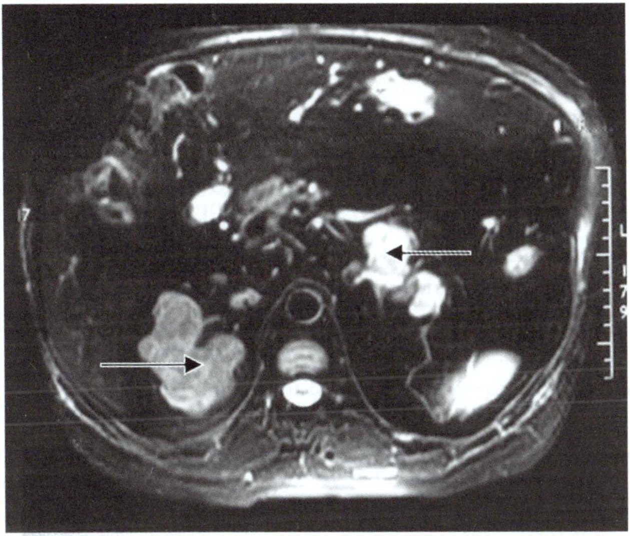

Fig. 63.2: MRI showing bilateral macronodular adrenal hyperplasia (arrows)

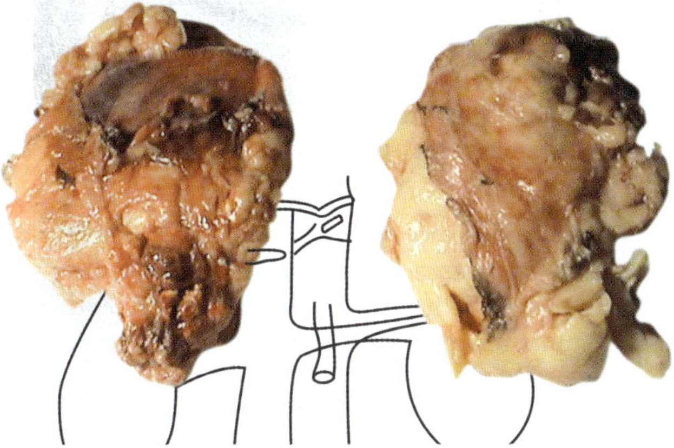

Fig. 63.3: Operative specimen of bilateral adrenalectomy

BP: 160/100 mm Hg, with postural drop 10 mm in systolic pressure. He had round facies, centripetal obesity with a BMI of 29, thinned skin, ecchymotic patches, taenia corpori, taenia unguim in toes along with bilateral pitting pedal edema. Fundus examination revealed grade 1 hypertensive changes. He did not have voilaceous striae, buffalo hump/ supraclavicular pad of fat, cataract or hyperpigmentation. CVS and respiratory system were within normal limits. He had protuberant abdomen and truncal obesity. Nervous system examination revealed proximal muslce weakness in lower limb. Clinical impression of Cushing's disease was made and following investigations were done:

Basal cortisol - 749.1 nmol/L

LDDST - 786.4 nmol/L

HDDST - 868.3 nmol/L

ACTH (11:00 PM) - 6.824 pg/ml.

Based on above investigations a diagnosis of ACTH independent Cushing's syndrome was made.

USG: 6.3 × 7.2 solid mass superior to right kidney? adrenal mass.

CT Scan bilateral multilobulated suprarenal masses with moderate enhancement.

MRI bilateral macronodular adrenal hyperplasia.

He was put on ketaconazole but could not tolerate the drug, had severe nausea, loss of appetite and the drug was withdrawn. He was than taken up for surgery and open transabdominal bilateral adrenalectomy was performed.

QUESTIONS

What are causes of bilateral Cushing's syndrome?

Approx. 10% of ACTH-independent CS results from bilateral lesions and the two most important causes are bilateral macronodular adrenal hyperplasia and Primary Pigmented Nodular Adrenal Hyperplasia (PPNAD).

What is AIMAH?

The various synonyms used are:

- Massive macronodular adrenocortical disease (MMAD)
- Autonomous macrondular adrenal hyperplasia (AMAH)
- ACTH independent macronodular adrenal hyperplasia (AIMAH)
- Giant or Huge macronodular disease

AIMAH is entirely different from the diffuse bilateral adrenals found in chronic ACTH stimulation state of Cushing's disease or ectopic ACTH secretion states. Differential diagnosis also includes bilateral diffuse adrenal hyperplasia seen in Cushing's associated with Mc Cune-Albright syndrome and in MEN-1(usually non-functional).

How do you make a diagnosis of AIMAH?

- Patients are usually older as compared to unilateral Cushing's adenoma
- More frequently seen in males
- Most frequent presentation is Cushing's syndrome
- Diagnosis is usually suspected on imaging studies–CT or MRI- the typical appearance of adrenal is like a " bunch of grapes" wherein the adrenal are replaced by numerous nodules upto 4 cm or more; on T1–weighted MRI the signal intensity is equal to muscle while on T2–weighted images they are hyperintense as compared to liver.

What is the macro and microscopic picture?

Combined adrenal weight is > 60 gm and can reach upto 200 gm. Nodules are composed of two types of cells- those with clear cytoplasm (lipid-rich) forming nest-like structures, and those with a compact cytoplasm (lipid-poor) that form island like structures. Overall, steroid hormone synethesis in AIMAH is an inefficient process. In AIMAH different stages of a common multistep tumoral processs are present in different locations at the same time, as suggested by heterogeneous clonal pattern.

Is the cortisol production in AIMAH autonomous?

Though cortisol production is by and large autonomous, in a significant proportion of cases of AIMAH, the cortisol production may be under the control of aberrant (ectopic or eutopic) hormone membrane receptors. Cortisol secretion becomes driven by a hormone that escapes cortisol-mediated feedback. The various aberrant receptors could be:

i. ***GIP-dependent CS:*** Adrenal expression of GIP receptor causes food-dependent cortisol production where plasma levels of cortisol are relatively low during fasting but increase following meals. Hypersecretion of GIP is not the cause but it is the aberrant hypersensitivity of adrenal gland to this peptide that results in this response.

ii. ***Vasopressin-responsive CS:*** Cortisol secretion increases with upright posture or other physiologic stimuli of endogenous vasopressin

iii. ***Beta-adrenergic responsive CS:*** In patients with AIMAH and CS, plasma cortisol and aldosterone levels are elevated during increase in endogenous catetcholamine levels (upright posture, insulin-induced hypoglycemia and exercise).

iv. *Aberrant receptor for LH/hCG:* Increase in cortisol levels in women during sequential pregnancies.
v. Serotonin (5HT4) receptors.
vi. Leptin receptors.

What are investigation protocols for evaluating the presence of aberrant adrenal hormone receptors?

DAY 1 : postural test
Standard mixed meal test
ACTH stimulation test
DAY 2 : GnRH
TRH
DAY 3 : Glucagon stimulation test
Cisapride stimulation test

Increase in plasma cortisol by ≥ 50% is considered positive for aberrant receptor tested.

What is the treatment of AIMAH?

Surgical treatment in the form of bilateral adrenalectomy has been recommended as the treatment of choice, especially in patients with severe CS resulting in hypertension, diabetes, osteoporosis, apparent brain atrophy, and neuro-psychological manifestations. In subclinical AIMAH perhaps follow-up with CT and biochemical assessment is sufficient.

Identification of aberrant adrenal hormone receptors in AIMAH provides new opportunities to use specific pharmacological therapies as an alternative to adrenalectomy:

- In GIP dependent CS: Somatostatin or Octreotide
- In catecholamine dependent CS: Beta blockers
- In LH/hCG dependent CS: Leuprolide
- In VI-AVPR dependent CS: V1-AVPR antagonists

Chapter 64

Adrenal Cyst

CASE STUDY

A 29-year-old male presented to the department of ganstroenterology with complaints of flank pain for 2 years. A screening ultrasound was suggestive of a liver cyst/right kidney cyst. There was no other contributory history. On examination, he was of average built and looked healthy. Examination of abdomen was non-contributory as well. A subsequent CECT revealed that it was indeed an adrenal cyst. On examination he was not hypertensive and he did not have any Cushingoid features. He did not give any history of episodic headaches, palpitations or increased sweating. Hormonal evaluation revealed normal basal cortisol (27.59 nmol/L) and normal 24 hour urinary metanephrine. In view of large size of adrenal cyst (> 6 cm) he was advised to undergo surgery.

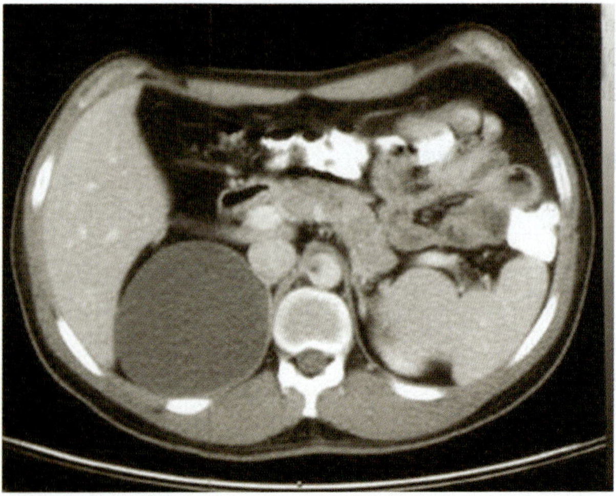

Fig. 64.1: CECT showing low-density mass with smooth borders and thin walls

QUESTIONS

How can you classify adrenal cysts?

They can be functional or non-functional (more common). Based on histopathology they can be divided into: pseudocyst, epithelial cyst, endothelial cyst (commonest) and hemorrhagic cyst, vascular cyst and sometimes cystic lymphangiomas and parasitic cysts.

How would you evaluate these cysts?

The differential includes a pancreatic pseudocyst on the right side and liver cyst on the left side. CECT is the imaging procedure of choice to differentiate from the liver or pancreatic cyst- adrenal cyst appear as low-density masses with smooth borders and thin walls. Calcification may sometimes be present. All cysts should undergo hormonal evaluation in the form of 24 hour urinary metanephrine and LDDST and in an hypertensive patient serum potassium or aldosterone-renin ratio.

Can adrenal cyst be malignant also?

Rarely the adrenal cyst can be associated with malignancy; the incidence is approximate 7%.

What are management issues in adrenal cysts?

All functional cysts should be excised by way of unilateral adrenalectomy. Smaller (<6 cm) and non-functional cyst can be followed up. Large (>6 cm) cyst with its potential for malignant change and complications like hemorrhage, and pressure effects should undergo unilateral adrenalectomy, espescially laparoscopic approach. The utitiliy of FNAC, both diagnostic or therapeutic is doubtful.

Chapter 65

Adrenal Myelolipoma

CASE STUDY

A 35-year-old male patient was found to be hypertensive when he developed epistaxis 6 months back and was put on beta blockers. Subsequently he developed nonspecific chest pain and was evaluated with an echocardiogram which was normal. An ultrasound done during this evaluation found a 12 cm right adrenal echogenic mass. Examination did not reveal anything significant. A clinical diagnosis of adrenal incidentaloma was made and he underwent hormonal work-up including 24-hour urinary metanephrine, overnight dexamethasone suppression test and serum potassium. He was further evaluated by CT which revealed a right adrenal mass with a HU > –50

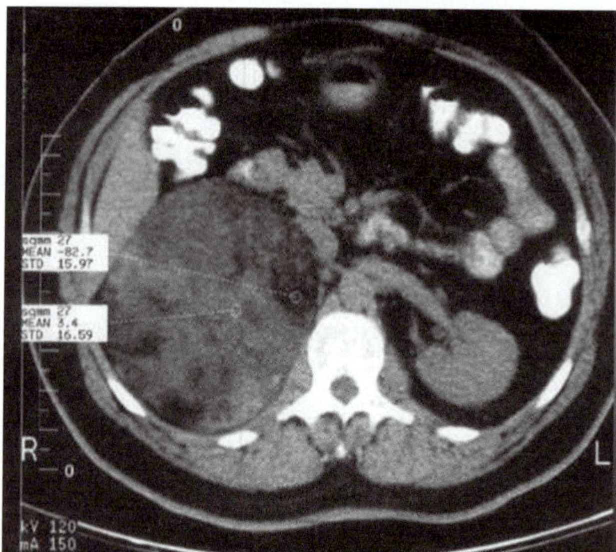

Fig. 65.1: CT showing an adrenal mass with a HU> –50

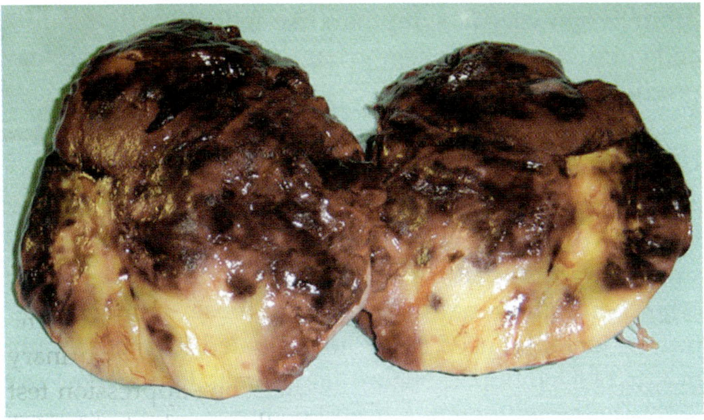

Fig. 65.2: Bisected adrenalectomy specimen showing haemorrhagic and fatty areas

suggestive of adrenal myelolipoma.The patient was taken up for surgery via the open transperitoneal approach and at operation a 15 × 14 cm mass weighing 950 gm was removed. The cut section revealed yellow fatty areas with foci of hemorrhage. The postoperative period was uneventful and he was discharged on 6th postoperative day. The histopathology was reported as adrenal myelolipoma.

QUESTIONS

How do adrenal myelolipomas present?

Myelolipomas are benign lesions with a variable mixture of myeloid and fat components. Majority of these are asymptomatic and nonfunctional and are usually discovered at autopsy. Now a days because of more frequent use of imaging they are being commonly discovered as adrenal incidentalomas. When they attain large size they may produce non-specific symptoms like abdominal discomfort, and vomiting. Rarely haemorrhage and tumor necrosis may produce acute symptoms.

How do you diagnose adrenal myelolipoma?

The presence of gross fat on CT (< –30 to –200 HU) is virtually diagnostic of myelolipoma. However, those with small amounts of fat may be difficult to differentiate from other benign adrenal masses while those with a greater proportion of fat need to be differentiated from other fatty masses of the retroperitoneum like lipomas, liposarcoma and renal angiomyolipoma. A useful pointer is identification of a pseudocapsule between the myelolipoma and the adjacent retroperitoneal fat, which represents a thin rim of residual adrenal cortex around the lesion.

Do all myelolipoma require surgical management?

After a confirmed diagnosis of myelolipoma on CT scan, those tumors which are less than 4 cm and asymptomatic can be followed-up while large and symptomatic myelolipomas should be surgically removed by adrenalectomy. Bleeding is likely to occur in large lesions and those which are predominantly composed of myeloid tissue. Since these tumors are very soft, adequate care should be taken during surgery to avoid rupture and spillage.

Section 4

ENDOCRINE PANCREAS DISORDERS

Chapter 66

Organic Hypoglycemia: Insulinoma

CASE STUDY

An 18-year-old boy was referred with complaints of episodes of fainting attacks for last several years. The attacks were more frequent in the morning and were relieved by taking glucose solution or with biscuits. The frequency of attacks has been increasing so much so that he had difficulty in getting up in the morning and he continued to sleep for many days continuously and had only sugar containing foods in between. He did not give any history of seizures, headache or excessive sweating. On intense questioning, it became evident that he did not have any access to oral hypoglycemic agents or to insulin injections. There were no medical or para medical personnel in his family. He was hospitalized for supervised 72 hr prolonged fasting test which was

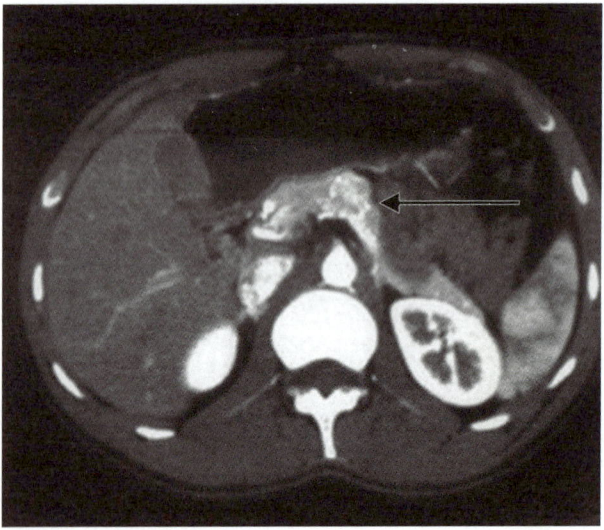

Fig. 66.1: Angio CT showing enhancing lesion in body of pancreas (arrow)

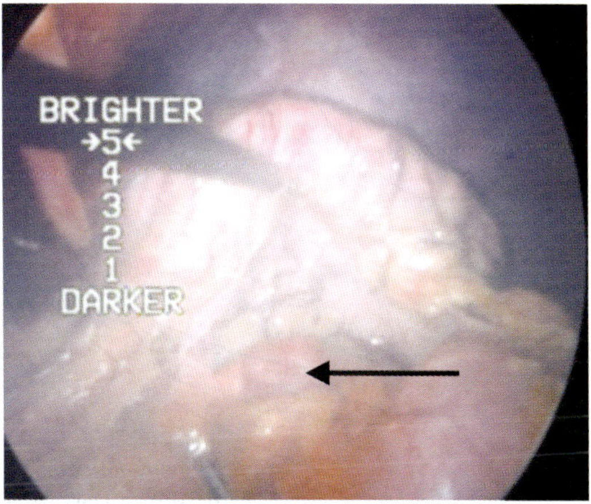

Fig. 66.2: Endoscopic view showing the bright red adenoma in the body of pancreas (arrow)

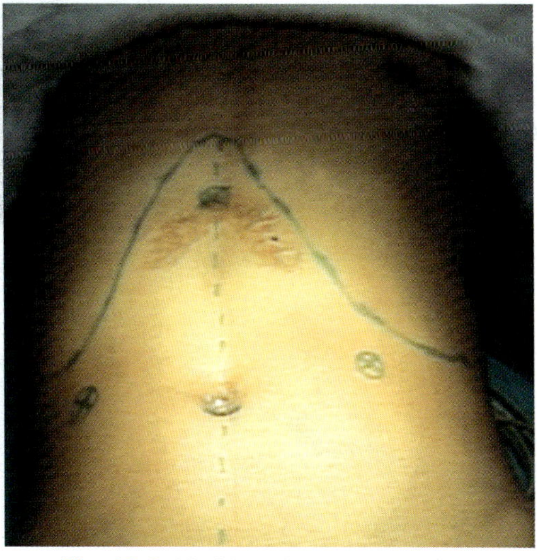

Fig. 66.3: Markings for port placement

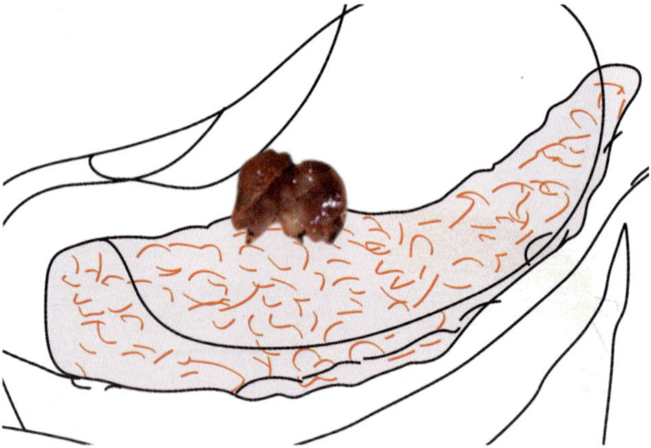

Fig. 66.4: Surgical specimen of laparoscopic enucleation

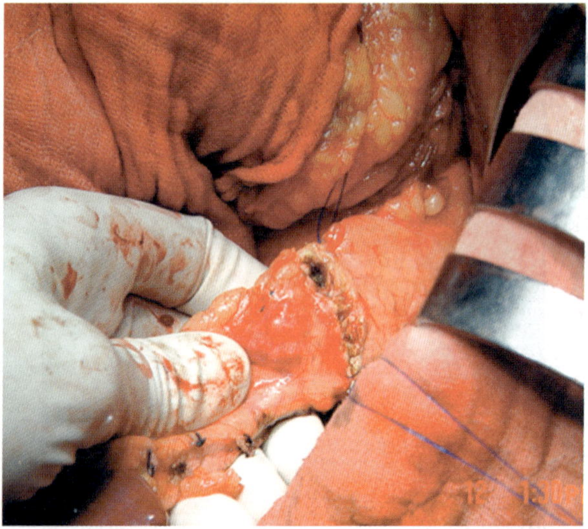

Fig. 66.5: Distal pancreatectomy in progress in another patient

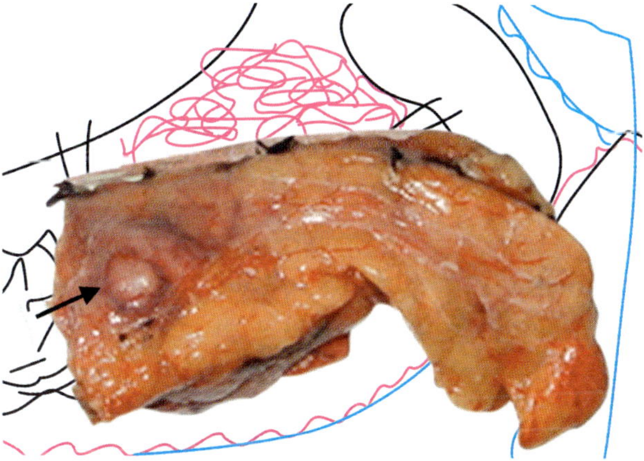

Fig. 66.6: Surgical specimen showing the insulinoma (arrow)

terminated after 4 hours when his blood sugar fell down to 24 mg% and corresponding insulin values were 16.2 ng/dl and C-peptide values were elevated to 2.2 ng/ml (0.7 to 1.9 ng/ml). After confirming the biochemical diagnosis of insulinoma, localization was done with CT angio which revealed a enhancing lesion in the body of the pancreas. Work-up for MEN was done which revealed normal calcium level. He underwent laparoscopic enucleation utilizing 6 ports and a 2.8 × 1.8 cm hypervascular tumor, which weighed 1.8gm was enucleated from the body of the pancreas. Following enucleation, fibrin glue was injected in the tumor bed percutaneously. The postoperative period was uneventful and serial ultrasound did not reveal any peripancreatic collection or formation of pseudocyst. Post-operatively he was able to maintain his blood sugar levels without the need for dextrose infusion. The histopathology showed was a tumor tissue displaying cells arranged in sheets and nests. These cells show round to oval mildly anisomorphic nuclei, salt and pepper chromatin, conspicuous nucleoli and moderate amount of cytoplasm. Any obvious mitotic activity was not seen.

QUESTIONS

When would you suspect insulinoma?

The manifestations of patients with insulinoma can be grouped into:

1. ***Neuroglycopenic symptoms:*** Light headedness, blurred vision, diplopia, confusion, amnesia, abnormal behavior; seizures may occur in one-third of patients. Sometimes, the symptoms may progress to loss of consciousness.
2. ***Sympathetic symptoms:*** Hypoglycemia results in release of catecholamine which produces symptoms such as weakness, sweating, tremor, nausea, anxiety and palpitations.

Symptoms occur in variable combinations, though for an individual patient, the symptom complex follows a stereotypic pattern. Symptoms generally occur after a fast in the morning (because of long over night fast), after skipping a meal, or after exercise. This fact should be kept in mind as women in our country keep day-long fasts due to various religious/culture practices. Another point to be remembered is that since the symptoms of insulinoma are primarily behavioral, patients are often misdiagnosed and definitive diagnosis is delayed by an average period of 15 month to 3 years. Because these patients often learn to avoid the symptoms related to prolonged periods of fast by eating small meals frequently or having snacks, they tend to put on weight and by the time the diagnosis of insulinoma is made, they may be very obese.

How would you confirm the biochemical diagnosis?

Traditionally the diagnosis of insulinoma is suggested by the presence of "Whipple's triad"-symptoms of neuroglycopenia and of catecholamine excess that occur during fasting or exercise, accompanied by a serum glucose level lower than 45 mg/dl which resolve after administration of glucose.

Supervised 72 hour fasting test

At present, demonstration of an insulin level that is inappropriately high for the serum glucose during an episode of severe hypoglycemia makes the diagnosis. Prolonged fasting may provoke this. Patients are fasted, and plasma levels of glucose, insulin, and C-peptide are measured every 6 hours. When plasma glucose level fall below 40 mg/dl or symptoms of hypoglycemia develop, the test is terminated. Approximately 33% become hypoglycemic within 12 hours, 65% within 24 hours, 84% within 36 hours, 93% within 48 hours and 99% within 72 hours.

Measurement of C-peptide levels: C-Peptide is secreted in equimolar amounts as insulin by Beta cells and is an accurate marker for endogenous insulin secretion. Its measurement is useful in two situations. In the diabetic patient, anti-insulin antibodies may interfere with plasma insulin measurements while C-peptide is unaffected. Additionally, normal C-peptide levels in the setting of elevated blood glucose levels and hyperinsulinemia point towards accidental or surreptitious use of insulin or sulfonylurea.

Additional tests

1. ***Measurement of pro-insulin:*** In patients with borderline fasting insulin levels, measurement of pro-insulin is useful.
2. ***C-peptide suppression test:*** This involves the infusion of exogenous insulin (beef or pork) to suppress endogenous insulin secretion. In healthy subjects, when hypoglycemia is induced by exogenous insulin, endogenous insulin (measured as C-peptide secretion) is suppressed by 50-70%. Elevated C-peptide after infusion suggests presence of insulinoma.
3. ***Measurement of plasma or urinary sulfonylurea:*** Some oral hypoglycemic agents produce an elevation of insulin, C-peptide and pro-insulin, similar to Insulinoma, and in these instances, detection of sulfonylurea in blood or urine should alert the physician of this possibility.

How would you localize the tumor?

This is undertaken only once the biochemical diagnosis of insulinoma is confirmed.The desire to localize the insulinoma is universally accepted and certainly facilitates the operative procedure. In spite of lower sensitivity of USG, CT and MRI, these imaging studies give essential information about presence of metastases, and identify patients with large malignant tumors.

However, a negative preoperative imaging should not deter the surgeon from operation if the biochemical diagnosis is certain because the use of intraoperative ultrasound (IOUS) and bi-digital palpation have to an extent reduced the need for a positive preoperative localization. In most situations, we feel that more invasive and expensive localization studies can be avoided.

A wide range of localization methods are available viz:

Noninvasive imaging

1. Transabdominal ultrasound is operator-dependent to a large extent and localization rates very widely from 13 to 65%.
2. Lower localization rates have been reported for CT scan and MRI.

Invasive imaging

1. ***Somatostatin receptor scintigraphy (SRS):*** This represents a major advance in preoperative tumor imaging. However, unlike gastrinomas, only 30-50% Insulinoma have Type 2 Somatostatin receptors to be detected by SRS.
2. ***Endoscopic ultrasound (EUS):*** Results are very good with overall sensitivity of 88% and specificity of 100% but tumors located distally in the pancreas or projections from the surface are not easily localized.

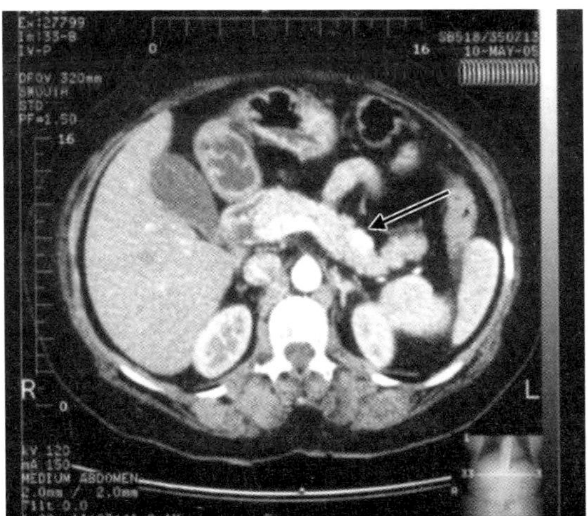

Fig. 66.7: Angio CT showing enhancing lesion in body of pancreas (arrow)

3. Selective arterial stimulation and venous sampling (ASVS) has largely replaced portal venous sampling (PVS). This is a regionalization modality and suggests the possible region of pancreas likely to harbor the tumor. It involves functional localization by hormone measurement in the hepatic vein after sequential superselective intra-arterial injection of calcium.This procedure is based on the premise that like many other apudomas, insulinomas can be stimulated to secrete their hormone when the serum concentration of calcium is raised. In spite of the excellent published result, this technique is technically demanding, invasive and not widely available.
4. *Selective angiography:* Historically selective angiography was the method of choice for pancreatic insulinomas. However, because of its cost and invasiveness it is no longer done.

How would you prepare the patient for surgery?

Objective: to optimize the physiologic condition of the patient

1. IV infusion of 10% dextrose is given overnight while fasting to avoid the risk of hypoglycemia.
2. To control severe hypoglycemia in the preoperative period octreotide or diazoxide may be given. However, in that case, measurement of intraoperative blood glucose following excision of insulinoma to know the completeness of excision cannot be utilized.
3. Prophylactic antibiotics.
4. Limited bowel preparation.

What is the surgical management of these patients?

Incision

The abdomen is explored through a bilateral subcostal incision. Use of fixed retractors to elevate the costal margins, provides excellent exposure.

Initial exploration

The abdomen is initially explored for evidence of metastatic disease especially the liver and subsequently the pancreas is exposed and mobilized in a stepwise manner for performing the bi-digital palpation and IOUS.

Exposure of the pancreas

This may be accomplished through the lesser sac by division of gastrocolic ligament or by reflecting the greater omentum cranially off the transverse colon utilizing the generally avascular cleavage. The omentum and the stomach are retracted superiorly, and congenital adhesions between the posterior wall stomach and pancreas are divided.

Mobilization of head of pancreas

To facilitate bimanual palpation of the head of the pancreas, a generous/extended Kocher maneuver is performed, after retraction of the hepatic colon flexure, if necessary, that is carried distally to the superior mesenteric vessels. The mobilization of the pancreatic head should be complete until the aorta can be palpated with the fingers.

Mobilization of the uncinate process and neck of pancreas

The uncinate process is then mobilized by dividing its small vascular attachments to the superior mesenteric vessels, allowing their full medial retraction. To gain optimal exposure of the neck and uncinate process of the pancreas, the gastroepiloic artery along the greater curvature of the stomach and the gastro-epiploic vein as it joins the gastrocolic venous trunk, which empties into the superior mesenteric vein at the inferior border of the pancreas, can be sacrificed safely. This is frequently required if an adenoma is being palpated at the uncinate process.

Mobilization of body and tail of pancreas

By incising the peritoneum along the inferior border of the pancreas, the body and the tail of the pancreas are mobilized.

Exposure of the posterior surface of pancreas

By gently dissecting beneath the entire posterior surface of the pancreas, with care being taken to avoid injury to the underlying adrenal gland, the entire body and tail of pancreas can be rotated around the axis of splenic vessels. Alternatively, when the tail of the pancreas extends deep into the splenic hilum, the short gastric vessels are divided and spleen is freed from its peritoneal attachment, allowing the body and tail to be lifted up together with the spleen which can then be rotated medially to visualize the posterior surface of pancreas.

Bidigital palpation and visual inspection

Proper exposure should allow full bimanual palpation and visual inspection of both anterior and posterior surface. Gentle bi-digital palpation of the entire gland permits at least 90% of tumors to be identified as the tumor is firmer than the surrounding soft pancreatic parenchyma. Uncommonly, the reddish purple or white tumors are actually exposed on the surface, but more commonly they are covered by a variable thickness of normal pancreatic parenchyma. Thus, even if an insulinoma is found early in the course, the whole pancreas should be examined to avoid missing multiple tumors.

What intraoperative aids you can use to have good outcome?

Intraoperative ultrasound (IOUS)

At this point of time we recommend IOUS, preferably by a radiologist. The objectives of IOUS are:

1. To detect occult insulinomas–IOUS is superior to simple bi-digital palpation alone.
2. To define the relationship of the tumor to the pancreatic duct and vessels.

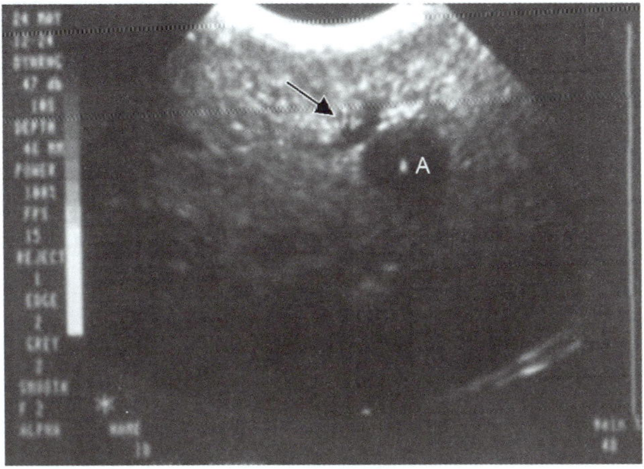

Fig. 66.8: Intraoperative ultrasound showing the adenoma (A) close to pancreatic duct (arrow)

3. To locate or exclude the presence of additional tumors as seemingly sporadic cases with multiple tumors have been reported.

Intraoperative hormone measurements (IHM)

With the development of rapid immunoreactive insulin (IRI) assays, intraoperative hormone measurements may be used to confirm the completeness of surgery. This is based on the fact that insulin, like most peptide hormones, have very short half lives in the systemic circulation. Serum levels decrease rapidly after resection of insulinoma. The overall accuracy of this test is 85%.

In addition, the intraoperative use of secretin stimulation can confirm the excision of all autonomous tissue. Researchers have shown that secretin stimulates beta cell insulin secretion in normal tissue but not in tumor cells or in the case of nesidioblastosis. Therefore, an increase in serum insulin 2 min. after injection of secretin occurs only after complete resection of tumor tissue, when inhibition of alpha-cell secretion by the autonomous tumor has stopped.

Blood sugar levels also begin to increase in most patients within 15 min of removal of an insulinoma. However, in very thin patients, the increase in blood sugar levels may take longer. An hours delay in the hyperglycemic response may be noted in more than 20% of patients.

Which resection procedure would you use for insulinoma?

Selecting the resection procedure

For pancreatic head tumors it is important to define the relationship of the pancreatic and bile ducts and the vessels to the tumor. If the tumor is well away from these structures.

enucleation is the method of choice. Otherwise, a pancreaticoduodenectomy (Whipple's procedure) can be performed, even for benign disease. Recent improvement in surgical techniques, postoperative care, and surgical expertise have made this operation possible with minimal morbidity and mortality. A higher risk of fistula formation after enucleation of tumors in the pancreatic neck/uncinate process have been noticed, possibly because of the oblique course of pancreatic duct and the confluence with the accessory duct of Santorini in this part of pancreas. Majority of tumors in the uncinate process of the head, neck, as well as body of pancreas may be enucleated. In the rare case of a tumor of the midpancreas that cannot be enucleated, resection of the body and tail has generally been recommended, but an extensive resection may result in pancreatic insufficiency. A technique of central pancreatectomy with distal pancreaticogastrostomy as an alternative to left pancreatectomy in an effort to preserve pancreatic function has been described. At the same time, improvements in the treatment of diabetes have lessened the concern of postoperative pancreatic insufficiency. Tumors in the pancreatic tail may also be enucleated, especially the ones close to the body or protruding from the margins of the pancreas. However, a liberal attitude towards a spleen-preserving left-sided pancreatic resection is suggested in lesions of the tail.

Enucleation

Small, benign tumors lying away form the pancreatic duct (as revealed on IOUS) can be enucleated. Meticulous technique is the key to safe enucleation. Generally, a plane can be developed between the tumor and the softer normal pancreas because of the presence of a pseudo capsule around the insulinomas. Enucleation is accomplished by dissecting immediately adjacent to the tumor, bluntly separating the tumor from normal pancreas with fine instruments and a sucker. Fine bridging vessels are managed with clips or bipolar cautery. Additional maneuver that helps is the use of left hand with the fingers behind and pushing forward the gland and the thumb placed anteriorly to provide counter traction on the tumor; alternatively one can lift the pancreas with one hand and pull the tumor upwards with a stitch placed through it.

Maneuvers to decrease the risk of pancreatic leak: No effort is made to close the defect, but a drain (preferably a soft silicone drain) is routinely placed as fistula formation is not uncommon. Biological sealants, such as fibrin glue, are used to limit the occurrence of a pancreatic fistula. If there is suspicion of injury to the pancreatic duct, intravenous secretin will visualize extravasations of pancreatic fluid from the resected area. An injured duct may be closed using fine sutures, or, alternatively, the operation is converted to a resection.

Left-sided pancreatic resection

A spleen preserving left side pancreatic resection is a safe procedure. The pancreatic tail is mobilized from the splenic vessels, often by dividing several smaller branches. The pancreas may be cut with a scalpel according to the "fish mouth" technique. Smaller bleeders should be suture ligated with polypropylene 5-0 or 6-0. Alternatively harmonic scalpel is particularly useful in resection of caudal pancreas, where the hemostatic effect and limited tissue destruction are appreciated. A thorough search for the main pancreatic duct in the remaining pancreas is suggested, since ligation of the duct presumably reduces risk of postoperative leakage.

In case no tumor is identified how will you proceed ?

Very rarely, careful exploration along with the use of IOUS may fail to reveal a tumor. In this case, blind distal pancreatectomy is to be avoided, though it was recommended in the past. Because, at least 50% of impalpable, occult insulinomas are located in the head or uncinate process of the pancreas, blind distal pancreatectomy would seem often to be destined to failure. Some recommend that pancreatic biopsy should be done to exclude adult onset nesidioblastosis.

Patients in whom an insulinoma has not been identified at the first operation should be referred to an experienced unit. The diagnosis must be reconfirmed and subsequent study with SASI, if not previously done, and selective venous sampling for insulin and pro-insulin may redirect subsequent exploration. Surgical re-exploration is often more difficult. Dissection is hampered by scarred tissue planes and the pancreas is firmer compromising the surgeon's ability to palpate a small tumor.

What are the complications of pancreatic surgery for insulinoma ?

The three main complications of pancreatic surgery are:

1. Intraperitoneal leak of pancreatic fluid
2. Pancreatic fistula, and less commonly
3. Pseudocyst formation

With the use of IOUS, fistula formation is not so common after enucleation. Nevertheless, as mentioned earlier, closed suction drains are used to control fistula output. Most authors have reported that postoperative drainage containing high amylase concentrations in almost all cases resolve spontaneously. In some cases one may leave the drain in place while the patient is fed. Because a drain may be required for a significant length of time, a soft material such as silicone is preferred. Also, special care should be given to fixing the drain to the skin.

Octreotide and Somatostatin analogues have been suggested both as a prophylactic means as well as in postoperative setting of a fistula. However, recent evidence shows no obvious benefit.

SPECIAL SITUATIONS

Malignant insulinoma

Account for only 5-10% of all insulinomas. They may be discovered preoperatively or more commonly intraoperatively by finding of metastases (liver or lymph node) or tumor infiltration and postoperatively by the pathological finding of microscopic infiltration. Reports of elevated levels of proinsulin or chorionic gonadotropin and its subunits have been correlated with malignancy, though with poor sensitivity. Patients with malignant insulinomas present with the same but more troublesome hypoglycemic symptoms as compared to patients with benign disease. Primary tumors are usually single and large, averaging 6 cm. Intra-operatively malignancy should be suspected if the tumor is hard and causes puckering of surrounding soft tissue, or appear to be infiltrating or causing distal dilatation of the pancreatic duct.

Management

Treatment of primary: Unless the tumor is widely spread, involving major vascular structures, tumor resection is indicated to reduce troublesome hypoglycemia and to improve outcome. One may consider enucleation including a rim of normal pancreatic tissue in cases where the pseudo capsular margin is unclear or the size is > 2 cm. Otherwise aggressive attempts at resection are recommended as these tumors are much less virulent than their malignant ductal exocrine counterparts.

Treatment of liver metastases: Because metastases usually also maintain hormonal hypersecretion, only complete resection alleviates the symptoms completely. Thus, palliative resection should be considered only when at least 90% of the tumor bulk can be excised. The liver metastasis can be treated with any one or a combination of the available methods; surgical resection, radiofrequency ablation, liver embolization and chemotherapy. Cytoreductive hepatic surgery for malignant insulinoma can be performed with a mortality of less than 3% to provide effective palliation and probably prolong survival. Doxorubiein and streptozocin chemotherapy has been associated with an encouraging 70% tumor regression rate, and remission from hypogly-cemic symptoms has extended to 18 months. Unfortunately, this combination of drugs is also associated with considerable toxicity.

Prognosis: Median disease free survival after curative resection was 5 years, but recurrence will develop in 63% at a median interval of 2-8 years. Median survival with recurrence tumor is only 19 months. Palliative resection yielded a median survival of 4 years, but biopsy only 11 months.

Adult onset nesidioblastosis

This disease is widely debated, as some researches and clinicians have questioned its presence. Though rare, it is an important cause of hypoglycemia and hyperinsulinemia in adults. It has a characteristic histopathological picture of diffuse hyperplasia or hypertrophy of islet cells which are also seen budding off the ductular epithelium. Nesidioblastosis may be suspected in cases of negative preoperative localization attempts, negative intraoperative ultrasound and bi-digital palpation. In such as situation, almost all clinicians agree that the abdomen be closed and invasive imaging like intra-arterial calcium angiogram should be done. If insulin levels rise after each selective calcium injection, nesidioblastosis is the likely diagnosis. Surgical management of this entity is also controversial. Various surgical approaches include 70% distal pancreatectomy and near total pancreatectomy.

Chapter 67

Insulinoma and Hyperparathyroidism as Part of MEN-1

CASE STUDY

A 45-year-old lady presented with complaints of episodes of vertigo for last 6 months. These attacks were initially once a day but later became more frequent. The attacks usually occurred in the morning and few of these were accompanied by seizures. The attacks persisted for 1-2 hours and were relieved by taking glucose in water. She also gave history of persistent bone pains for last 5 years and was infact diagnosed as a case of hypophosphatemic osteomalacia and was put on calcium and vitamin D supplementation since then. A clinical impression of organic hypoglycemia was made and she was hospitalized for supervised 72-hour prolonged fasting test which was terminated after 3 hours when her blood sugar fell to 22 mg% with corresponding

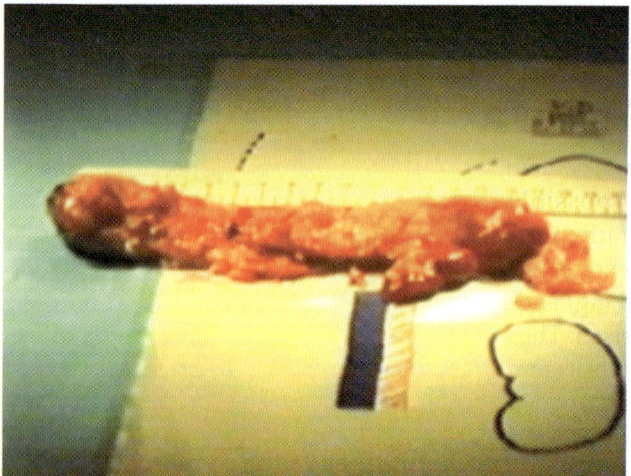

Fig. 67.1: Subtotal pancreatectomy specimen showing multiple adenomas in the body and tail

insulin values of 15.11 ng/dl. Her biochemistry also revealed high serum calcium values (11.2 and 11.5 mg%) and subsequently her PTH was also found to be elevated (543 pg/ml). USG abdomen was done which showed 3.2 × 1.5 cm hypoechoic area in the body of the pancreas. USG neck revealed right parathyroid mass measuring 2.3 × 1.7 cm. Subsequent CECT revealed multiple hypervascular tumors in the body and tail of the pancreas and also bilateral adrenal hyperplasia. CT of the pituitary region did not reveal any lesion in the pituitary. A working diagnosis of MEN-1 was made due to presence of two components of MEN-1: multiple insulinoma and hyperparathyroidism. She was taken up for exploratory laparotomy and on finding multiple tumors in the body and tail, subtotal distal pancreatectomy to the left of SMV was performed and the pancreatic stump was closed with mattress sutures after closing the cut end of the pancreatic duct with figure of eight prolene suture. The postoperative period was uneventful and after 12 days she was taken up for bilateral neck exploration. Three parathyroid glands were found to be enlarged but the 4th gland could not be identified even after extensive dissection of possible ectopic sites. Two and half gland parathyroidectomy was performed- right inferior gland adenoma (weight: 12 gm), left superior gland adenoma (wt: 700 mg) and half of normal appearing superior gland was excised. The histopathology was suggestive of parathyroid hyperplasia. Unfortunately, in the postoperative period she developed peripancreatic collection and subse-quently succumbed to multiple organ failure.

QUESTIONS

When should you suspect MEN-1 in a patient of insulinoma?

According to English literature, nearly 10-15% of insulinomas are a component of MEN-1. Infact, the possibility of MEN-1 should be considered in all patients of insulinoma, particularly if they are young and if multiple tumors are present. This is particularly important because surgical strategy differs between tumors with MEN-I and sporadic cases. Presence of hyperparathyroidism in a patient of insulinoma is virtually diagnostic of MEN-1, and therefore, liberal policy of serum calcium determination is recommended. Recent characterization of MEN-1 tumor suppressor gene menin on chromosome 11q13 allows MEN-1 to be diagnosed in patients with apparently sporadic insulinomas.

What should be the management strategy for insulinoma in MEN-1 patients?

Insulinomas that occur in the setting of MEN-1 usually require a different surgical approach. This is based on the fact that MEN-1 patients usually demonstrate multiple pancreatic tumors and more importantly, these tumor range from microscopically small tumors spread all over the whole pancreas to large and sometimes malignant tumors in the same patient. Further, these tumors may produce a variety of hormones. Thus, the insulinomas in a patient of MEN-1 may occur with tumors producing other hormones such as gastrin. The surgical strategy in MEN-1 should be guided by two principles: total removal of gross disease and adequate prophylactic resection to minimize recurrence without causing endocrine and exocrine pancreatic insufficiency. The best way to achieve this is routine distal subtotal pancreatectomy (to the level of portal vein), with enucleation of tumors in the head (guided by IOUS for safe removal).

What are the features of HPT associated with MEN-1 syndrome?

HPT is the most frequent (90%) endocrine disorder associated with the MEN-1 syndrome. Most have multiple abnormal parathyroid glands. HPT antedates the appearance of other endocrine disorders by as much as 10 years. One must, therefore, consider MEN-1 syndrome in any patient with HPT caused by parathyroid hyperplasia.

What are operative considerations in HPT associated with MEN-1?

HPT associated with MEN-1 presents a clear challenge to surgeons because the rate of persistent and recurrent disease is much higher in this group. The two therapeutic options are: Subtotal parathyroidectomy with B/L thymectomy or Total parathyroidectomy with autotransplantation (a more aggressive approach).

In patients with MEN-1 syndrome and an apparent solitary parathyroid tumor, the recommendations are removal of the normal and abnormal parathyroid glands, thymectomy, careful inspection for supernumerary glands and biopsy, marking and frozen section of 2 normal appearing parathyroid glands on the other side.

What is the cause for persistent or recurrent HPT in MEN-1?

Most common cause for failed operations is not overgrowth of the small hyperplastic parathyroid remnant, but failure to remove one or more supernumerary glands.

Why is long-term follow-up necessary in these patients?

Long-term follow-up of these patients is necessary because of late recurrence of HPT and development of other endocrine tumors.

Section 5

OTHER ENDOCRINE DISORDERS

Chapter 68

Gonadal Dysgenesis

CASE STUDY

A 15-year-old girl was evaluated for primary amenorrhea. She did not attain menarche but had breast development for last one year. She had no dysmorphic features. There were no evident Turner's features. There was no ambiguous genitalia; hernial sites were normal and urethral opening was normal, with no clitoromegaly. Since there was no progress of puberty she was investigated by:

FSH	:	85 m IU/L (3.3-8.8)
LH	:	9.5 (1.1-8.2)
Testosterone	:	0.74
Estradiol	:	< 20
PRL	:	11.0 ng/ml (3.6-18.9)
TSH	:	5.1 m IU/L

An USG pelvis was asked for which revealed hypoplastic uterus and absent ovaries with normal kidneys.

Karyotyping was ordered which revealed 46XY.

A working diagnosis of pure XY gonadal dysgenesis was made. She underwent diagnostic laparoscopy with possible prophylactic laparoscopic removal of streak gonads if present. Laparoscopy revealed two streak gonads with a hypoplastic uterus. Both streak gonads were excised.

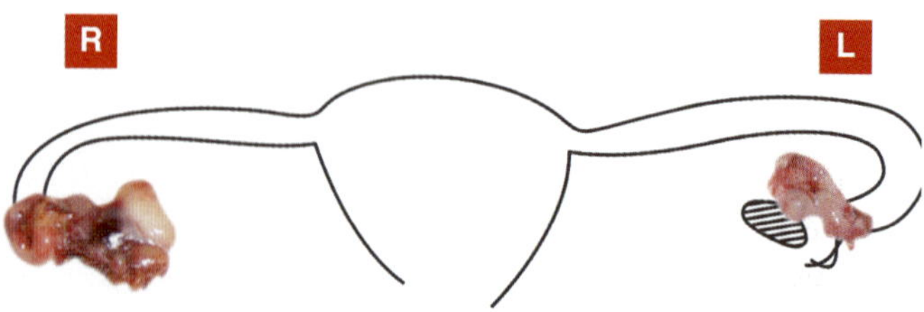

Fig. 68.1: Bilateral streak gonads along with a tumor (gonadoblastoma) in right streak gonad

Pathology revealed bilateral streak gonads along with a mixed germ cell sex cord-stromal tumor (gonadoblastoma) in right streak gonad.

QUESTIONS

What is gonadal dysgenesis (GD)?

GD is characterized by defective testis determination. These patients have steak gonads that do not secrete testosterone or antimullerian hormone, and thus, mullerian duct structures develop. This syndrome is therefore, an association of female phenotype, female internal genitalia, normal or tall stature, sexual infantilism and primary amenorrhea.

What is the clinical presentation of such patients?

Patients with pure gonadal dysgenesis have a female phenotype. Primary amenorrhea with sexual infantilism is the most frequent presenting symptom in a child reared as a female. They have a normal or tall stature with no stigmata of Turner's syndrome.

How do you evaluate such patients?

i. Sex steroid levels are extremely low.
ii. Progressive and marked elevation of gonadotrophins
iii. Ultrasound of pelvis normally reveals a hypoplastic uterus with absent gonads.
iv. Karyotyping is usually 46XY.
v. Spontaneous breast development may be the first evidence of development of gonadoblastoma.

What is the pathology of streak gonads in such patients?

At laparotomy or laparoscopy usually two streak gonads are found. In majority (> 95%) of the streak gonads, ovary-like stroma is found though there are no ovarian follicles or seminiferous tubules. A frequent finding is presence of Leyding–type cells and calcification. In more than 50% of streak gonads, a gonadoblastoma or dysgerminoma may be found.

What is the management of such patients?

Pubertal development is initiated by estrogen replacement therapy like Primarin. A prophylactic gonadectomy during diagnostic laparoscopy is indicated because all these patients are at high risk of development of gonadoblastoma, dysgerminoma or seminoma.

Chapter 69

Klinefelter Syndrome with Gynecomastia

CASE STUDY

A 20-year-old boy presented with progressive enlargement of both breasts for last three years. On examination, bilateral tender gynecomastia of 5-6 cm was present. He had eunuchoid body proportions with bilateral firm testes and a testicular volume of 2 ml, along with decreased pubic hair. There was no history of drug intake and there were no associated diseases like diabetes. A clinical diagnosis of Klinefelter's syndrome was made which was confirmed on relevant investigations:

i. *Serum FSH* : 72 IU/L EL (elevated)
ii. *Serum testosterone* : 7.3 mIU/L (low)
iii. *Serum prolactin* : 236 mIU/L (normal)
iv. *Serum TSH* : 3.2 mIU/L (normal)
v. *Karyotyping* : 47 XXY (abnormal)
vi. Ultrasound revealed bilateral concentric glandular enlargement of breasts.

He was put on testosterone replacement. He subsequently underwent reduction mammoplasty for bilateral gynecomastia.

QUESTIONS

What are the forms of gynecomastia?

Gynecomastia is defined as generalized enlargement of male breast. It is the most common benign breast condition in men. There are two main forms of gyneomastia : pubertal and adult.

Pubertal gynecomastia

Beginning at age 11, gynecomastia may develop in 30% of boys and by age 14 may be seen in 66% of boys. It may be unilateral to start with. Spontaneous regression occurs in most of them by 1-2 years and treatment is rarely indicated.

Adult gynecomastia

Upto 30% of men may develop gynecomastia during middle age and the incidence increases with advancing age. By seventh decade more than 60% men may have gynecomastia.

What are the etiologic factors?

i. Excess of estradiol
ii. Deficiency of testosterone
iii. Imbalance in the ratio of estradiol to testosterone
iv. Abnormalities of regulatory hormones
v. Drugs
vi. Idiopathic

How would you evaluate a case of gynecomastia?

The most important thing is to make a distinction whether one is dealing with a physiological or a pathological gynecomastia. The gynecomastia is considered pathological when the palpable tissue is more than 4 cm in diameter, or palpable tissue is greater than 2 cm but is tender, or palpable tissue is greater than 2 cm but is increasing in diameter on follow-up. A gynecomastia is considered physiological if it is less than 2 cm in diameter or between 2-4 cm but nontender and is not increasing in size.

Confirmation of gynecomastia

A hallmark of gynecomastia is its location directly under the nipple and its concentric distribution unlike the eccentric hard mass of malignancy. The technique for confirming the presence of gynecomastia is as follows: walk the fingers-start palpating from outside to inside with tips of fingers, flexed at MCP joint and the appreciation of "flipping an edge" of tissue at the interface of normal and glandular tissue confirms the presence of gynecomastia.

Detailed clinical history

Use of medications, presence of chronic diseases, any testicular swelling, history of chest trauma, etc.

Physical examination

Determine percentage of ideal body weight, signs of hypogonadism, testis should be palpated carefully and one should look for any signs of diseases like acromegaly, thyro-toxicosis, Cushing's syndrome or liver disease.

Simon classification of gynecomastia

Grade	*Description*
I	Small but visible breast development with no redundant skin
IIa	Moderate breast development with no redundant skin
IIb	Moderate breast development with redundant skin
III	Marked breast development with much redundant skin

FNAC

Yield of cells in gynecomastia is not satisfactory because gynecomastia is a predominantly fibrous lesion. Hence FNAC is not recommended as a first line investigation and should be confined to older men.

Radiology

Ultrasound is the best imaging modality to confirm the presence of gynecomastia, to distinguish the presence of fat (pseudogynecomastia) from glandular tissue and to characterize it so as to differentiate from malignancy. The utility of mammography is limited in the evaluation of gynecomastia.

Laboratory investigations

Routine tests in all patients include thyroid function tests, DHEAS, estradiol, LH, hCG – Beta, testosterone.

What are the management options?

i. Majority of patients of gynecomastia evaluated on OPD basis will fall into the idiopathic category after hormonal evaluation is done.
ii. Stop the offending drug or medication
iii. Reassurance in cases of pubertal and physiological gynecomastia
iv. In patients in whom intervention is required options may be either hormonal or surgical
v. ***Medical management:*** Medical therapy in the form of danazol, tamoxifen or testolactone (an aromatase inhibitor) produces a reduction in size in significant number of patients.
vi. ***Surgical therapy:*** When breast tissue diameter is more than 5 cm and persists for more than 3 years (persistent pubertal gynecomastia) the only therapeutic option is reduction mammoplasty. In adults with recent onset idiopathic gynecomastia, persistence of glandular enlargement or pain after a trial of tamoxifen or danazol is an indication for surgery.

Is there a increased risk of malignancy in gynecomastia?

Historically it was thought that frequency of breast carcinoma is higher in Klinefelter syndrome but this has not been observed in few recent series. On the other hand, germ cell tumors are 50 times more common in this syndrome.

Index

A

Adrenal cysts 487
- evaluation 487
- management 487

Adrenal incidentaloma 464
- biochemical tests 466
- characteristics 468
- evaluation 465
- natural history 466
- pathologies 465

Adrenal myelolipomas 491
- diagnosis 492
- surgical management 492

Adrenocortical carcinoma 349
- clinical presentation 351
- prognosis 357

AIMAH 481
- diagnosis 481
- treatment 483

Amyloid goiter 66
- histological features 68
- preoperative diagnosis 67
  - CT scan 67
  - FNAC 67
  - thyroid function tests 67

Anaplastic thyroid carcinoma 249
- clinical presentation 252
- diagnosis 252
- prognosis 255
- role of chemotherapy 254
- role of immunohistochemistry 253

B

Benign adenomas 348

Bilateral adrenal masses 471
- causes 473
- evaluation 473

Bilateral Cushing's syndrome 481

Bone metastases 215

C

Calcified adrenal masses 347

Cardiovascular disorder associated with thyrotoxicosis 63
- definitive management 63
- emergency management 63
- risk of thromboembolism 63

Central compartmental dissection 230

Clitoromegaly 367

Completion thyroidectomy 188

Cushing's disease 337

D

De Quervain's thyroiditis 85
- clinical diagnosis 88
- diagnostic investigations 90
- differential diagnosis 89
- etiopathogenesis 87
- management 91

Distant metastases 227

Dyshormonogenetic goiter 107
- clinical manifestations 110
- diagnosis 111
- role of surgery 112

E

Ectopic ACTH syndrome 326

Ectopic Cushing's syndrome 328

Euthyroid multinodular goiter 9
- clinical features 12
- etiopathogenesis 11
- evaluation 12
- treatment 13

Extra-adrenal pheochromocytoma 445
- characteristics 449
- precautions 449

F

Familial isolated hyperparathyroidism 287
- clinical features 291
- diagnosis 291
- genetic analysis 291

Familial pheochromocytoma 408

Follicular neoplasm 199
- frozen section evaluation 200

Follicular variant of papillary carcinoma 177
- diagnosis 179

G

Gonadal dysgenesis 525
- clinical presentation 525
- management 526

Graves' disease 36
- clinical features 36
  - pretibial myxoedema 37
  - thyroid acropachy 37
- diagnosis 37
  - antibody measurement 37
  - hormonal assay 37
  - thyroid scan 37
- management options 38
  - medical management 38
  - RAI therapy 40
  - surgical management 40

Graves' eye disease 48
- local management options 51
- local measures 50
- management options 50

Gynecomastia 528
- classification 528
  - adult gynecomastia 529
  - pubertal gynecomastia 528

etiologic factors 529
evaluation 529
management options 531

H

Hashimoto's disease 81
diagnosis 82
clinical observation 82
FNAC 82
serology 82
thyroid function tests 82
differential diagnosis 82
Graves' disease 83
subacute thyroiditis (SAT) 83
treatment 84
Hirschsprung's disease 237
Hodgkin's lymphoma 260
Hurthle cell neoplasm 203
clinical and histological characteristics 203
optimal management 204
postoperative management 204
prognostic factors 205
Hyperaldosteronism 321

I

Insulinoma 500
biochemical diagnosis 501
Insulinoma in MEN-1 patients 518
features 519
management strategy 518

J

Juvenile Graves' disease 55
initial management 55

K

Klinefelter syndrome 532

L

Laparoscopic adrenalectomy 318
Laparoscopic surgery in ACC 378
Large goiter 93
clinical presentation 97
intraoperative problems 97
anterior jugular veins 97
incision 97
intubation 97
look for tracheomalacia 98
middle thyroid vein 97
parathyroids 98
RLN 98
Ryle's tube 97
SCM 97
superior pedicle 98
tubercle of Zuckerkandl 98
precautions in postoperative 98
preoperative work-up 97
Lateral aberrant thyroid 156

Lingual thyroid 103
  clinical presentation 105
  evaluation 106
  management 106
Locally invasive papillary carcinoma 157
  management options 161
  routes 160
  symptoms 160
Lung metastases 168
  management 168, 169

M

Malignant insulinoma 512
Malignant pheochromocytoma 400
  features 400
Management of glucocorticoid 320
Marine-Lenhart syndrome 101
Mc Cune-Albright syndrome 481
MEN 2A 233
  causative gene 237
  characteristics 238
  clinical features 238
  components 237
Metastatic adrenocortical carcinoma 359
  medical management 362
  newer modalities 364
Multiple liver metases 227

N

Nelson's syndrome 330
Normotensive pheochromocytoma 459
  pathophysiology 459

O

Occult papillary carcinoma 154
  investigations 155
Organ of Zuckerkandl 450
Orthostatic hypotension 438
  pathophysiology 439

P

Pancreatitis in PHPT 284
Papillary microcarcinoma 148
  detection 148
  surgical management 149
Papillary thyroid carcinoma 138
  adverse prognosis 141
  diagnosis 139
  etiopathogenesis 139
  histological features 142
  molecular biology 140
  optimal management 141
Paragangliomas 454
  clinical presentation 454
  management 455
Parathyroid crisis 298
  evaluation 299
  management 299

Parathyroid cyst 32
management 32
Persistent hungry bone syndrome 301
Persistent hypercalcitoninemia 243
postoperative management 246
Pheochromocytoma 383
anesthetic considerations 394
biochemical diagnosis 388
complications 385
hemodynamic characteristics 384
hypertension 385
management 390
metabolic abnormalities 387
pathophysiology 383
phenoxybenzamine (PXB) 391
prazosin 392
preoperative α-blockade 390
selective alpha-1 antagonists 392
Pheochromocytoma of the bladder 427
biochemical diagnosis 428
prognosis 429
surgical management 428
Primary hyperaldosteronism 312
characteristics 312
diagnosis 313
Primary hyperparathyroidism 265
biochemical diagnosis 273
clinical features 272
differential diagnosis 273
operative considerations 276
postoperative considerations 278

R

Reoperative thyroidectomy 187
Retrosternal goiter 113
complication in surgery 124
consequence 130
diagnosis 130
management 131
risk factors 130
tracheomalacia 129
treatment options 121
types 119
Role of iodine deficiency 12
Role of radio-iodine therapy 14
Role of thyroxine suppressive therapy 13

S

Skeletal metastases 212
Solitary thyroid nodule 3
clinical evaluation 4
investigations 5
FNAC 5
serum TSH 5
ultrasonography 5

management 6
levothyroxine
suppressive therapy 7
other treatments 7
surgery 6
Sporadic MTC 217
clinical behavior 225
microscopic pathology 225
origin 225
postoperative management 231
Stroke pheochromocytoma 420
etiology 420
pathophysiology 421

T

Tall cell variant 171
biological characteristics 175
clinical characteristics 174
diagnosis 174
management 175
Technique of tracheostomy 131
Test for adrenal insufficiency 475
Thoracic duct fistula 156
Thyroglossal duct cyst 74
clinical features 74
differential diagnosis 75
branchial cyst 75
lymph node enlargement 75
midline epidermoid cyst 75
evaluation 75
histological picture 76
operative procedure 77
Thyroid cancer in children 191
clinical presentation 193
histopathological characteristics 193
management 195
preoperative evaluation 194
Thyroid cyst 29
management 31
aspiration 31
ethanol sclerotherapy 31
levothyroxine suppression 31
Thyroid lymphoma 257
clinical presentation 260
incidence 260
palliative surgery 261
pathological diagnosis 260
sub-types 260
treatment 261
Thyrotoxic periodic paralysis 59
clinical features 59
management 59
Total thyroidectomy 166
Toxic adenoma 23
diagnosis 25
clinical features 25
differential diagnosis 26
laboratory diagnosis 25
ultrasound 26

management options 26
radio-iodine therapy 27
surgical management 26
percutaneous ethanol injection 27
Toxic multinodular goiter 17
diagnosis 19
management options 20
anti-thyroid medications 20
RAI 21
surgery 21
pathogenesis 19

U

Unexplained shock 441
management 443
pathophysiology 442
Unilateral hyperplasia 320

V

Vertebral metastases 214
VHL gene 410
von Hippel Lindau disease 405
von Recklinghausen's disease 408